Minor Ailments in Primary Care – An Evidence-based Approach

For Butterworth-Heinemann:

Commissioning Editor: Heidi Harrison

Development Editor: Kim Benson

Production Manager: Yolanta Motylinska

Design/Production: Helius and Kneath Associates

Minor Ailments in Primary Care – An Evidence-based Approach

Edited by

Just A. H. Eekhof

Arie Knuistingh Neven

Theo J. M. Verheij

Consultant editor

Keith Hopcroft

ELSEVIER
BUTTERWORTH
HEINEMANN

EDINBURGH LONDON NEW YORK OXFORD PHILADELPHIA
ST LOUIS SYDNEY TORONTO 2005

ELSEVIER
BUTTERWORTH
HEINEMANN

ISBN 0 7506 8837 8

British Library Cataloguing in Publication Data
A catalogue record for this book is available from the British Library.

Library of Congress Cataloging in Publication Data
A catalog record for this book is available from the Library of Congress.

Note
Knowledge and best practice in this field are constantly changing. As new
research and experience broaden our knowledge, changes in practice,
treatment and drug therapy may become necessary or appropriate. Readers
are advised to check the most current information provided (i) on procedures
featured or (ii) by the manufacturer of each product to be administered, to
verify the recommended dose or formula, the method and duration of
administration, and contraindications. It is the responsibility of the practitioner,
relying on their own experience and knowledge of the patient, to make
diagnoses, to determine dosages and the best treatment for each individual
patient, and to take all appropriate safety precautions. To the fullest extent of
the law, neither the publisher nor the editors assumes any liability for any
injury and/or damage.

ELSEVIER your source for books,
journals and multimedia
in the health sciences

www.elsevierhealth.com

The
publisher's
policy is to use
**paper manufactured
from sustainable forests**

Printed in China

CONTENTS

Body

FOREWORD

It is a great pleasure to write a Foreword for this important book, which has been such a success in The Netherlands and which is now being made available to a much wider audience. I have no doubt that primary care workers around the world will turn again and again to this comprehensive, thoughtful, scholarly and practical guide to the management of a range of ailments frequently encountered in primary care, but which often escape the attention of textbooks focusing on the major medical problems. It also seems likely to me that many others, including first-aid workers, non-medical community workers and, indeed, the literate public, will find a great deal in this textbook to guide their work and to support self-care of minor disorders.

Primary medical care is characterized by a number of dimensions, which include continuity (the provision of personal or organizational care to the same individual or groups of patients over time, the coordination of services and, critically, comprehensiveness) and the ability of the primary care physician to deal with whatever 'comes through the door'. And, of course, what comes through the door can be almost anything, and the practitioner (or nurse practitioner, or community worker) will find himself or herself more or less well prepared to deal with it. The extent of preparedness will, in turn, depend on the education and training that the individual has received – undergraduate teaching in medicine and post-graduate training in general practice, nursing and allied professions. It is unlikely that much attention will have been paid to minor ailments during the undergraduate years, with the possible exception of attachments to GPs' surgeries in the clinical phase of training. More likely, the spotlight, during vocational training, will have been on the management of the acute presentations of illness seen in primary care, the management of the major chronic non-infective diseases and the psychosocial aspects of individual and population healthcare. Practice-based nursing staff are also unlikely to be familiar with many of the common, minor problems encountered in primary care. Minor ailments can get squeezed out of education for general practice at every turn of the way, particularly at a time when GPs in many countries are seeking to redefine their role and to emphasize the importance of primary care in a cost-effective healthcare system and, also, when governments, seeking value for money from their health services, introduce performance-related payments linked to easily measurable criteria of preventive care and chronic disease management. In both these scenarios it is hardly surprising that, on the one hand, GPs will emphasize their role in the management of life-threatening disorders in the primary care setting and, on the other, that quality measures will be linked to the serious, chronic disorders (cardiovascular risk factors, diabetes, asthma, obstructive pulmonary disease, etc.) for which structured care is increasingly being provided in general practice. Nursing staff in primary care are, similarly, increasingly concerned with chronic disease management, although there is plenty of scope to develop expertise in other areas of patient care. Hardly surprising then, that teaching and training in the management of the minor ailments seen in general practice gets squeezed out of the curriculum and off the political agenda.

However, a GP (or nurse practitioner or other healthcare professional) needs to be able to respond appropriately to all of the conditions presented in primary care, and whenever possible to manage them in a way which contains costs and, in most healthcare systems, avoids referral to expensive secondary and tertiary care specialists. The ability to make a diagnosis, to inform and reassure the patient and to provide appropriate management for minor ailments is at the core of providing comprehensive primary care. Indeed, patients will be just as appreciative of a GP's ability to relieve a painful condition through a brief intervention in the surgery as his or her skill in manipulating antihypertensive drugs to control what is an essentially an asymptomatic condition.

This book has a number of strengths. It is extremely well produced and accessible, and the template used for each of the conditions described makes reference very easy. Each section contains a useful box of Key Points, summarizing the important issues that have been covered. The writing is clear yet scholarly, and the relevant literature is cited at the end of each section. The authors and editors are to be congratulated on their efforts to assemble an evidence base for the treatment of minor ailments in general practice and the success of this enterprise can be judged by the inclusion of this textbook alongside the practice guidelines published by the Royal Dutch College of General Practitioners.

One of the great clichés of medical textbook reviewing is to conclude by saying that this book should find a place in every practice library. On this occasion, of course, the book has already found a place in every practice library in The Netherlands. It deserves to be widely used in general practice and primary care around the world and to inform the teaching and training of healthcare professionals working in the community.

Roger Jones
Wolfson Professor of General Practice
Guy's, King's & St. Thomas' School of Medicine
London

INTRODUCTION

Although minor ailments form a large part of the work of a GP, relatively little is known about them – a fact highlighted as long ago as 1902.[1] Important and life-threatening diseases and syndromes receive a lot of attention during medical education, whereas minor ailments, which form a much larger part of the GP's daily routine, get hardly any. When trying to look up information on minor ailments GPs often end up with articles from non-peer-reviewed magazines and websites of unknown standing.

The authors of this book have described the most frequently encountered complaints and disorders that do not pose a serious health threat and often have a good prognosis, but which receive little attention during medical education or in scientific papers.

Only a small percentage (about 10%) of patients with a minor ailment visit a GP with their problem. The rest either wait until it disappears of its own accord or buy their own medication, perhaps after consulting a pharmacist. Alternatively, they learn to live with the symptoms – despite the fact that they can be a significant burden to the patient.

In our view, diagnosing and treating minor ailments should be based on scientific data whenever possible. Unfortunately, such information is not easily accessible by the GP, if indeed it exists at all. As a result, practising in an evidence-based way is difficult in this field of medicine. This book will help to resolve that problem, as it aims to provide relevant and reliable information on minor ailments. The available evidence is used wherever possible, and key references are listed at the end of each chapter.

In The Netherlands, *Minor Ailments in Primary Care* has an accepted place beside the well-known Guidelines of the Dutch College of General Practitioners (NHG). While the NHG Guidelines cover about 80 major subjects (e.g. diabetes, asthma, ankle sprains, the menopause, deafness, shoulder symptoms), *Minor Ailments in Primary Care* has become *the* reference book for GPs for the treatment of minor ailments in general practice.[2] Areas for which an NHG Guideline is published are not covered in this book. This UK edition of *Minor Ailments in Primary Care* retains the overall philosophy of the book and its key evidence base, but orients the information towards UK primary care professionals and, where appropriate and possible, highlights UK epidemiological data. This task was aided by some key resources – in particular, the *British National Formulary*, *Clinical Evidence* (BMJ Publishing Group) and General Practice Notebook (http://www. gpnotebook.co.uk).

In The Netherlands, far more copies of the 4th edition of the book have been sold than there are GPs. Almost all Dutch GPs have their own copy, and it has found its place in the training programme for GPs as well as in examinations during vocational training. It is also useful for other medical professionals, medical students and practice nurses. Even interested patients may use it as a reference book, as they usually do not consult the GP for these disorders.

The Editors

References

1. A plea for the study of minor ailments. *The Lancet* 1902;**159**(4098):757.

2. Information about the Guidelines of the Dutch College of General Practitioners (NHG): http://www.nhg.artsennet.nl

CONTRIBUTORS (THE NETHERLANDS)

I. A. Arnold – *Leiden*
Dr B. J. M. Aulbers – *Delft*
Dr J. L. Baggen – *Ransdaal*
A. M. Bakker – *Budel*
Dr G. H. de Bock – *Haarlem*
F. J. Böhm – *Leiden*
Prof. Dr W. J. H. M. van den Bosch – *Lent*
F. S. Boukes – *Schoonhoven*
J. H. Brenninkmeijer – *Amstelveen*
J. A. Brienen – *Delft*
M. Bruinsma – *Roderesch*
J. P. Cleveringa – *Oosterhesselen*
Dr E. Crone-Kraaijeveld – *Rotterdam*
Dr C. F. Dagnelie – *Rotterdam*
Dr J. H. Dekker – *Amsterdam*
H. J. van Duijn – *Katwijk*
M. Dijk – *Leiden*
Dr J. A. H. Eekhof – *Leiden*
R. Glotzbach – *Delft*
V. J. F. van Gool – *Amsterdam*
A. F. M. Haverkort – *Beuningen*
W. M. Hoekstra – *Leidschendam*
J. M. Hollander – *Purmerend*
P. P. Hoogwater – *Best*
E. de Jager – *Leiden*
R. Jamin – *The Hague*
D. Janssen – *Leeuwarden*
T. O. H. de Jongh – *Gouda*
S. Jonkers – *Leiderdorp*
Dr A. Knuistingh Neven – *Krimpen aan de Lek*
I. A. Kuiper – *Heemstede*
Prof. Dr A. L. M. Lagro-Janssen – *Nijmegen*
H. M. Lam – *Aalsmeer*
J. van der Leden – *Leiderdorp*

Dr P. L. B. J. Lucassen – *Bakel*
Dr H. W. J. van Marwijk – *Oegstgeest*
M. Matthijsen – *The Hague*
J. S. Meijer – *Amsterdam*
Dr W. A. Meyboom – *Dedemsvaart*
Prof. Dr J. D. Mulder – *Noordwijk*
A. M. Muysken-Du Saar – *Maastricht*
J. M. Th. Oltheten – *Noordwijk*
Ch. H. Phaff – *Maastricht*
T. A. L. Polman – *Franeker*
B. P. Ponsioen – *Brielle*
R. A. van Randeraat – *Leiden*
F. J. N. Rijkée – *Delft*
Dr E. Y. R. Roeleveld-Kuyper – *The Hague*
P. L. Schoonheim – *Amsterdam*
W. Schuurman – *Bergen aan Zee*
B. E. van der Snoek – *Maarn*
J. Stolk – *Leiden*
A. van Stralen-Bohlmann[†] – *Leiden*
Dr J. G. Streefkerk[†] – *Hoofddorp*
J. Theunissen – *Breukelen*
Dr A. W. C. van Veelen – *Biddinghuizen*
M. Venema – *de Wijk*
A. A. A. Verheij – *Budel*
Prof. Dr Th. J. M. Verheij – *Noordwijk*
P. A. Verstappen – *The Hague*
N. G. van Vliet – *Waddinxveen*
A. Voorhoeve – *Deventer*
Prof. Dr Th. B. Voorn – *Oosterhout*
Dr H. de Vries – *Amsterdam*
I. Wagenaar – *Utrecht*
Dr E. P. Walma – *Schoonhoven*
B. S. Wanrooy – *Diemen*
Dr H. C. P. M. van Weert – *Amsterdam*
Dr F. H. Weisz – *Amsterdam*
J. J. van Wijngaarden – *Vlaardingen*
Dr S. Zwart – *Kampen*

GENERAL

I

PARTIAL THICKNESS BURNS

DEFINITION

Partial thickness burns can be epithelial, dermal or deep dermal – the first two are referred to as first degree, the last as second degree. In first-degree burns, erythema occurs. Superficial second-degree burns, with only little loss of dermis, are characterized by blisters and a uniform pinkish-red colour of the skin.

As the depth of a burn is the most important parameter for prognosis and therapy, full-thickness burns are also defined here. Deep second-degree burns, in which only the deeper dermis structures remain intact, show an alternately red and waxy white discoloration. In full-thickness burns, also known as third-degree burns, the entire dermis is destroyed; the appearance is whitish-yellow to brownish-black.

AETIOLOGY/PATHOGENESIS

Thermal injuries are caused by local contact with solids, liquids or gases, electricity or open fire. Sunlight, hot water, food prepared with hot water (coffee, tea, soup) and short-term direct contact with hot objects are the most common causes of superficial burns. It is helpful to have information about the cause of the burn, as this is of great importance for the diagnosis of the depth and seriousness of the burn.

PRESENTATION

The patient attending the GP with a burn may have a number of concerns. The first is usually whether the injury can be treated by the GP or requires specialist attention. The burn is generally painful, and the patient is often quite scared and wants to know how serious it is and what the prognosis is (e.g. the time for recovery and the likelihood of scarring).

EPIDEMIOLOGY

In the UK, 0.4–1% of the population will suffer a burn each year. One study revealed that approximately 4% of children under 5 years old who attended an accident unit presented with a burn. In general practice in The Netherlands, there is an incidence of 2–4 per 1000 patients per year. This means that burns represent 1 in 200 new consultations, these being approximately equally divided between men and women and relatively more common in young children (0–4 years) and those over 75 years old.

Based on the available data, it can be estimated that approximately 80–90% of cases involve superficial (first-degree and superficial second-degree) burns. Undoubtedly, the so-called 'tip of the iceberg' phenomenon also plays a role: many burns are not reported to the GP and are therefore not recorded.

HISTORY

This, like the examination, is concerned with determining whether the injury is indeed only a superficial burn, or if there is a significant risk of a deep second- or third-degree burn. The GP should ask:

- about the cause of the burn
- when the burn occurred
- about the duration of the burn itself
- whether the patient cooled the burn and for how long
- whether the patient tried another treatment and, if so, what.

With sunburn (also from a tanning bed), the greatest risk is of a superficial burn. In the case of burns due to water, oil, a hot object or open fire, the risk of a deep burn is higher.

EXAMINATION

The following diagnostic aids are used to distinguish between deep and superficial burns.

The pin-prick test helps to distinguish between superficial burns, which bleed quickly after being pricked and which are very painful, and deeper burns, which are less sensitive or painless due to the loss of sensitive nerve endings, and which bleed less quickly. The capillary refill is intact for superficial burns, and is less or not present at all for deeper burns.

This distinction is important, because spontaneous recovery of deep second- and third-degree burns can occur only in the sweat glands or hair follicles or at the edges of the burn, while regeneration of superficial burns can occur in the remaining epithelial tissue. This has implications for prognosis and treatment. In particular, deep second-degree burns that are not recognized as such can later lead to scarring. This can cause functional as well as cosmetic problems.

Burns from scalding require special attention and account for the majority of burns in children. The seriousness of scalding is too often underestimated. The greatest risk is the occurrence of hypertrophic scars. For children, it is important to pay particular attention to the chest area: they often pull hot liquids onto themselves from a table, countertop or cooker.

The surface area of the burn is also very important with regard to possible systemic complications, such as shock, sepsis and even multi-organ failure. An estimate is made of the surface area based on the familiar 'rule of nine'. The critical percentage for hospital admittance is 15% of the body surface area for adults and 10% for children, regardless of the depth of the burn.

For the sake of completeness, the 'rule of nine' used to determine the percentage of the total body surface area is as follows: the head is 9%, each arm is 9%, the front of the torso is 2 × 9%, the back of the torso is 2 × 9%, each leg is 2 × 9%, and the genital/perineum area adds the last 1%, to give a total of 100%.

Finally, the location of the burn is important. For burns to the eyes, ears, face, hands and perineum, there is a risk of functional problems later, as well as a higher risk of infection. For burns to the face, it is important to consider the possibility of inhalation trauma resulting from smoke inhalation.

All these factors play a role in the GP's decision to either offer treatment and provide a follow-up consultation, or to refer the patient to hospital. Arranging purely primary-care follow-up is only suitable for burns that will be able to regenerate from the remaining epithelial tissue, and for which the surface or site of the burn, or the general condition of the patient, do not make it necessary to refer the patient to a specialist.

If doubt exists with regard to the depth of the burn, one should always consult a colleague with more experience, or contact the local burns unit.

TREATMENT

In the acute situation, cool the burn as quickly as possible, if possible with running water (or at least frequently refreshed water) for at least 15 minutes. This shortens the duration of thermal trauma, and slows the release of toxic substances from irreversibly damaged cells, to ensure that no more cells die than is necessary. Furthermore, this method combats the formation of oedema, which allows the circulation to the viable remaining epithelial tissue to remain intact.

Tetanus vaccination should be considered, as appropriate.

First-degree burns generally recover spontaneously within 1 week. A soothing skin cream may be applied to prevent the burn from drying out. Moist compresses may also be used. Analgesics are appropriate if pain is a problem.

Conservative therapy for superficial second-degree burns can be classified as follows: open-wound treatment, half-closed-wound treatment and closed-wound treatment.

The *open-wound treatment* involves letting air heal the burn: serous wound fluid dries up and forms a crust that seals the injury, protecting it against dehydration and infection. However, this is only possible if the injury is localized, so that it can be constantly exposed to air.

The *half-closed-wound treatment* consists of covering the wound with ointments and creams, followed by gauze and/or a bandage. Infected or easily infected wounds should be treated this way, in addition to burns that, due to their position, cannot be treated in any other way. The preferred course of treatment involves using 1% silver sulfadiazine cream (very effective against *Pseudomonas aeruginosa*), applied on hydrophilic gauze that must be changed daily. The temporary white-yellow discoloration of the burn makes it difficult to assess its depth; it is important to be sure that the burn is superficial. If in doubt, begin with a neutral ointment (possibly after cleaning the wound) or with semipermeable membranes (see below). Povidone iodine ointment 10% is indicated for possible contamination with Gram-positive bacteria (usually *Staphylococcus aureus*). The creams have a limited shelf-life once opened.

The *closed-wound treatment* can only be used for burns that are sterile. If there is a blister, it is easiest to leave this intact. Paraffin gauze can be used to support the blister top. Puncturing the blister is often not necessary; however, the blister top must be removed after 3–5 days and the treatment continued according to the half-closed-wound method.

Another closed-wound treatment with excellent results involves hydroactive or biosynthetic bandages, which consist of semipermeable (i.e. allows gases and water to evaporate through, but not bacteria) polyurethane film on the outside and a layer of hydrocolloid on the inside. The inner layer seals the wound off and enables the formation of a gel, so that no damage is done when the bandage is removed; in other words, it forms an 'artificial skin' under which re-epithelialization can take place. The dressing must be changed once every 1 or 2 days. It has been observed that healing takes place faster using this method than, for example, using silver sulfadiazine cream. Unfortunately, this method is relatively expensive and cannot be used for every wound site, given the limited diversity and shape of the bandages. The gel that is formed (which looks and smells like pus) can make the patient think something is wrong; therefore, inform the patient and the caregivers about this.

Very clear agreements should always be made with regard to further treatment. A superficial second-degree burn must be fully healed in a maximum of 3 weeks. If the GP considers the parents or caregivers to be sensible and reliable, he can ask them to contact the surgery if the wound has not completely healed after this time. Alternatively, a specific follow-up appointment could be arranged. In the case of more extensive lesions, the healing process should be monitored by the GP in the first 2 weeks. The patient must also be told how to deal with complications, such as infection of the wound.

PREVENTION AND ADDITIONAL INFORMATION

Permanent damage, such as hypertrophic scars, can be prevented by good follow-up.

The prevention of burns is a huge subject, which falls outside the remit of this book.

Key points

- The depth of a burn is the most important parameter for prognosis and therapy.
- Burns from scalding require special attention and account for the majority of burns in children. The seriousness of scalding is too often underestimated.
- If doubt exists with regard to the depth of the burn, one should consult a colleague with more experience, or contact the local burns unit.

Literature

Arnold IA, Eekhof JAH, Knuistingh Neven A. Kleine kwalen: Oppervlakkige brandwonden. [Minor ailments: partial thickness burns]. *Huisarts Wet* 2004;**47**:207–10.

Morgan ED, Bledsoe SC, Barker J. Ambulatory management of burns. *Am Fam Physician* 2000;**62**(9):2015–26.

Werner MU, Lassen B, Pedersen JL, Kehlet H. Local cooling does not prevent hyperalgesia following burn injury in humans. *Pain* 2002;**98**(3):297–303.

2

PRICKLY HEAT/POLYMORPHIC LIGHT ERUPTION

DEFINITION

Prickly heat/polymorphic light eruption is characterized by an erythematous, itchy rash with papules and/or vesicles, especially on parts of the skin exposed to the sun. The rash develops several hours after exposure to the sun and is usually seasonal (late spring, early summer). It disappears spontaneously after several days or weeks; there are no remaining symptoms.

AETIOLOGY/PATHOGENESIS

UVA rays in particular, and UVB rays to a lesser extent, or a combination of the two, have a role.

A distinction must be made between:

- polymorphic light eruption (PLE) – in effect, a 'sun allergy'
- phototoxic dermatitis – an intensified reaction to sunlight resulting from oral medication (such as penicillin, tetracyclines, psoralens with PUVA)
- photo contact-allergic dermatitis – a contact dermatitis from certain substances (such as plants) which, after previous sensitization, cannot occur without UV rays
- metabolic light oversensitivity – such as cutaneous porphyria and xeroderma pigmentosum.

PLE is usually delayed – the rash develops several hours after exposure to sunlight.

PRESENTATION

The patient presents with an itching rash, usually on the hands, arms or face. Patients are bothered mainly by the itch or the cosmetic effects, particularly if the rash is on the face. They will want to know the cause of the symptom: the connection with exposure to sunlight is not always obvious. They also want to know what they can do about it – in particular how to prevent itching before they fly off to a sunny destination.

EPIDEMIOLOGY

This complaint occurs in 10–20% of primarily young, female adults; men are affected to a considerably lesser extent. The problem recurs when the skin is intensively exposed to sunlight, i.e. every sunny spring.

HISTORY

The GP should ask the patient:

- how the rash came about (the link with exposure to the sun)
- about any previous episodes
- about external contact with chemical substances (e.g. working in the garden), ointments or cosmetics (sunscreen can also cause a phototoxic reaction)
- about the use of medicines
- for information on the worsening of the rash after indirect exposure to sunlight (behind glass or in the shade), to help differentiate between UVA and UVB oversensitivity – a positive response points to UVA oversensitivity.

EXAMINATION

When inspecting the affected skin – primarily the hands, arms and face – a polymorphic pattern with red papules and erythema is apparent, as well as eczema-like dry skin and small vesicles.

Characteristically, the body parts exposed to the sun are the most affected. The hands are more often affected than the face. In the case of facial redness, the chin triangle and the area underneath the eyebrows are not affected.

Generally, no additional examination is necessary. Contact-allergy testing may occasionally be required.

TREATMENT

The problem will disappear on its own after a few days or weeks
if there is no further exposure to the sun. Over the course of the
summer, habituation will occur. The first course of action is to
reassure the patient and offer an explanation. A neutral lotion
(e.g. calamine lotion) or a corticosteroid cream (1% hydrocortisone
cream) can be advised if itching is a problem.s

Newer sunscreens offer, in addition to a high UVB protection factor,
protection against UVA rays. However, the protection factor against
UVA rays is lower (factor 7–8) than that against UVB (factor 15 or
higher).

Sunscreen recommendations are as follows: apply an ample amount
of cream half an hour before exposure to the sun. Reapply after
2–3 hours, and also after swimming or heavy perspiration. Substances
that act as sunblocks (titanium dioxide 2–5%) also protect to a certain
degree against UVA rays, but have cosmetic drawbacks.

PREVENTION AND ADDITIONAL INFORMATION

The most important action to take is to advise patients to expose
themselves very gradually to sunlight in the spring (e.g. 15 minutes
on the first day, and then 30 minutes more on each subsequent day)
and to cover the skin as much as possible. If there is a phototoxic
or photoallergic reaction, the substances responsible for this should
be avoided.

Key points

- The rash develops several hours after exposure to the sun and is
  usually seasonal.

- Characteristically, the body parts exposed to the sun are the most
  affected.

- The problem will disappear on its own after a few days or weeks, if
  there is no further exposure to the sun. Over the course of the
  summer, habituation will occur.

Literature

Ling TC, Gibbs NK, Rhodes LE. Treatment of polymorphic light eruption. *Photodermatol Photoimmunol Photomed* 2003;**19**(5):217–27.

Ossenkoppele PM, Van Vloten WA, Van Weelden H. Licht op foto-allergy en fototoxiciteit [Shining a light on photoallergy and phototoxicity]. *Ned Tijdschr Geneeskd* 1992;**32**:1540–4.

Polman TA.L, Eekhof JAH, Knuistingh Neven A. Zonneallergie [Prickly heat/polymorphic light eruption]. *Huisarts Wet* 2004;**47**:242–5.

Van de Klaauw JW, Gill K. Zonverbranding [Sunburns]. *Huisarts Wet* 1988;**31**:212–14.

3

ACUTE HIVES/ACUTE URTICARIA

DEFINITION

Urticaria, also called hives or nettle rash, is characterized by clearly defined, rapidly developing (and generally equally rapidly disappearing) severely itchy bumps on the skin. One version of this is the rash that develops after contact with stinging nettles (hence the alternative name 'nettle rash'). There are two types: an acute form, which is by far the most common (80% of cases), and which disappears within 4 weeks; and a chronic or recurring form, which can last longer than 4 weeks.

AETIOLOGY/PATHOGENESIS

The disorder is caused by local oedema in the skin, resulting from modified permeability of the smaller blood vessels. On parts of the body covered primarily with loose connective tissue (e.g. eyelids, lips, scrotum), there is a more diffuse swelling, known as angio-oedema. The underlying problem is usually immunological or allergic.

Various triggers have been reported, such as direct contact with the skin (e.g. dermographism), absorption through the stomach/intestinal system (medicines or food), inhalation (chemical or natural substances) and exertion. Connective tissue disorders and viral illnesses may also cause urticaria. However, the precise cause often remains obscure.

PRESENTATION

The patient suffers from an itchy skin rash, or spots varying in size from several millimetres to the size of a hand. Over time, these spots change location, and they may have disappeared by the time the patient visits the GP. In angio-oedema, there is no itching, but the patient suffers from swelling of the eyelids, lips or tongue, or even the glottis (accompanied by shortness of breath).

EPIDEMIOLOGY

Overall, 4–6% of the total population will suffer from urticaria, usually the acute form, at some time. The average GP sees more than 10 cases of urticaria or angio-oedema annually. Most of these resolve by 4 weeks, and thus, on average, one new case of chronic or recurring urticaria will appear in a GP's practice each year.

HISTORY

For acute urticaria (present for less than 4 weeks), a short history is sufficient, focusing on the likely trigger. The GP should ask:

- when the problem began
- if the patient has experienced urticaria before and, if so, when, and whether a cause was determined
- about unusual foods eaten
- about any medication taken
- about any other symptoms.

The cause may be a combination of different factors (e.g. cold urticaria can be triggered by preceding alcohol use, physical exertion, overly thin clothing, or alternating exposure to heat and cold). Recording this information can be helpful, particularly if the urticaria persists or recurs.

EXAMINATION

The physical examination for acute urticaria is limited to inspection. Additional examination at the first episode is not usually necessary. In uncomplicated cases, investigations are not required. Particular allergens may be identified by RAST (radioallergosorbent test) and skin-prick testing, but this is a consideration only in dramatic, persistent or recurrent cases.

TREATMENT

Acute urticaria is a minor problem that usually disappears by itself. The main role of the GP is to reassure the patient. In some cases it is possible to determine the cause. The condition can recur, even after a long time, and is sometimes associated with symptoms of anaphylaxis. Antihistamines, such as loratadine (10 mg once daily) and cetirizine (10 mg once daily), which have only a minor sedative effect, are preferred.

'Acute' urticaria can also recur chronically. Careful taking of the history each time is the best way to determine the cause.

Referral to a specialist is indicated in troublesome chronic or recurrent cases, or where there are anaphylactic reactions. In such situations, urticaria is no longer considered a 'minor ailment'.

PREVENTION AND ADDITIONAL INFORMATION

Preventing urticaria is difficult as long as the cause is unknown, which is generally the case for the first manifestation of acute urticaria.

Key points

- The precise cause of urticaria often remains obscure.
- Most cases of acute urticaria resolve by 4 weeks.
- 'Acute' urticaria can also recur chronically. Careful taking of the history each time is the best way to determine the cause.

Literature

Dubertret L, Aguttes MM, Tonet J. Efficacy and safety of mizolastine 10 mg in a placebo-controlled comparison with loratadine in chronic idiopathic urticaria: results of the MILOR study. *J Eur Acad Dermatol Venereol* 1999;**12**:16–24.

Greaves MW, Sabroe RA. ABC of allergies. Allergy and the skin. I: Urticaria. *BMJ* 1998;**316**:1147–50.

Lee EE, Maibach HI. Treatment of urticaria. An evidence-based evaluation of antihistamines. *Am J Clin Dermatol* 2001;**2**(1):27–32.

4

INSECT BITES AND STINGS

DEFINITION

There are several possible culprits. These include wasps, hornets and bees (which use their stings to pierce the skin), and mosquitoes, horseflies, fleas and ticks (blood-sucking insects that use their mouths to make an opening in the skin and then suck out the blood of their victim).

AETIOLOGY/PATHOGENESIS

While stinging or biting, an insect can transfer certain substances from their poison sac (wasps and bees) or salivary glands (mosquitoes, horseflies, fleas, ticks) into the wound. The adverse effects for humans can be classified into three groups:

- toxic effects on tissues
- allergic reactions (systemic or local)
- transmission of infectious diseases.

The substances transmitted from the insect can have a *toxic effect on human tissue*. There is an immediate local reaction at the site of the bite or sting, with vasodilatation, cell destruction and mast-cell degranulation, with the release of histamine. This causes local erythema, oedema, itching and pain – an inflammatory reaction around the wound. All insect bites cause this local reaction. The bite or sting may also become infected with bacteria from the skin.

All insects can cause a *local allergic reaction* after sensitization, but only wasps, hornets, bees and bumblebees can cause a *systemic allergic reaction*. The poison contains various substances, according to the insect. For bees, these are primarily mellitine, phospholipase A and hyaluridonase; for wasps and hornets, histamine, several quinines, phospholipase A and B, and hyaluridonase. If the person stung has already had contact with substances (particularly peptides) from the same insect in the past, sensitization can develop and an allergic reaction can occur.

Allergic reactions can be divided into four types. In this context, two are important. For severe symptoms occurring after wasp and bee stings, *type 1 (immediate, humoral type) allergic reactions* play an important role. In this reaction, immunoglobulin E (IgE)–allergen complexes activate mast cells and basophils, which release mediators and chemotactic factors. They also activate eosinophils and neutrophils, macrophages, monocytes and lymphocytes. The result is that within a few minutes there is an extensive local reaction, or a systemic reaction, possibly with anaphylactic shock. If the allergic reaction develops later, it is usually a delayed type-4 reaction and not an IgE-mediated one.

Blood-sucking insects can *transmit infectious diseases*. Lyme disease is caused by ticks infected with *Borrelia burgdorferi*. Malaria only occurs as an imported illness in patients who have visited the tropics. Typhus fever (from lice) and the plague (from fleas) are serious diseases, but are very rarely encountered.

PRESENTATION

The patient complains of a red spot or bump that may itch or be painful, and which may have developed after an insect bite or sting. The redness and/or swelling can also extend beyond the sting/bite site, so the symptoms may increase over time.

Some patients visit the GP with symptoms of a generalized reaction, such as itching and a rash over the entire body, swollen eyelids and/or lips, or shortness of breath. Such symptoms can sometimes increase within a few minutes, resulting in fainting, breathing problems, loss of consciousness and (very rarely) death.

Other patients see their GP to ask if they have been bitten by a tick and, if so, whether the GP can remove it. They may also ask about the risk of developing Lyme disease.

Sometimes, the patient does not present with an insect bite or sting, but has symptoms typical of an infection. *B. burgdorferi* causes erythema migrans, an expanding erythema near the site of the tick bite.

EPIDEMIOLOGY

A GP with an average practice is consulted around 20 times a year for an insect bite or sting. In about 10% of these cases there is a generalized reaction, consisting of widespread itching, urticaria and a minor degree of bronchospasm. Anaphylactic shock is rare: one UK study revealed that about 1 person per 10,000 per year presents with loss of consciousness or collapse secondary to anaphylaxis; this figure rises to 3 in 10,000 per year for respiratory difficulties caused by anaphylactic reactions. It is estimated that about 11% of cases of anaphylaxis are caused by insect venom.

HISTORY

The GP should ask:

- how long ago the patient was stung or bitten
- when the symptoms began
- whether an insect was seen in the area, and whether it was recognized or caught
- whether a sting was left behind in the wound by the insect, and whether it was removed
- about local symptoms (redness, itching, swelling, pain) and symptoms of a generalized reaction (itching, rash over the entire body, swollen eyelids and lips, vomiting or diarrhoea, shortness of breath or loss of consciousness)
- about reactions to previous insect stings or bites
- about relevant work activities (e.g. beekeeper, gardener, cattle farmer, forest ranger) or leisure and lifestyle factors (outdoor recreation, poor accommodation and hygiene, pets)
- for tick bites, about how long the tick was present on the body and where the tick bite took place.

EXAMINATION

In the case of a local reaction, the examination is focused on the site of the sting or bite: the GP looks for redness, swelling, a sting, the effects of scratching, and signs of a secondary bacterial infection, with this possibly extending to the regional lymph nodes.

If symptoms of a general reaction are present, the entire body should be examined for urticaria, oedema and erythema, and also to check for evidence of respiratory or circulatory problems (inspiratory stridor, threat of collapse). If the symptoms of a generalized reaction develop within 15–20 minutes of the sting, it is essential to check the pulse, blood pressure and breathing. Following a serious generalized reaction, extensive allergy tests should be conducted by an allergist.

TREATMENT

For a local reaction, if the bee sting is still present it must be removed very carefully. Near the base of the black sting is a white poison sac, which can secrete more poison in the wound if touched. The best way to remove the sting is to scratch it out of the wound using a sharp object (knife, credit card, fingernail).

If there is a tick present, it must be completely removed using special tick tweezers. Grip the tick as close to the skin as possible, and carefully remove it with a slight twisting motion. The longer the tick remains on the skin, the greater the risk of infection (5% during the first 24 hours, 100% after 3 days). In the presence of erythema migrans, or if the tick has been present on the body for more than a day (and therefore is larger due to the sucked blood) give doxycycline 100 mg twice daily for 14 days, or amoxicillin 500 mg four times daily for 2 weeks (if the patient is allergic to penicillin, give erythromycin 250 mg four times daily for 3 weeks).

Pain and swelling can be treated by icing the local area (e.g. applying ice in a plastic bag to the skin). If the patient has been stung in the throat, sucking on an ice cube can help prevent glottal oedema. Oral painkillers (e.g. paracetamol, ibuprofen) can also be taken.

The effect of local application of antihistamine creams has not been proven. Besides, such creams can cause sensitization.

Oral antihistamines can be prescribed for an extensive local reaction (e.g. cetirizine 10 mg once daily, or loratadine 10 mg once daily). Histamine is the most important mediator, especially in the initial hours of an allergic reaction; antihistamines are most effective at this time. Later, other mediators play a significant role, and antihistamines have no effect on these.

Secondary infection should be handled with proper wound care, such as a moist bandage or povidone iodine ointment gauze for exudating wounds; if necessary, a local antibiotic ointment (e.g. fusidic acid) can be used.

For a generalized reaction, the most important thing is to determine whether there is a threat of anaphylactic shock. If the symptoms of a generalized reaction develop within 15–20 minutes of the bite or sting, the patient should be observed for the first hour. An anaphylactic reaction rarely occurs later than this. If the patient develops respiratory or circulatory problems, he should be taken to hospital as soon as possible. In the meantime, 0.5 ml of adrenaline 0.1% should be given intramuscularly. Next, an antihistamine must be injected intravenously; an intravenously injected corticosteroid does not provide immediate improvement, but does prevent further deterioration as a result of a delayed-type allergic reaction. The patient should also be given oxygen in the acute phase, if possible.

In the case of inspiratory stridor due to glottal oedema, it is best to administer a few puffs of a β_2 sympathomimetic in spray form (salbutamol or terbutaline aerosol).

Resuscitation is carried out if breathing or circulation stops; adrenaline doses can then be repeated. The most serious reaction will generally have passed after 20 minutes.

PREVENTION AND ADDITIONAL INFORMATION

Pets must be treated for fleas. In the summer, additional vacuuming must be performed to combat fleas (for every flea seen on an animal, there are 10–100 in the surrounding area). When using insecticides, care should be taken to avoid intoxication of children, pets and pregnant women. Screens can be used to keep flying insects out of the house, and a mosquito net can be used in the bedroom.

Insect repellents such as diethyltoluamide do help, but must be applied frequently to the skin, as they evaporate after several hours, especially in warm weather. In rare cases, even when used according to the instructions, serious neurological side-effects can occur. The classic smouldering spiral (popular in the tropics), which spreads smoke that insects find unpleasant, is an effective and inexpensive preventive aid.

Most stings and bites can be treated at home; however, the patient should contact a physician in the case of a sting in the throat or a generalized reaction. Luckily, life-threatening allergic reactions occur only very rarely; direct stings in the neck and the throat are probably more often the cause of problems.

Preventing serious (anaphylactic, generally IgE-mediated) reactions by means of hyposensitization using pure insect poison appears to be effective. If a serious reaction occurs after a bee or wasp sting, it is sensible to refer the patient to an allergist or other specialist for preventive immunotherapy. Children seldom have a repeat occurrence of a serious reaction. Patients who have had serious reactions should be prescribed adrenaline for self-administration, and they (and their close contacts) should receive instruction on how to use it.

Key points

- There are three types of adverse effects to insect bites or stings: direct local effects, allergic reactions and the transmission of infection.

- Only wasps, hornets, bees and bumblebees can cause systemic allergic reactions.

- Antihistamines are most effective in the first few hours of an allergic reaction to a bite or sting.

- An anaphylactic reaction rarely occurs later than the first hour after the incident.

- Patients who have had serious reactions should be prescribed adrenaline for self-administration, and they (and their close contacts) should receive instruction on how to use it.

Literature

Balit CR, Isbister GK, Buckley NA. Randomized controlled trial of topical aspirin in the treatment of bee and wasp stings. *J Toxicol Clin Toxicol* 2003;**41**(6):801–8.

Dick L. Travel medicine: helping patients prepare for their trips abroad. *Am Fam Physician* 1998;**58**:383–98.

Ewan P. ABC of allergies: anaphylaxis. *BMJ* 1998;**316**:1442–5.

Hunt KJ, Valentine MD, Sobotka AK, Benton AW, Amodio FJ, Lichtenstein LM. A controlled trial of immunotherapy in insect hypersensitivity. [The Cochrane Controlled Trials Register (CCTR/CENTRAL)]. *The Cochrane Library*, Issue 2. Oxford: Update Software, 2004.

Sheikh A, Alves B. Hospital admissions for acute anaphylaxis: time trend study. *BMJ* 2000;**320**:1441.

Stanck G, Strle F. Lyme borreliosis. *Lancet* 2003;362:1639–47.

Visscher PK, Vetter RS, Camazine S. Removing bee stings. *Lancet* 1996;**348**(9023):301–2.

5
LICE/PEDICULOSIS

DEFINITION

Infestation with head lice (*Pediculus humanus* var. *capitis*), pubic lice (*Phthirus pubis*) and/or body lice (*Pediculus humanus* var. *corporis*) is characterized by itchy papules, the presence of nits (lice eggs) on the hair shaft, and possibly the visible presence of the lice themselves between the hairs, on the skin or in the clothes of the patient.

AETIOLOGY/PATHOGENESIS

Lice are parasites, which occur only in humans: they are transmitted at schools, boarding schools and in overpopulated houses (i.e. places where there is close contact between people), or by direct physical contact.

Head and body lice look the same and are the same length (2–3 mm). Pubic lice (also known as 'crabs') are a little larger and visible to the naked eye.

Head lice are transmitted by normal contact between children (particularly at school), and by borrowing a comb or putting on a hat that belongs to someone who has head lice. Pubic lice are generally transmitted via infested clothing or bed linen, or intimate physical contact. Body lice are caught by wearing clothes infested with lice. In contrast to head and pubic lice, body lice and their nits are only rarely found on the body: this insect is only present on the skin when feeding. Body lice can transmit typhus, relapsing fever and trench fever.

PRESENTATION

Cases of head lice – or anxiety about possible infestation – are usually presented by the parents of schoolchildren, often after warnings from other parents, teachers or the school nurse. Scalp itching is the other common reason to consult. Pubic lice infestation is generally presented as an itchy skin rash in the pubic region; the patient may have seen the lice. Body lice infestation is presented as severe itching on the body, with papules and scratching effects, or as impetiginized skin lesions.

EPIDEMIOLOGY

School nurses are familiar with head lice as a regularly recurring problem; there is apparently no clear increasing or decreasing trend in recent decades. GPs may see this complaint less often because of school-based treatment or because of the use of over-the-counter treatments. For head lice, the incidence is 1 per 1000 patients per year. Pubic lice are seen several times a year by GPs. Body lice are seen only rarely.

HISTORY

If head lice are suspected, the GP asks:

- about the reason for the consultation (usually contact or itching)
- whether head lice are currently a problem at the child's school.

In possible pubic lice, the GP asks:

- about the patient's sexual contacts, if the patient has not already volunteered this.

If body lice are suspected, the GP asks:

- about the social conditions (unless these are already clear).

EXAMINATION

The physical examination is generally focused on the symptomatic part of the body. If head lice are suspected, the scalp is examined to see if nits are present. These look like small white dots attached to the hair shaft close to the skin. In contrast to dandruff, the nits are firmly attached. Microscopic examination can provide confirmation: put the suspect hair in a drop of water on a glass slide, place the coverslide on top and examine with a 4× or 10× objective lens.

The nit will appear as an elongated oval attached to the hair. Nits are found mainly in the hair of the softer areas of the scalp above the ears or on the neck. Head lice themselves are seen less frequently. The examination is also aimed at ruling out other disorders, such as seborrhoeic eczema. However, treatment should not be started unless live lice are found – nits are not a sign of active infestation.

In the case of pubic lice, both the lice and nits can be seen in the pubic area, while the lice can also sometimes be found elsewhere, such as in the eyebrows and on the scalp. The skin has excoriated erythematous papules. Close examination can rule out the presence of scabies (the lesions are usually elsewhere, and there may be the characteristic tunnels) and other skin disorders.

In the case of body lice, the skin is examined for papules and the effects of scratching and possible impetiginization. Body lice are rarely found on the body itself. Instead, the GP should look for body lice and their eggs in the seams and hems of the patient's clothing.

If the diagnosis of head, pubic or body lice is certain, additional examination is not necessary. Otherwise, further examination can be carried out based on the possible differential diagnoses, considering, for example, seborrhoeic dermatitis, scabies, fungal infection or impetigo.

TREATMENT

Infested clothing, hairbrushes, pillowcases, etc., must be cleaned thoroughly.

Malathion and permethrin are the preferred treatments. A single application of malathion lotion can be used for head and pubic lice. Malathion may be washed off after 12 hours; it has an unpleasant odour. If the itching continues or returns, treatment must be repeated: any eggs that are unfortunately still alive will hatch 8–9 days later. Reinfestation should also be considered. Permethrin (the lotion for head lice, and the cream for pubic lice) is at least as effective as malathion. In 97–99% of cases, a single treatment is sufficient. Permethrin can be washed out after 10 minutes, remains on the hair for at least 10 days, and does not have an unpleasant smell.

The treatment has been successful if the itching does not return. The treated, dead nits will disappear by themselves over time without causing problems, even without the use of a special comb.

The treatment for body lice is simple: wash the clothes well.

PREVENTION AND ADDITIONAL INFORMATION

Preventing head lice in schoolchildren seems to be an endless task. In the event of an outbreak, the entire class should checked by parents, teachers or the school nurse so that all infested children can be treated at the same time. Family members should also be checked. The goal of the GP is to make clear that having head lice is not, by definition, a sign of poor hygiene on the part of the child, their classmates or parents.

The prevention of pubic lice is hindered by both infested bed linen and human inability to use common sense during intimate contacts with strangers! In this case, the GP may use the subject of preventing pubic lice to enable discussion of other, more serious, sexually transmitted diseases.

The prevention of body lice is a matter of social care. For the homeless and vagrants, an initial measure to prevent body lice is simple clothes-washing.

Key points

- Treatment for head lice should not be started unless live lice are found – nits are not a sign of active infestation.
- In contrast to dandruff, nits are firmly attached to the hair shaft.
- In the case of pubic lice, both the lice and nits can be seen in the pubic area.
- Body lice are rarely found on the body itself. Instead, the lice and their eggs may be seen in the seams and hems of the patient's clothing.

Literature

Brown S, Becher J, Bradt W. Treatment of ectoparasitic infections: review of the English-language literature 1982–1992. *Clin Infect Dis* 1995;**20**(Suppl 1): 104–9.

Chodidow O. Scabies and pediculosis. *Lancet* 2000;**355**:819–26.

Dodd CS. Interventions for treating headlice (Cochrane Review). *Cochrane Library*, Issue 2. Oxford: Update Software, 2004.

Meinking TL, Clineschmidt CM, Chen C, Kolber MA, Tipping RW, Furtek CI, Villar ME, Guzzo CA. An observer-blinded study of 1% permethrin creme rinse with and without adjunctive combing in patients with head lice. *J Pediatr* 2002;**141**(5):665–70.

Van der Stichele RH, Dezeure EM, Bogaert MG. Systematic review of clinical efficacy of topical treatment for head lice. *BMJ* 1995;**311**:604–8.

6

SCABIES

DEFINITION

Scabies is a contagious skin infestation caused in humans by the scabies mite *Sarcoptes scabiei* var. *hominis*. Animals (dogs, cats, horses, rabbits, pigs, etc.) have their own varieties that, in theory, cannot live on human skin, but which can sometimes cause problems in people if there is long-term close contact with an infected animal.

AETIOLOGY/PATHOGENESIS

The scabies mite is usually transferred through intensive skin contact (more intensive than shaking hands). It is transmitted only rarely by sleeping in an infected bed or by wearing infected clothing.

The mite can only live away from the human body for 3 hours. When it finds a new host, the mite can burrow into the stratum corneum within an hour. The male mite dies soon after fertilizing the female; the female can live for 30–40 days. The female mite digs tunnels by consuming skin cells, and by using the sharp 'jaws' on her front legs and lytic enzymes. She deposits three or four eggs in the burrow each day; the larvae, which hatch in 3 days, grow into adult mites after 2 weeks.

The symptoms develop due to an allergic reaction to the mites. The distribution of the allergic response usually does not match up with where the mite is located at that time.

After infestation, the following four stages are distinguished:

- *Incubation period*. In a first-ever infestation, the symptoms only develop after 4–10 weeks. In a subsequent infection, the symptoms develop almost immediately.
- *Primary sensitization period*. At each burrow, there is an itching papule, or sometimes vesicles or bullae. The total number of female mites on a patient can vary from 20 (in a healthy patient) to

thousands (in a patient suffering from the extremely contagious Norwegian scabies). In this last rare case, there is an inadequate immune response due to, for example, an immune or neurological disorder, or poor hygiene.

- *Secondary sensitization period*. After, or at the same time as, the local symptoms develop, there is a more generalized symmetrical and intensely itchy eruption. This is a cell-mediated occurrence, primarily on the wrists, elbows, underarms and sides of the body, and sometimes on the waist, buttocks, upper legs or ankles.
- *Delayed reactions*. In chronic cases, very diverse skin abnormalities can occur, varying from superficial vesicles or erythematous nodes, to hyperpigmented, tumour-like lesions; impetiginization is also possible.

Serious and even lethal complications of scabies can develop in the case of immunosuppression (e.g. HIV infection, corticosteroid use) or due to extensive secondary impetiginization (poor hygiene).

PRESENTATION

Itching is the first and most important complaint. This usually develops gradually and is almost unbearable at night or in warm conditions. The back, the middle of the chest and the head are almost never affected, except in young children.

EPIDEMIOLOGY

Prevalence and incidence figures in the UK are unreliable. Many patients treat themselves with over-the-counter remedies. Also, affected contacts are not documented.

Figures quoted for the incidence of scabies vary from 2.2 to 3.8 per 1000 patients per year. It is known that epidemics of scabies are related to living conditions. There may be a periodicity of 15–20 years in the virulence of the scabies mite, which is linked to the build-up of immunity in the population after infestation.

HISTORY

In any patient complaining of itching, consider scabies. The GP asks:

- when the itching started

- where on the body the itching is the worst
- if the itching is worse at night or when it is warm
- whether there are people in the environment who are experiencing itching or who have scabies (remember that the incubation period can be up to 10 weeks)
- whether bed partners, family members or friends at school are also experiencing itching
- whether there is regular contact with (house) pets.

It should also be established whether there are pointers in the history of other skin disorders, such as eczema or urticaria.

EXAMINATION

Scabies causes a polymorphic skin eruption with papules, vesicles, the effects of scratching, and sometimes also pustules, nodules and bullae. The epidermal burrows are pathognomonic; these can be recognized as greyish-white linear tracks 0.5–1.5 cm long. These tunnels are present, with decreasing frequency, on the sides of the fingers, the flexor side of the wrists, the lateral side of the foot, the penis and the scrotum, the extensor side of the elbow, the area around the navel and the folds of the underarm. However, these tunnels are only visible in less than half of cases. The polymorphic skin eruption is symmetrical; the head, back and the front of the thorax are not affected. There may also be secondary impetiginization due to scratching. Other symptoms develop in children, the elderly and patients with an immune-system disorder. They have less itching and skin symptoms, but the mite still reproduces. In infants, scabies can occur on the face, the soles of the feet and the palms of the hands. The severity of infection is influenced by the immune status of the host, the state of hygiene and any treatment.

A diagnosis can only be made with certainty by detecting the mite or eggs. Using a drop of ink (or oil) that is then wiped off, it is easy to follow the course of a tunnel; sometimes, using a magnifying glass, a thicker area can be seen where the mite is located. The mite can be 'caught' by opening the end of the tunnel with a needle; the mite and the eggs will stick to the needle. A scalpel can also be used to scrape off the oiled tunnel, and the material can be examined under a microscope to check for mites and eggs.

TREATMENT

The usual treatments are permethrin or malathion. All household members and other significant contacts should be treated. The treatment should be applied diligently to the whole body, not forgetting finger and toe webs and under the nails. Two applications, 1 week apart, are required; malathion should be washed off after 24 hours, permethrin after 12.

Bed linen and underclothes also need to be washed: blankets, duvets and other clothes need to be shaken out. Ritualistic cleaning, such as vigorously scrubbing the skin or boiling clothes and linens, is not necessary.

In the case of significant impetiginization, antibiotics are necessary (flucloxacillin, adult dose 250–500 mg four times daily for 7 days); milder infections clear by themselves after the mite has been eliminated (see Chapter 13 on impetigo). If scabies was transmitted through casual sexual contact, tests for other sexually transmitted diseases should also be discussed.

After appropriate treatment, the patient may still experience itching for several days or weeks, due to toxic decomposition substances. In this case, a persistent or new infection must be ruled out; the itching can be treated with local corticosteroids or an oral antihistamine.

Referral to a dermatologist is indicated if there is doubt about the diagnosis, if the treatment fails, or if there are complications. In the case of an epidemic in a closed community, the help of a dermatologist or a public health doctor is often required to manage the situation.

PREVENTION AND ADDITIONAL INFORMATION

Scabies can be transmitted even by hand-holding for a certain period of time; it is therefore not only a result of poor hygiene. However, the number of mites is decreased by washing. If scabies is not treated properly, or the infected person's contacts are not traced, the mite can spread quickly.

Key points

- The scabies mite is usually transferred through intensive skin contact (more intensive than shaking hands). It is transmitted only rarely by sleeping in an infected bed or by wearing infected clothing.

- The symptoms develop due to an allergic reaction to the mites.

- In any patient complaining of itching, consider scabies. The itching usually develops gradually and is almost unbearable at night or under warm conditions.

- All household members – and other significant contacts – should be treated.

- After appropriate treatment, the patient may still experience itching for several days or weeks.

Literature

Chosidow O. Scabies and pediculosis. *Lancet* 2000;**355**:819–26.

McCarthy JS, Kemp DJ, Walton SF, Currie BJ. Scabies: more than just an irritation. *Postgrad Med J* 2004;**80**(945):382–7.

7

DOG AND CAT BITES

DEFINITION

A bite from a dog or a cat results in micro-organisms from the animal's mouth entering the wound. Because of the way they bite and the anatomy of their teeth, dogs usually cause tearing wounds and crushing injuries; cats cause deep, penetrating wounds.

AETIOLOGY/PATHOGENESIS

In a bite wound there are, on average, three different types of micro-organisms that are transmitted from the mouth of the animal. These are usually three of streptococci, *Staphylococcus aureus*, *Pasteurella multocida* and *Capnocytophaga canimorsus*. Jagged and/or deep bite wounds form the ideal breeding ground for these micro-organisms.

A scratch wound has a lower chance of infection than a bite wound. 'Cat-scratch disease' can have more causes than the name suggests. It can also be caused by a cat bite, and sometimes a dog bite. A regional lymphadenopathy with micro-abscesses develops proximal to the scratch or bite.

PRESENTATION

Patients often know that a bite wound is 'dirty' and ask whether antibiotics are required. In the case of a tearing injury or flap wound, patients also often ask whether stitches are necessary. In the case of superficial wounds, the patient sometimes only asks for advice by telephone.

EPIDEMIOLOGY

The incidence in Dutch general practice is 3.2 per 1000 patients per year. Of these, 90% of bites are caused by dogs and 6% by cats.

Overall, 3% are referred to secondary care. It is striking that three-quarters of people bitten are younger than 30 years old. In children up to 4 years of age, the consequences can be serious; they are bitten more often in the face than adults. Three-quarters of dog bites are located on the arm or the hand.

HISTORY

The health of the animal and the person bitten are most important. The GP asks:

- where (home or abroad) and when the incident took place, and whether the animal was sick when it bit the victim
- whether the patient is a 'YOPI' – does the patient belong to the risk groups 'young' (<5 years old), 'old' (>65 years old), 'pregnant' or 'immunocompromised' (corticosteroid use, diabetes mellitus, malignancy)
- whether the patient has a heart valve problem or a joint prosthesis.

EXAMINATION

It is very important to estimate the extent of tissue damage. The depth of a cat bite is difficult to determine. Sensation and movement should be tested, because damage to nerves, tendons, bone and joints is possible. If the patient attends late (after one or more days) the GP must check for signs of cellulitis around the wound, and for fever. In cat-scratch disease, painful regional lymph nodes are present.

TREATMENT

Two controversies emerge when studying the literature. They concern whether or not to close gaping wounds and whether or not to administer antimicrobial prophylaxis. In general, it is thought that stitches may make the problem worse and increase the risk of infection. Only if the bite is on the face should the edges of the wound be approximated (i.e. sutured loosely).

The least controversial element is the basis of treating every bite: cleaning the wound. Thorough rinsing and, where necessary, debridement reduces the risk of infection by a factor of 20. Local anaesthesia can help with proper cleaning.

Applying a moist bandage for 2 days also reduces the risk of infection, probably through a combination of improved circulation and drainage.

Administering antibiotics can sometimes prevent infection. Nonetheless, bearing in mind the risk of promoting resistance, the general advice is not to use antibiotic prophylaxis for a dog bite. The exceptions are delayed presentation, deep wounds that are difficult to clean, bites on the face and the patient with lowered resistance to infection. A cat bite has a much greater risk of infection (25–50%) than a dog bite (5–15%) and administering antibiotics is advisable for cat bites.

Amoxicillin/clavulanic acid 625 mg three times daily for 7–10 days is the preferred treatment, in view of the sensitivity spectrum of the likely micro-organisms. In a person with penicillin allergy, doxycycline is a suitable alternative; for children and pregnant women clarithromycin is a good choice. If there is a significant risk of infection, the patient should have the wound checked by the GP or practice nurse 1–3 days later. Finally, the patient should be protected against tetanus, following the guidelines in the Department of Health's book *Immunisation against Infectious Disease*.

If underlying structures have been damaged, referral should be made to secondary care. In the extremely rare situation of suspected rabies, advice should be sought from the Health Protection Agency (http://www.hpa.org.uk; tel. 0207 7339 1300).

PREVENTION AND ADDITIONAL INFORMATION

Make clear to the patient why a tetanus injection may be necessary and that this does not protect against wound infection. General recommendations for preventing bites are as follows: do not pet animals or pets you do not know; do not touch animals when they are eating or when they are playing with other animals; be careful with a female and her young; and do not leave a young child alone with a pet.

Key points

- A scratch wound has a lower chance of infection than a bite.
- Only if the bite is on the face should the edges of the wound be approximated.
- Thorough rinsing and, where necessary, debridement reduces the risk of infection by a factor of 20.
- The general advice for a dog bite is not to use antibiotic prophylaxis, although there are exceptions. A cat bite has a much greater risk of infection (25–50%) than a dog bite (5–15%), so administering antibiotics for cat bites is advisable.

Literature

De Melker HE, De Melker RA. Hondenbeten: publicaties over risicofactoren, infecties, antibiotica en primaire wondsluiting [Dog bites: publications on risk factors, infections, antibiotics and primary wound closure]. *Ned Tijdschr Geneeskd* 1996;**140**:709–13.

Department of Health. *Immunisation against infectious disease 1996*. London: DoH, 1996.

Medeiros I, Saconato H. Antibiotic prophylaxis for mammalian bites (Cochrane Review). *Cochrane Library*, Issue 2. Oxford: Update Software, 2004.

Moore F. I've just been bitten by a dog. *BMJ* 1996;**314**:88–90.

Van de Lisdonk EH, Van Deijck RHPF. Au! Over zelfbehandeling van schaaf-, snij- en bijtwonden [Ow! About treating scrapes, cuts and bite wounds yourself]. *Huisarts Wet* 1998;**21**:410–12.

Wiggins ME, Akelman E, Weiss AP. The management of dog bites and dog bite infections to the hand. *Orthopedics* 1994;**17**(7):617–23.

8

ABRASIONS

DEFINITION

Abrasions are superficial wounds in which usually only the epidermis and small parts of the dermis are damaged.

AETIOLOGY/PATHOGENESIS

When the skin is scraped along a rough surface, the epidermis is damaged. This can happen in traffic accidents, in and around the house, and while doing sports. When sports (such as hockey) are played on artificial grass, participants can suffer ugly abrasions on the knees, elbows and hands; the intense friction means these will feel like burns. The extensive abrasions seen in cycling accidents are often contaminated with, for example, dirt, gravel and grit. Iatrogenic abrasions refer to 'donor sites': the abrasion that remains after taking off the skin used for a graft.

PRESENTATION

The usual reason for a consultation is to get the wound treated and dressed. Patients may also attend for pain relief and a tetanus vaccine. Other injuries may also require attention.

EPIDEMIOLOGY

Little is known about the incidence of abrasions. GPs probably only see the tip of the iceberg: most patients with these minor injuries are not likely to consult.

HISTORY

The history is usually short. The GP asks:

- how the abrasion happened (knowledge about how it occurred helps when estimating the extent of the damage to the deeper structures and the degree of contamination of the wound)
- when the abrasion occurred (significant lesions older than 6 hours must be considered as infected)
- about factors that could negatively affect wound healing, such as a systemic illness (e.g. diabetes mellitus), atherosclerosis, chronic venous insufficiency and medication (anticoagulants, corticosteroids, cytotoxics)
- about tetanus cover.

EXAMINATION

This consists primarily of local inspection, unless damage to deeper structures is suspected.

An abrasion is characterized by point-shaped (petechial) bleeding from the dermis. Extensive abrasions, however, can lead to significant blood loss. The lesion can be very painful as a result of damage to superficial nerve endings, which are present in great numbers in the skin. The depth, size, site and extent of contamination and the likelihood of foreign bodies should be assessed. It is important to remember that, in the case of additional contusion, damage to the underlying soft structures can be greater than might appear on the outside.

TREATMENT

First of all, abrasions must be cleaned thoroughly. The wound can be rinsed out with running tap water. Adding other substances to the water (such as soap) is not necessary.

Foreign bodies (such as dirt or gravel) must be removed with a sterile gauze to prevent infection and unattractive 'tattoo' scars. If the wound is very dirty, it may have to be cleaned using a brush (and perhaps tweezers). Because this can be very painful, it is a good idea to use a local anaesthetic. After cleaning, the abrasion must be disinfected with povidone iodine or chlorhexidine 1%.

Depending on the site, size and depth, the abrasion may be left to air dry. As the wound fluid dries, a scab develops that seals it; this keeps it from drying out and becoming infected. The process of healing (epithelization) takes place under the protective scab. This falls off spontaneously once the epithelial tissue has recovered.

Wound covering is important for skin areas under clothing and for deeper abrasions. One can choose between dry wound healing and moist wound healing.

Non-occlusive dressing (dry wound healing). The abrasion can be covered with paraffin gauze or non-adherent absorbent compresses. For older and/or seriously contaminated abrasions, povidone iodine ointment gauze may be used or an antibiotic ointment (fusidic acid) may be applied locally. In dry wound healing, a crust forms on the wound. This protective crust, however, also has disadvantages. It is vulnerable and rather inflexible. Impregnated gauze and non-adherent absorbent compresses can stick to the crust, and can disrupt the healing of the wound when the dressing is removed (it needs to be changed at least once a day); this can also be painful.

If, despite proper cleaning and disinfection, the wound still becomes infected, it must be cleaned again. Subsequently, a povidone iodine ointment gauze may be used or an antibiotic ointment (fusidic acid, three times daily for 1 week) may be applied locally. For extensive infections, regional lymphadenopathy and fever, oral antibiotics are indicated (such as flucloxacillin in standard doses).

Occlusive covering (moist wound healing). Here the function of the crust is taken over by a synthetic occlusive wound bandage/covering. The wound stays wet/moist, which speeds up the healing process and is less painful for the patient. If necessary, the bandage can be changed after a day; it can remain on the wound for another 3–5 days. Synthetic occlusive bandages are mainly indicated for tender and inflexible crusts (sportsmen, on moving parts: knees, elbows, etc.). These synthetic bandages are relatively expensive.

Tetanus vaccine should be administered if appropriate.

PREVENTION AND ADDITIONAL INFORMATION

Explanation and hygiene advice is usually sufficient. The prognosis for abrasions is good; they are sometimes troublesome wounds, but usually heal without complications or scarring.

Abrasions occurring during sport can be prevented by the use of protective clothing or equipment (e.g. cycling gloves, elbow and knee pads).

Key points

- Remember to check tetanus status.
- Extensive abrasions can lead to significant blood loss. The lesion can also be very painful as a result of damage to superficial nerve endings, which are present in great numbers in the skin.
- Do not overlook important damage to deeper structures.

Literature

Afset JE, Maeland JA. Susceptibility of skin and soft-tissue isolates of *Staphylococcus aureus* and *Streptococcus pyogenes* to topical antibiotics: indications of clonal spread of fusidic acid-resistant *Staphylococcus aureus*. *Scand J Infect Dis* 2003;**35**:84–9.

Bryan J. Moist wound healing: a concept that changed our practice. *J Wound Care* 2004;**13**:227–8.

Jonkman MF. Occlusief wondverband [Occlusive wound dressing]. *Ned Tijdschr Geneeskd* 1991;**135**:1905–8.

Smeenk G, Sebens FW, Houwing RH. Nut en gevaren van op de huid toegepaste antibiotica en desinfectantia [Use and adverse reactions of local antibiotics and disinfectants on the skin]. Ned Tijdschr Geneeskd 1999;**143**:1140-3.

9

HAEMATOMAS (IN AND AROUND MUSCLES)

DEFINITION

A haematoma is a localized collection of blood that has leaked from the blood vessels. This broad definition means that a haematoma can occur in every part of the body where blood vessels are present; this is (nearly) everywhere. Thus, for example, haematosalpinx, haematopericardium, haematomediastinum, haemarthrosis and subdural haematoma fall within this definition. These disorders, however, go beyond what is covered in this chapter.

The focus here is on the concept of an 'effusion of blood' (sometimes, if visible, also called a 'bruise'): an accumulation of blood from the blood vessels, which is generally localized subcutaneously, inside muscle fascia or between muscle and bone. A slight to moderately painful swelling develops, which is usually easily palpable. The swelling changes colour at a later stage.

AETIOLOGY/PATHOGENESIS

A haematoma can occur in two ways. First, *from outside* due to blunt trauma. The size of the haematoma depends on the intensity and site of the force. For example, blunt trauma to the skull will cause a haematoma that manifests in a very visible, painful swelling. This haematoma develops very quickly because of the damage to the many blood vessels in the vessel-rich area. The size is limited due to the high resistance of the area – there is little space between the bone and the skin, causing the pressure to rise quickly, the bleeding vessels to be squeezed shut, and the leak of blood to be 'plugged'. In other areas of the body, such as the calf, the bleeding experiences much less resistance, is usually less visible or palpable, and, if left untreated, can be profuse.

Second, a haematoma can occur *from inside*. This is usually caused by an acute overload of locomotor structures (muscles, tendons, ligaments): a rupture develops which results in blood vessel damage and bleeding. This is seen frequently in sports, but also in daily life (e.g. as a result of slipping or stumbling). The patient may have forgotten the incident by the time he attends complaining of swelling or discoloration. These haematomas can be very extensive yet go unnoticed if they occur in soft tissue with little resistance.

The haematoma itself can move due to the influence of gravity and resistance from the surrounding area. As a result, after several hours to several days, the site of the haematoma will not necessarily be the same as the area of trauma. A well-known example involves a haematoma on the forehead resulting in a 'black eye'. This downward tracking also occurs in muscle ruptures.

Other factors can also play a role in the development of a haematoma. For example, people taking oral anticoagulants have a higher risk of a more extensive haematoma and will also develop a haematoma more quickly as a result of relatively minor trauma. The same applies to patients with coagulation disorders; frequent and easily developing haematomas can be the first sign of such a disorder. Haematomas are seen more frequently in the elderly than in young people. It is likely that the decreased strength and elasticity of small blood vessels play a role in this.

PRESENTATION

The patient is usually worried about the appearance and/or has pain. He will want to know if the haematoma needs to be treated and whether additional examination is necessary to rule out, for example, a fracture.

EPIDEMIOLOGY

No research data on the occurrence of haematomas are available. However, everyday – and clinical – experience suggests that they occur very frequently.

HISTORY

The GP asks:

- about the nature of the trauma
- about the use of anticoagulants or any coagulation disorder.

EXAMINATION

The size or extent of the haematoma is assessed. The GP assesses whether there is any significant underlying trauma (e.g. a fracture, muscle rupture) and checks that the appearance of the haematoma is consistent with the history. The colour and characteristics of the haematoma often develop as follows:

- 0–2 days: swollen and sensitive
- 0–5 days: red, blue, purple
- 5–7 days: green
- 7–10 days: yellow
- 10–14 days (or longer): brown
- 2–4 weeks: gone.

Alarm bells should ring if the haematoma is more extensive than expected, or if haematomas are recurrent (remember acquired coagulation disorders, arterial rupture and chronic excessive alcohol use).

For children with a haematoma, remember possible child abuse, especially in the case of recurrent problems. A haematoma resulting from abuse sometimes has a recognizable form, such as the imprint of a hand, belt or teeth, and is often found on unusual areas of the body. The history may also arouse suspicion if it does not tally with the nature, form and site of the haematoma.

TREATMENT

In general, the rule of thumb is to leave the haematoma alone. Resolving a haematoma by aspiration is not usually necessary and can lead to infection. Surgically opening the haematoma also has a high chance of secondary infection. An exception to this is a haematoma under a fingernail or toenail, which can be extremely painful. To relieve the pain, a small hole may be made in the nail (see Chapter 100). Massaging the muscle groups in which the haematoma is present is not advisable. Physiotherapy is only appropriate if it is necessary to expedite functional recovery at a later stage.

Most haematomas should be treated conservatively, with rest, ice and, possibly, pressure (using a pressure dressing), and elevating the relevant body part.

Ice the injury three or more times a day for the first day as follows: fill a plastic bag with ice cubes and wrap it in a towel; put this on the haematoma for half an hour. Icing also helps to decrease the pain. After 2–4 days, the patient needs to start moving the affected body part.

PREVENTION AND ADDITIONAL INFORMATION

To prevent haematomas due to external forces, accident prevention is the key. For other haematomas, measures to prevent injury should be taken (e.g. warming-up, cooling-down and stretching exercises).

Key points

- A haematoma can occur in every part of the body where blood vessels are present.
- Beware the haematoma that is more extensive than expected, or the patient with recurrent haematomas (remember acquired coagulation disorders, arterial rupture and chronic excessive alcohol use).
- For children with a haematoma, remember possible child abuse, especially in the case of recurrent problems.
- In general, the rule of thumb is to leave the haematoma alone.

Literature

Rooser B, Bengston S, Hagglund G. Acute compartment syndrome from anterior thigh muscle contusion: a report of eight cases. *J Orthop Trauma* 1991;**5**(1):57–9.

Schmitt BD. *The child with non-accidental trauma*. Chicago: University of Chicago Press, 1987.

10
WARTS

DEFINITION

The common wart is a round, clearly defined skin papule, with a diameter of several millimetres to a centimetre, from skin colour to yellowish-grey, with a rough, cauliflower-like surface.

AETIOLOGY/PATHOGENESIS

Warts are small, benign tumours of the skin or mucous membranes. There are many different types of viral wart, such as the common wart, plane wart, filiform wart and verruca. Senile or seborrhoeic keratoses are sometimes described as 'seborrhoeic warts', although they are not viral.

Viral warts are caused by the human papillomavirus (HPV). Different varieties of HPV cause different types of warts (for more information, see the related chapters). For a number of types of HPV (HPV-16, -18 and -38), research is underway to examine their relationship with cancer. However, HPV-1 and -2 are not regarded as potentially carcinogenic. This chapter covers the common wart. Verrucas are covered in Chapter 119.

Common warts are caused by HPV-2. If warts are to develop, the individual must be infected with this virus – but other conditions must also be present, such as the weakening of local skin resistance due to a minor injury. This is demonstrated by the familiar distribution on the hands (80%), the knees (of children) and the beard area (in men). Developing immunity during life is apparently also a factor, because warts occur most often in young people, primarily in school-going children. The fact that various warts on the same individual can all disappear spontaneously in a short time confirms the role of immunity. In addition, immunosuppression can result in the development of large numbers of warts.

PRESENTATION

Children usually attend with one of their parents. The reasons for the consultation vary. People often think warts are dirty or ugly: other people comment on them or show their aversion. It is often asked whether a wart is contagious. A rapid increase in the number of warts, or pain or cosmetic worries about warts are also reasons for attendance.

EPIDEMIOLOGY

Quoted prevalence rates vary hugely (from 0.84% in the USA to 12.9% in Russia). In the UK, the prevalence amongst 4- to 6-year-old children is 12%.

Approximately 80% are common warts. In an average practice, a GP can expect approximately 20 new cases per year.

HISTORY

The GP asks:

- how long the wart has been present
- whether the patient has already tried to treat it
- if there are warts on other parts of the body
- if the patient is bothered by the wart.

If the patient has a lot of warts, the GP should consider whether immune factors might be of any relevance.

EXAMINATION

When examining the lesion, the diagnosis is usually immediately clear. If a wart does not have the normal appearance, the differential diagnosis might include: molluscum contagiosum, skin carcinoma and amelanotic melanoma.

TREATMENT

Appropriate treatment first involves providing an explanation about the natural course and the advantages and disadvantages of the therapeutic options. Treatment sometimes makes matters worse. For small warts, or those that are not particularly troublesome, the patient can be advised to let nature take its course. As 80% of warts disappear within 2 years by themselves, waiting for a spontaneous cure is a realistic option.

If it is decided to treat the wart, the following are possibilities.

Self-treatment with salicylic acid. Dab the wart once a day with salicylic acid, using a cotton bud or a matchstick; make sure the solution does not spread out onto the surrounding healthy skin, as this may cause blisters. The skin around the wart may be protected with Vaseline. After each application, cover the wart with an adhesive plaster. Make sure the bottle is kept out of children's reach.

Freezing with liquid nitrogen. The centre of the wart must be firmly dabbed with a cotton bud well moistened with liquid nitrogen. The freezing appears as a white discoloration. A margin of 3 mm around the wart should be frozen at the same time. The treatment takes 10–20 seconds and may be repeated after a month if necessary. With this treatment, two-thirds of warts disappear in 1–3 months. The application of the liquid nitrogen is painful for several seconds. GPs may provide this service in-house or may refer the patient to the local minor surgery facility.

Curettage. The wart may initially be frozen with ethyl chloride spray, although this may be painful. Local anaesthesia with 2% lignocaine is an alternative. Heavy bleeding can sometimes occur after thawing.

PREVENTION AND ADDITIONAL INFORMATION

People probably are regularly infected with HPV-2 through normal hand contact. However, only a minority of those infected actually develop warts, so the individual's immune response is important. It has not been proved that common warts can be spread via swimming pools. Because the complaint is harmless, there are no good reasons to advise the patient to take socially isolating measures (from not shaking hands to not going swimming). There is no effective vaccine.

Key points

- If warts are to develop, the individual must be infected with HPV, but other conditions must also be present, such as the weakening of local skin resistance due to a minor injury.
- Treatment sometimes makes matters worse.
- 80% of warts disappear within 2 years by themselves.
- It has not been proved that common warts can be spread via swimming pools.

Literature

Gibbs S, Harvey I, Sterling JC, Stark R. Local treatments for cutaneous warts (Cochrane Review). *Cochrane Library*, Issue 1. Oxford: Update Software, 2003.

Koning S, Bruijnzeels MA, Van der Wouden JC, Suylekom-Smit LWA. Wratten: incidentie en beleid in de huisartsenpraktijk [Warts: incidence and treatment in general practice]. *Huisarts Wet* 1994;**37**:431–4.

Kuykendall TD, Johnson S. Evidence-based review of management of non-genital cutaneous warts. *Cutis* 2003;**71**:213–22.

Sterling JC, Handfield-Jones S, Hudson PM. Guidelines for the management of cutaneous warts. *Br J Dermatol* 2001;**144**:4–11.

11

MOLLUSCUM CONTAGIOSUM

DEFINITION

Molluscum contagiosum is a skin infection characterized by waxy papules with a central umbilication, usually no larger than 2–5 mm, which generally disappear spontaneously without scarring.

AETIOLOGY/PATHOGENESIS

Molluscum contagiosum is caused by a pox virus. The infection probably takes place through direct skin contact. The incubation period is 2–7 weeks. In young adults, this infection sometimes appears in the anogenital area, which suggests that the infection can be sexually transmitted. The lesions are often seen on eczematous skin. It is not known whether the eczema develops secondarily to the mollusca, or vice versa. Illnesses and/or medication that lower a person's resistance or suppress the immune system can cause widespread infection. An intact immune system provides life-long immunity after infection. As a result, given time, molluscum contagiosum always disappears spontaneously and permanently. As is the case for common warts (see Chapter 10), molluscum contagiosum is therefore usually a childhood illness.

PRESENTATION

Because this infection often affects children, the patient attends with one or both parents. The usual query relates to what the problem is and what course it will take. The GP is also consulted for aesthetic reasons, and often with a request for active treatment. Less frequent reasons for a consultation are itching (usually when the infection occurs at the same time as eczema) or pain due to secondary infection. The patient may also visit with the fear that the problem will spread or be passed on to others.

Occasionally, adults will present with this infection in the anogenital area. Very rarely, the lesions will be present on the conjunctivae, which can result in chronic conjunctivitis.

EPIDEMIOLOGY

In The Netherlands, the incidence is 2.4 per 1000 patients per year. Approximately 16% of children up to age 15 visit their GP at least once for molluscum contagiosum, the peak incidence being between the ages of 6 and 10. Around 2% of the patients are young adults with the infection in the anogenital area. For this group, the infection can be considered a sexually transmitted disease (STD). Molluscum contagiosum occurs in people of all races and all over the world. Small epidemics have been described in schools and children's homes.

HISTORY

Depending on the site of the problem, the GP asks:

- about pointers of reduced resistance or immunosuppression
- about the development of the infection over time
- about close contacts who also have this infection.

For young adults with molluscum contagiosum in the anogenital region, the sexual history should be taken. For children with the infection in the same region, the possibility of sexual abuse should be considered.

EXAMINATION

The physical examination consists of inspection of the affected skin, paying attention to the typical appearance of molluscum contagiosum: domed papules with a central umbilication, a waxy transparent colour, a diameter of 2–5 mm (sometimes up to 10–15 mm), usually found in groups on one or more places on the body. There may be signs of secondary infection, and the mollusca may be surrounded by eczema. If necessary, all the patient's skin should be examined, including the conjunctivae, mouth and anogenital area.

The appearance is so typical that no additional investigation is needed. If the mollusca are localized to the anogenital area, other STDs should be considered and investigated appropriately.

TREATMENT

In principle, it is sufficient to wait for the infection to disappear spontaneously. Molluscum contagiosum resolves without scarring, usually taking between 6 months and 3–4 years. If the papules show signs of inflammation (not caused by a secondary infection or scratching), then spontaneous healing usually soon follows.

Occasionally, because of the long duration and contagiousness of the ailment, it is deemed necessary to treat the infection actively. Depending on the site and number of lesions, the following options can be considered. First, an optional anaesthetic ointment may be applied, and then a few lesions squeezed between thumbnails until empty. The parent(s) can be instructed in how to do this. Other alternatives are curettage, after numbing the area (with lidocaine ointment) if necessary, and making a superficial incision in the papule, followed by squeezing out the contents and, perhaps, applying povidone iodine solution (10%) or iodine tincture (1%). Treating the lesions with liquid nitrogen is considerably less effective than for common warts. In the case of secondarily infected papules, the infection must be treated first. Fusidic acid cream three times daily for 1 week is the preferred treatment.

Secondary eczema will disappear after treatment of the mollusca. Pre-existing eczema, in which molluscum contagiosum thrives, must be treated properly.

PREVENTION AND ADDITIONAL INFORMATION

The main method of infection is direct skin contact. This is generally not preventable in children. It should always be explained that this is a harmless infection that inevitably disappears in time by itself. If the lesions are present in the anogenital area, a condom offers some protection in sexual contact.

Key points

- Molluscum contagiosum always disappears spontaneously and permanently.
- For young adults with molluscum contagiosum in the anogenital region, a sexual history should be taken.
- For children with the infection in the same region, the possibility of sexual abuse should be considered.

Literature

Lewis EJ, Lam N, Crutchfield CE. An update on molluscum contagiosum. *Cutis* 1997;**60**:29–34.

Ordoukhakian E, Lane AT. Warts and molluscum contagiosum: beware of treatments worse than the disease. *Postgrad Med* 1997;**101**:223–6.

Silverberg N. Pediatric molluscum contagiosum: optimal treatment strategies. *Paediatr Drugs* 2003;**5**(8):505–12.

Stulberg DL, Penrod MA, Blatny RA. Common bacterial skin infections. *Am Fam Physician* 2002;**66**:119–24.

Stulberg DL, Hutchinson AG. Molluscum contagiosum and warts. *Am Fam Physician* 2003;**67**(6):1233–40.

12

BOILS/FURUNCLES

DEFINITION

A furuncle or boil is an acute abscess of a hair follicle, usually caused by *Staphylococcus aureus*. A carbuncle is a conglomeration of furuncles with necrosis and abscesses. Furunculosis is the presence of large numbers of furuncles at the same time or repeatedly.

AETIOLOGY/PATHOGENESIS

A furuncle develops from folliculitis – a superficial infection of a hair follicle. A furuncle is a deeper seated infection, where an infiltrate forms, accompanied by necrosis and pus. In a carbuncle, there is more extensive and even deeper infiltrate. A combination of different furuncles together is also referred to as a carbuncle. The difference between a furuncle and carbuncle cannot always be clearly defined.

A local predisposing factor for the development of these lesions is the blockage of a hair follicle from chemicals or oil. Local irritation of the skin, for example due to chafing clothing, can also lead to these infections. This is often the case in the groin area, on the neck and on the buttocks (for cyclists). General predisposing factors are: a lowered general resistance to infection, anaemia, diabetes mellitus, poor hygiene, obesity and hyperhidrosis. Usually, however, there are no such factors. In the majority of cases, the pathogenic micro-organism is *S. aureus*; exceptionally it is *S. epidermidis*.

PRESENTATION

Most people do not immediately see their GP when they have a furuncle. A consultation is usually prompted by pain or the general symptoms of infection, such as fever and general malaise (for carbuncles), or for questions about preventive measures.

EPIDEMIOLOGY

The incidence in general practice for these infections is 5.7 per 1000 patients per year, with the highest incidence being in men aged 15–29 years. The GP probably only sees the tip of the iceberg.

HISTORY

The GP asks:

- how long the problem has been present
- how it has developed over time
- about symptoms of diabetes mellitus or reduced resistance to infection
- about other people in the immediate environment with skin infections
- about cardiac valve lesions or joint prostheses.

EXAMINATION

The physical examination for a furuncle is usually limited to local inspection. It may be palpated to check if it has reached the stage of fluctuation. They are usually found on hairy areas of the body, such as the neck, face, underarms and buttocks.

A culture is only considered necessary if a furuncle does not respond to the recommended treatment, and for patients with immunodeficiency. In the case of furunculosis (e.g. when more than four furuncles are present at the same time and/or more than four times within a year) it is worth establishing whether the patient is a carrier of S. aureus by taking swabs of the nasal mucous membrane and the perineum – these areas can be a source of repeated self-infection. However, culture results are of limited value: 70–90% of the Dutch population are transient carriers of S. aureus, while approximately 10% are permanent carriers. In the case of furunculosis, up to 50% of people are carriers.

Further tests are not usually required unless there are pointers to other pathology such as diabetes.

TREATMENT

For people who are generally healthy, a furuncle or carbuncle is a troublesome and contagious, but harmless, complaint. In most cases, they are managed by the GP; no more than 6% of patients are referred to hospital.

In the case of single small furuncles, an explanation and recommendations about hygiene are usually sufficient. The GP can recommend hot compresses, which may help it come to a head. Apart from that, the patient should leave the furuncle alone to prevent the bacteria from spreading. Lancing and drainage can promote the healing process, as long as the furuncle is 'pointing' and fluctuation is present. In most cases, however, lancing is not necessary, as the furuncle discharges pus spontaneously. The pain disappears immediately after this, as does the redness after a few days.

A furuncle that recurs in exactly the same place can be permanently cured by excising the relevant hair follicle.

Because antibiotics cannot penetrate an abscess, antimicrobial therapy is not advised for low-risk patients with minor furuncles. However, antibiotic therapy is indicated in certain situations that predispose to complications. These include: furunculosis and carbuncles, lesions on the lips or nose, the immunosuppressed, and patients with valve lesions or joint prostheses.

As 80% of the *S. aureus* strains produce penicillinase, the recommended treatment is a penicillinase-resistant antibiotic, preferably flucloxacillin 500 mg four times daily. In the case of penicillin allergy, an alternative is erythromycin 500 mg four times daily for 7 days.

For patients who have a furuncle more than four times a year, the possibility of underlying illness and staphylococcal carriage must always be investigated.

PREVENTION AND ADDITIONAL INFORMATION

Patients with a furuncle must always be informed about its contagiousness, both for themselves and people in the surrounding environment. Preventive measures mainly involve promoting proper hygiene and good health.

Rubbing the skin should be avoided, because this can encourage bacteria to enter. The patient should be advised to wash using soap and water, and to wash clothes and bed linens daily, with the hottest water possible. As a supplementary measure, mupirocin ointment 2% can be applied to the nasal mucous membranes twice daily for 5–7 days. In addition, some sources have recommended treating the perineum with, for example, fusidic acid cream, 2–4 times daily every fourth week, for 4–15 months.

The prognosis of furuncles and carbuncles is good; they are troublesome complaints but generally heal without complications, although at times with some scarring. Of patients with furunculosis, 75% are free of problems after 2 years, if the exacerbations are treated. A quarter of patients continue to have complaints, despite an initial good response to the treatment.

Key points

- In the case of furunculosis (when more than four furuncles are present at the same time and/or more than four times within a year) investigate whether the patient is a carrier of *S. aureus*.

- In most cases, lancing is not necessary, as the furuncle discharges pus spontaneously.

- Antibiotic therapy is indicated in certain situations that predispose to complications, such as: furunculosis and carbuncles, lesions on the lips or nose, the immunosuppressed, and patients with valve lesions or joint prostheses.

- Of patients with furunculosis, 75% are free of problems after 2 years, if the exacerbations are treated. However, a quarter of patients continue to have complaints.

Literature
Bukman A, De Jongh TOH. Kleine kwalen in de huisartsgeneeskunde; furunkel, carbunkel en furunculose [Minor ailments in general practice; furuncle, carbuncle, and furunculosis]. *Ned Tijdschr Geneeskd* 1990;**134**:2432–3.

13

IMPETIGO AND IMPETIGINIZATION

DEFINITION

Impetigo is a contagious skin infection caused by staphylococci and/or streptococci. Impetiginization occurs when a pre-existing dermatosis (often eczema, sometimes an insect bite, prurigo or scabies) becomes infected and an impetigo-like rash develops.

AETIOLOGY/PATHOGENESIS

Impetigo is usually caused by *Staphylococcus aureus* and/or *Streptococcus pyogenes*. It usually starts with a small blister surrounded by a red ring. This fragile blister pops quickly, releasing fluid (exudate) and drying into yellow crusts. As various patches come together, they form a cluster of crusty lesions. The usual sites are the face, especially around the nose and mouth.

Spontaneous healing without scarring can occur in 2–3 weeks.

Impetigo bullosa is a variation of impetigo (always caused by staphylococci), in which blisters predominate. This form is present in people of all ages; in infants, it can quickly spread and take very serious forms (e.g. scalded skin syndrome).

Impetiginization is a bacterial (super)infection of an existing skin disorder. *S. aureus* is generally the cause. The infection can exacerbate the underlying skin disorder.

Complications of impetigo are generally heralded by a fever and a general feeling of malaise, but are very rare (osteomyelitis, general sepsis, glomerulonephritis).

PRESENTATION

Often accompanied by their parents, patients will visit the GP because of a skin lesion that will not heal, or because more spots continue to appear. The parents themselves often wonder if the child has impetigo, or they may have been asked by someone at the child's school whether the child has impetigo.

EPIDEMIOLOGY

Impetigo primarily occurs in children, mainly those aged 4–7 years. It often occurs in minor epidemics in a family or at schools. The incidence in general practice is 19.5 per 1000 patients per year in the age group 0–14 years. It occurs most often in children aged 4–5 years (38 new cases per 1000 contacts per year). In adults, it usually occurs in an environment where people live closely together (e.g. in the military).

HISTORY

The GP asks:

- when the problem started
- what it looked like when it started
- whether a single spot or several spots on the body are affected
- whether there is itching or pain
- whether there is a fever or a general feeling of malaise
- whether the patient often has such skin infections
- whether others in the patient's immediate environment have the same symptoms.

EXAMINATION

The physical examination involves careful inspection of the skin. The extent of the skin infection is assessed. The GP examines the spot(s) to see if there are signs of infection (redness, swelling or heat) and determines whether there are blisters, pus, crusts or necrosis. The GP also checks for an underlying skin disorder or wound.

TREATMENT

Cleaning the skin with an antiseptic is the basis of treatment for minor lesions.

If the lesions are more extensive, local application of fusidic acid 2% three times daily for a maximum of 14 days is the preferred treatment. Local treatment with mupirocin and erythromycin is not more effective than fusidic acid. If after 14 days there has been no improvement or a deterioration, oral treatment with flucloxacillin (adults and children from 12 years, 500 mg four times daily for 5–10 days) is indicated. This also applies to patients with a lowered resistance or if the infection is accompanied by general symptoms of illness.

In the case of limited impetiginization of eczema, first the anti-eczema therapy is intensified. If this does not lead to improvement, 1 week of treatment is carried out with fusidic acid (see above), after which the anti-eczema therapy is started again. In the case of extensive impetiginization, flucloxacillin (see above) is used in combination with the anti-eczema therapy.

PREVENTION AND ADDITIONAL INFORMATION

Prevention of infections is not possible. However, healing can be promoted and the transfer of bacteria limited by providing information on hygiene measures (including washing the hands, cutting the nails, using one's own towel). Hygiene measures serve to reduce the number of bacteria on the skin. This combats the further spread of the infection and its transmission to others.

It has not been proven that excluding individual cases from schools or daycare centres has an effect.

Key words

- *S. aureus* is generally the cause. The infection can exacerbate an underlying skin disorder such as eczema.
- It has not been proven that excluding individual cases from schools or daycare centres is beneficial.
- Cleaning the skin with an antiseptic is the basis of treatment for minor lesions; more extensive problems require topical or oral antibiotics.

Literature

Boukes FS, Van der Burgh JJ, Nijman FC, et al. NHG-standaard: bacteriële huidinfecties [NHG standard: bacterial skin infections]. *Huisarts Wet* 1998;**41**(9):427–37.

Koning S, van Suijlekom-Smit LW, Nouwen JL, Verduin CM, Bernsen RM, Oranje AP, Thomas S, van der Wouden JC. Fusidic acid cream in the treatment of impetigo in general practice: double blind randomised placebo controlled trial. *BMJ* 2002:26;**324**(7331):203–6.

Koning S, Verhagen AP, van Suijlekom-Smit LWA, Morris A, Butler CC, van der Wouden JC. Interventions for impetigo (Cochrane Review). *Cochrane Library*, Issue 3. Oxford: Update Software, 2004.

Ruijs WLM, Van Steenbergen JE. Besmettelijk ziek en toch op school: weren van kinderen is zelden nodig [Contagious, yet still at school: excluding children is rarely necessary]. *Medisch Contact* 2000;**55**:348–50.

Van Amstel L, Koning S, Van Suijlekom-Smit LWA, Oranje AP, Van der Wouden JC. De behandeling van impetigo contagiosa. Een systematisch overzicht [The treatment of impetigo contagiosa. A systematic overview]. *Huisarts Wet* 2000;**43**(6):247–52.

14

PITYRIASIS VERSICOLOR/TINEA VERSICOLOR

DEFINITION

Pityriasis versicolor is a benign superficial yeast infection of the skin, caused by *Malassezia furfur*. The infection is characterized by separate or connected, usually lightly scaly macules, found primarily on the top part of the trunk, neck and upper arms.

AETIOLOGY/PATHOGENESIS

The normal skin flora contains two morphologically different yeasts: the spherical *Pityrosporum orbiculare* and the ovoid *Pityrosporum ovale*. These yeasts colonize in particular the hairy part of the head and the area between the shoulder blades. *P. orbiculare* organisms can develop into a pathogenic mycelium known as *Malassezia furfur*, which is found in pityriasis versicolor lesions. Hypopigmentation results from the damage to the skin.

For this to develop, several factors may be relevant: seborrhoeic skin, excessive perspiration, hereditary factors, systemic administration of corticosteroids, malnourishment and immunosuppression. Exogenous factors also probably play a role, such as high relative humidity in the air and a high ambient temperature. However, the problem often occurs in the perfectly healthy, and very often recurs. This is because *P. orbiculare* remain present on the head, or because other triggering factors persist.

PRESENTATION

Patients usually consult for cosmetic reasons, complaining of a patchy discoloration of the skin. Some patients also complain of light to moderate itching.

EPIDEMIOLOGY

Pityriasis versicolor is mainly a disease of young adults.
Epidemiological data are scanty – many cases are self-treated or
untreated.

HISTORY

The GP asks:

- about the distribution of the discoloration
- whether the patient has been bothered by it in the past
- if the patient is experiencing itching
- whether the patient was in the tropics recently or in the past
- whether corticosteroids or immunosuppressive medication is
  being used.

EXAMINATION

The skin lesions appear as clearly defined, round or oval macules of
various sizes. They can also merge together to form larger patches.
Typically, the lesions are slightly scaly – this is more noticeable on
scratching the patches. The infection is most commonly found on the
top half of the trunk, but can also spread to the upper arms, neck and
abdomen. It rarely spreads to the thighs, genitalia or legs. In the
tropics, the face and the scalp (hairy parts) may also be affected. The
patches vary in colour from yellow to brown, but can appear very
pale or have a red tint, depending on the skin colour of the patient.
On white skin, the affected areas are darker than the surrounding
skin, but because these hypopigmented spots do not react to
sunlight, they stand out somewhat in people with dark skin or on
tanned skin after sun tanning.

If a Wood's light is used for additional examination, the patches will
fluoresce yellowish-green.

TREATMENT

Because this is a harmless, non-contagious infection with a high rate
of recurrence, it is questionable whether treatment is necessary.

If treatment is desired, local therapy is preferred. Good results can be achieved with selenium sulphide (selenium sulphide suspension 2.5%): apply to the patches in the evening (not to the eyes or genitalia) and wash off thoroughly in the morning. The BNF recommends application 2–7 times over a fortnight and the course repeated if necessary. Alternatives are imidazole preparations (such as miconazole cream 2% or ketonazole 2% cream applied twice daily for at least 2–3 weeks).

In the case of very extensive pityriasis versicolor, the application of these preparations will be a problem. In such cases, or if local therapy produces inadequate results, oral therapy is possible (e.g. itraconazole capsules 100 mg, two capsules once daily for 7 days).

To limit the chance of recurrence, a selenium sulfide shampoo may be prescribed to wash the scalp once a week.

PREVENTION AND ADDITIONAL INFORMATION

It is important to inform the patient that it can take months for the hypopigmented patches to disappear. However, the fine flakiness should disappear more rapidly.

To reduce the chance of pityriasis versicolor recurring, it is important to know that excessive perspiration, a high degree of humidity in the air and a high ambient temperature are all predisposing factors.

Regularly washing the scalp with selenium sulfide shampoo can reduce the risk of pityriasis versicolor and prevent recurrence.

Pityriasis versicolor is not contagious.

Key points

- The infection is most commonly found on the top half of the trunk, but can also spread to the upper arms, neck and abdomen.
- To limit the chance of recurrence, advise a selenium sulfide shampoo to wash the scalp once a week.
- Pityriasis versicolor is not contagious.

Literature

Duinen CM, Feldmann CT. Kleine kwalen in de huisartsgeneeskunde; pityriasis versicolor [Minor ailments in general practice; pityriasis versicolor]. *Ned Tijdschr Geneeskd* 1990;**134**:331–3.

Gupta AK, Batra R, Bluhm R, Faergemann J. Pityriasis versicolor. *Dermatol Clin* 2003;**21**(3):413-29.

Gupta AK, Nicol K, Johnson A. Pityriasis versicolor: quality of studies. *J Dermatolog Treat* 2004;**15**(1):40-5.

Sillevis Smit, Van Everdingen JJE. De systemische behandeling van oppervlakkige huidmycosen [The systematic treatment of superficial skin mycoses]. *Geneesmiddelenbulletin* 1997;**31**:135–8.

15
INTERTRIGO

DEFINITION

Intertrigo is an erythematous eruption in a skin fold, caused by warmth, moisture and chafing. It occurs most often in the skin folds under the breasts and in the groin.

AETIOLOGY/PATHOGENESIS

Intertrigo is caused by a combination of warmth, moisture and chafing in a skin fold. Predisposing factors include heavy and hanging breasts, heavy upper legs, excessive perspiration, tight clothing, and, especially, poor hygiene. The skin can macerate, ulcerate and develop exudates. The inflamed skin fold can easily become infected, nearly always by *Candida*. It is often stated that diabetes mellitus can cause intertrigo; however, this does not appear to be the case.

PRESENTATION

Although GPs regularly see rashes in the skin folds, these are not always presented as a problem. Instead, the GP often finds the rash by accident during a physical examination. Often, patients are too embarrassed to mention the problem, either because they are afraid the doctor will think they are not clean, or because the groin and the female breasts are often considered taboo. If the patient does present the rash, it is usually for cosmetic reasons. Other reasons include itching, burning pain or an unpleasant odour.

EPIDEMIOLOGY

Intertrigo is a common complaint. Accurate epidemiological data are not readily available.

HISTORY

The history is usually short. The GP asks:

- about whether the patient wears tight clothing
- whether the patient perspires often or excessively
- about how the symptoms have progressed.

EXAMINATION

Examination of the skin provides a great deal of information. If the patches are not infected, intertrigo produces light-red coloured skin around the fold, often with some whitish, macerated patches; the area may also be rather moist. If there is itching, the skin may have been further damaged by scratching. In later stages, the skin in the fold can be bright red and damp.

In the presence of secondary infection with *Candida*, there may be fissures in the fold, which may be covered with a white coating. Outside the large red patch of intertrigo, there will be similar patches: 'satellite lesions'. Erythrasma (see Chapter 16) should be considered in the differential diagnosis, because the areas affected are the same.

TREATMENT

The treatment of intertrigo should first focus on the conditions that promote the rash, such as warmth, moisture and chafing. If the intertrigo is bright red or damp, an emollient can be applied after washing, and strips of linen or other suitable dressings can help in absorbing the moisture. In the case of a *Candida* infection, a locally applied antifungal (e.g. miconazole or clotrimazole) is indicated.

PREVENTION AND ADDITIONAL INFORMATION

Improved hygiene is the first requirement: daily washing, followed by thorough drying of the skin folds.

However, frequent washing with soap can increase the pH of the skin and create a favourable environment for the presence of fungal infection, so soap residue should always be rinsed off well. The use of a pH-lowering soap (baby soap) may decrease the chances of this problem occurring. Tight clothing should be avoided. If a person is overweight, losing weight will not have a significant effect, because the skin folds will not decrease as a result, but can instead become deeper.

Key points

- In the presence of secondary infection with *Candida*, there may be whitened fissures in the skin fold. Outside the large red patch of intertrigo, there may also be 'satellite lesions'.

- Erythrasma (see Chapter 16) should be considered in the differential diagnosis, because the areas affected are the same.

- Frequent washing with soap can increase the pH of the skin and thus encourage fungal growth, so soap residue should always be rinsed off well.

Literature

Bell-Syer SEM, Hart R, Crawford F, Torgerson DJ, Tyrrell W, Russell I. Oral treatments for fungal infections of the skin of the foot (Cochrane Review). *Cochrane Library*, Issue 2. Oxford: Update Software, 2004.

Crawford F, Hart R, Bell-Syer SEM, Torgonson DJ, Young P, Russell I. Topical treatment for fungal infections of the skin and nails of the foot (Cochrane Review). *Cochrane Library*, Issue 2. Oxford: Update Software, 2004.

Staats CCG, Vermeer BJ, Korstanje MJ. Zwemmerseczeem: intertrigo, erythrasma of een infectie met een gist of schimmel? [Athlete's foot: intertrigo, erythrasma or a yeast or fungal infection?] *Ned Tijdschr Geneeskd* 1994;**138**:2343–5.

16

ERYTHRASMA

DEFINITION

Erythrasma is an intertriginous skin disorder, characterized by clearly defined, dry, reddish-brown lesions, sometimes with fine flaking, and occasionally accompanied by itching or a burning sensation. The disorder usually causes no other symptoms. Erythrasma generally occurs in the axillae or groins, or sometimes between the fingers or under the breasts.

AETIOLOGY/PATHOGENESIS

The disorder is caused by *Corynebacterium minutissimum*, which is part of the normal skin flora. Under certain conditions it can become active and cause infection through growth in the stratum corneum. This happens most frequently in the presence of excess sweating, heat (in the tropics) and obesity. Other risk factors include maceration of the skin, poor hygiene, and the use of antiseptic soap and powder.

Patients with diabetes mellitus have a higher risk of developing erythrasma. These patients are sometimes affected by the (otherwise rare) generalized form of this disorder: disciform erythrasma.

Erythrasma is generally a harmless disorder, except in the case of immunosuppression, corticosteroid therapy and patients who need to undergo a local surgical procedure (e.g. angiography via the groin).

In very rare cases, *C. minutissimum* is found as the cause of deeper tissue infections, but it has never been established that this type of infection is a complication of an existing erythrasma. Once in a while, a case of sepsis due to *C. minutissimum* is described as a complication in a patient with chronic myeloid leukaemia.

PRESENTATION

The patient usually visits the GP because the patches are not
'normal', and sometimes because of itching or cosmetic worries.

EPIDEMIOLOGY

Epidemiological data are scanty. Because the disorder is not always
recognized – and in particular is misdiagnosed as a fungal infection –
any available figures would probably give a false impression. It may
be assumed that the average GP encounters this disorder a few times
a year.

HISTORY

The diagnosis is usually clinched by examination. The GP asks:

- if the patient has been exposed a great deal to hot weather (the
  tropics)
- about perspiration
- about symptoms of diabetes
- about lowered general resistance (due to a chronic illness).

EXAMINATION

The typical form is clearly defined, reddish-brown, and sometimes
with fine flakiness. It appears mainly in the folds of the body,
especially the groin, underarms, between the fingers and toes, and
under the breasts. Differential diagnosis includes candidiasis, tinea
corporis, tinea pedis (when the lesions are between the toes),
pityriasis versicolor (see Chapter 14) and intertrigo (see Chapter 15).

If in doubt about the diagnosis, examination using a Wood's light is
useful. Erythrasma shows a coral-red fluorescence, caused by the
porphyrins that are produced by *C. minutissimum*.

TREATMENT

The preferred initial treatment is a locally applied cream (imidazole
preparations), as is used for fungal infections. This is the first choice
because of the bactericidal effect. In comparative studies, no clear
differences between the imidazoles have been found. The cream is

applied twice daily and will usually clear up the disorder after 1 or 2 weeks. Compared to the imidazoles, benzoic acid (in Whitfield cream) has only a mild effect.

In the case of persistent, recurring or complicated infections, oral erythromycin 250 mg four times daily for 1–2 weeks can be prescribed.

At first glance, erythrasma is sometimes mistaken for a fungal infection. The usual treatment for this (an antifungal) is, as described above, also effective for erythrasma – this compounds the 'mistaken identity'.

PREVENTION AND ADDITIONAL INFORMATION

This is a harmless disorder for which general prevention is not really possible or useful. The only recommendations that can be provided for individual prevention after an infection has cleared up are to avoid excessive warmth and moisture (dry well after washing) and to avoid antiseptic soap.

Key points

- The disorder is caused by *C. minutissimum*, which is part of the normal skin flora.
- It results in clearly defined, dry, reddish-brown lesions in the intertriginous areas.
- If in doubt about the diagnosis, examination using a Wood's light is useful – erythrasma shows a coral-red fluorescence.

Literature

Hamann K, Thorn P. Systemic or local treatment of erythrasma? A comparison. *Scand J Prim Health Care* 1991;**9**(1):35–9.

Mesritz F, Streefkerk JG. Kleine kwalen in de huisartsgeneeskunde; erythrasma [Minor ailments in general practice; erythrasma]. *Ned Tijdschr Geneeskd* 1994;**138**:343–4.

17

ERYTHEMA INFECTIOSUM/ FIFTH DISEASE/SLAPPED-CHEEK SYNDROME

DEFINITION

Erythema infectiosum – also known as fifth disease or slapped-cheek syndrome – is a viral infection accompanied by a rash, which begins on the cheeks and then also appears on the extensor side of the arms and legs and on the buttocks. The disorder is also accompanied by light to moderate cold symptoms and generally occurs in children aged 4–10 years.

AETIOLOGY/PATHOGENESIS

The infection is caused by the human parvovirus B19. It is transmitted by airborne droplet infection. One week after transmission, viraemia occurs, which lasts approximately 5 days and may be accompanied by mild cold symptoms. Approximately 1 week after the viraemia, a second period of illness occurs, which is characterized by a rash, malaise, a slight fever and, occasionally, arthralgia. A sore throat and a blocked nose may also occur. These symptoms disappear again after several days, but the rash can recur for a short time, during a period of several weeks, provoked, for example, by sunlight or a hot bath. However, the infection can also progress subclinically or atypically. It can sometimes be difficult to distinguish this from other exanthematic childhood illnesses (see Chapter 18).

PRESENTATION

The main reasons for presentation are the rash, joint aches and any recurrence. The classic story is that the child was listless for a few days, then seemed to feel somewhat better, but then developed bright red cheeks and was listless and unwell again. After a short time, pinkish-red, somewhat itchy spots appear on the extensor side of the limbs and sometimes on the buttocks and the trunk. The child also often has a slight fever. In about 10% of cases, arthralgia occurs for 1–3 days. All the symptoms disappear again after several days, but can recur for a short time over several weeks.

Adults may have a slightly different set of symptoms, with not so much rash, but arthralgia as the main complaint. Over a short time, the patient experiences pain and stiffness in both hands and knees, which can quickly spread to other joints. This type of infection will usually disappear after a few days; once in a while, the patient will have painful joints for several months.

There are indications that this infection in pregnant women may lead to spontaneous abortion or intrauterine foetal death.

EPIDEMIOLOGY

Erythema infectiosum appears in localized epidemics every 3–5 years, usually in the winter and early spring. There are also isolated cases that appear between epidemics. Most people are infected between the ages of 4 and 10 years. Sixty per cent of adults have antibodies against this parvovirus. Incidence figures are not known.

HISTORY

The GP asks:

- whether the rash was preceded by a short period of general malaise
- whether there are joint symptoms and, if so, how long these have been present
- whether other children in the area have the same complaint.

EXAMINATION

The physical examination consists of inspecting the rash. Characteristics are bright-red raised erythema on both cheeks at the beginning of the illness, followed by a pinkish-red maculopapular rash that blanches, usually found on the extensor side of the limbs and on the buttocks, and sometimes also on the trunk.

Any painful joints should also be examined. The arthralgia can be unilateral or bilateral; the affected joint is stiff and painful, and very occasionally even swollen and warm.

TREATMENT

Specific medical treatment is not possible or necessary. In exceptional cases, a simple painkiller can be indicated to relieve the arthralgia.

PREVENTION AND ADDITIONAL INFORMATION

Parents and children can be reassured. This infection is a harmless childhood illness, which never results in complications. Parents should be warned that exposure of the child to direct sunlight or an overly hot bath in the ensuing 2 weeks can cause the rash to return.

It seems prudent to keep children with this illness away from pregnant women.

Key points

- Erythema infectiosum generally occurs in children aged 4–10 years.
- The rash begins on the cheeks, and then appears also on the extensor side of the arms and legs and on the buttocks
- The rash can recur for a short time, during a period of several weeks, provoked, for example, by sunlight or a hot bath.
- In about 10% of cases, arthralgia occurs for 1–3 days.
- In pregnant women, this infection may lead to spontaneous abortion or intrauterine foetal death.

Literature
Brown KE, Young NS. Parvovirus B19 in human disease. *Ann Rev Med* 1997;**48**:59–67.

Kirchner JT. Erythema infectiosum and other parvovirus B19 infections. *Am Fam Physician* 1994;**50**:335–41.

Wilterdink JB. Medische virologie [Medical virology]. Houten: Bohn Stafleu Van Loghum, 1992.

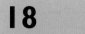

ROSEOLA INFANTUM/ SIXTH DISEASE/ EXANTHEMA SUBITUM

DEFINITION

Sixth disease, exanthema subitum or roseola infantum, is a harmless illness of very young children characterized by a high fever lasting approximately 3 days ('three-day fever'). After the child's temperature drops, a rash suddenly appears and lasts for 1–2 days.

AETIOLOGY/PATHOGENESIS

The human herpesvirus type-6 (HHV-6) that causes the illness is so contagious that almost all children have encountered it before their second year. Recently, a link was also found between roseola and the human herpesvirus type-7 (HHV-7). The exact incubation period is not known, but is estimated to be about 14 days. Infection probably takes place through droplet infection and oral contact. As for all herpesviruses, after infection, HHV-6 (and HHV-7) will remain present in the body for life.

PRESENTATION

It is likely that the GP sees only the tip of the iceberg of this illness. Not all cases are accompanied by rash, nor will the level or length of the fever always result in contact with the GP. Consultation may occur during one of the two stages of the illness: the fever or the rash.

EPIDEMIOLOGY

Roseola is the most common viral rash-producing illness in children under 3 years old. The average GP sees the illness three to four times a year. The annual incidence in children under 2 years old is 6–7%. A large part of the adult population appears to have antibodies against HHV-6. The risk of roseola in children older than 2 years is small. Boys and girls are affected equally; there are no clear seasonal differences; and the age distribution ensures that there is rarely more than one case in a family. Infections can also occur in older children and adults; these can appear to be symptoms of infectious mononucleosis, and a connection is often not made with a 'baby illness'.

HISTORY

Initially, the parent(s) will only notice a high fever. The GP asks:

- about symptoms of an upper respiratory infection, because these make roseola unlikely
- about symptoms of other possible causes of fever (e.g. gastroenteritis, ear–nose–throat infections).

EXAMINATION

During the fever stage, no other abnormalities are found. The rash consists of fine red macules and first develops on the neck and trunk, and later on the buttocks and thighs, and disappears over the extremities. The duration of the rash is usually no more than a couple of days. Distinguishing between this and other rash-producing illnesses, such as rubella and erythema infectiosum, is usually not difficult if account is taken of the patient's age, the characteristic history and the distribution of the rash. Further investigations are unnecessary.

TREATMENT

Roseola is a self-limiting disease, for which no treatment is known or necessary. The GP should immediately suspect the diagnosis if an infant or child under 2 years old has a fever without obvious signs of an infection to account for it. The GP can warn the parents of the expected rash; this will probably spare further consultations in the case of similar symptoms in the same family. Watchful waiting is indicated; it is helpful for the GP to reassure the parents and provide them with relevant information.

The fever can sometimes be so high that specific measures are necessary. As for every rapidly rising fever, febrile convulsions can occur with roseola. At present, it is thought that a relatively high percentage (30–40%) of (previously unexplained) febrile convulsions occur after an infection with HHV-6. How much benefit is obtained from the administration of paracetamol is unclear, but it is sensible to give the usual advice about cooling the child.

A common pitfall involves the use of an antibiotic in an infant with a fever, perhaps because of parental pressure – the subsequent development of a rash is often attributed to allergy when, in fact, it was caused by roseola.

PREVENTION AND ADDITIONAL INFORMATION

Prevention is not possible. Providing information about the nature of the illness and possible treatment of the symptoms is the only action required. It is not necessary to advise the parents to isolate the child due to contagiousness.

Key points

- Roseola is characterized by a fever that lasts for about 3 days, followed by a rash that begins as the fever subsides and which lasts for a couple of days.
- The risk of roseola in children older than 2 years is small – virtually all children have been infected by this age.
- The rash consists of fine red macules that develop first on the neck and trunk, and later on the buttocks and thighs, and which disappear over the extremities.
- The GP should immediately suspect the diagnosis if an infant or child under 2 years old has a fever without obvious signs of an infection to account for it.
- It is thought that a relatively high percentage (30–40%) of otherwise unexplained febrile convulsions occur after infection with roseola.
- If antibiotics are given in the febrile stage, the subsequent rash may well be misinterpreted as an allergy to the treatment.

Literature

Galama JMD. Humane herpesvirussen type 6 en 7; verwekkers van onder meer exanthema subitum [Human herpesviruses type 6 and 7; the causes of exanthema subitum and other illnesses]. *Ned Tijdschr Geneeskd* 1996;**140**:124–8.

Levy JA. Three new human herpesviruses (HHV 6, 7, and 8). *Lancet* 1997;**349**:558–63.

Ihira M, Yoshikawa T, Enomoto Y, Akimoto S, Ohashi M, Suga S, Nishimura N, Ozaki T, Nishiyama Y, Notomi T, Ohta Y, Asano Y. Rapid diagnosis of human herpesvirus 6 infection by a novel DNA amplification method: loop-mediated isothermal amplification. *J Clin Microbiol* 2004;**42**(1):140–5.

Van den Bosch WJHM (ed). Exanthema subitum. *Huisarts Wet* 1987;**30**:389–90.

19
CHICKENPOX/VARICELLA

DEFINITION

Chickenpox, or varicella, is a viral – usually childhood – illness. Red macules form on the trunk, limbs and head. These develop into papules, then vesicles, which contain a clear fluid. These vesicles in turn develop into pustules, and subsequently dry out; the crusts fall off in 1–2 weeks. Typically, the various stages (macules, papules, vesicles, pustules and crusts) are present at the same time. The vesicles may also be present, as ulcers, on the mucous membranes of the mouth, throat, vulva and penis.

The illness often causes itching and sometimes pain. In children, chickenpox is usually accompanied by a slight fever and general malaise for a maximum of a week. In the rare case of infection in adults, the general symptoms are more pronounced.

AETIOLOGY/PATHOGENESIS

Chickenpox is caused by a primary infection with the varicella-zoster virus. It is transmitted via personal contact or droplet spread, as the virus also multiplies in the throat. The illness is very contagious, from 1 day before the first skin abnormalities until the vesicles are dry. The incubation period is 12–21 days.

Complications occur in 5% of cases – most commonly a secondary infection of the blisters caused by scratching. Scarring is rare. In approximately one in 400 cases, a mild meningoencephalitis develops, accompanied by a temporary ataxia and tremor. Pneumonia develops very rarely.

After the illness, the virus remains present in the dorsal root ganglia for life. It can become active again later, giving rise to an attack of shingles (see Chapter 20). In people with a compromised immune response and in newborns, an infection with the varicella-zoster virus can be very serious.

The virus passes through the placenta. Pregnant women who develop chickenpox are at risk of having a baby with congenital defects (congenital foetal varicella syndrome). This risk is 1% in the first 12 weeks and 2% between weeks 13 and 20. Maternal infection up to 1 week before and 1 week after delivery is also a problem – it can result in severe chickenpox infection in the neonate. The pregnant woman herself is at risk of complications, especially pneumonia.

PRESENTATION

Most parents diagnose the illness themselves, but want to know what further action they should take. Children often need something to combat the itching. Lesions in the mouth and/or throat also can cause localized pain.

EPIDEMIOLOGY

Chickenpox is endemic, and occurs sometimes in local epidemics. There is a seasonal variation that peaks between March and May. The incidence is by far the highest in children aged 0–4 years: approximately 20 new cases per 1000 children per year. By the time they reach adulthood, 90% of people have been infected. Chickenpox only occurs in isolated cases in adults; it occurs in about 3 per 1000 women in pregnancy.

HISTORY

The GP asks:

- whether the immune system is compromised
- whether the patient (in the case of a woman of child-bearing age) is pregnant
- whether any contacts have chickenpox.

EXAMINATION

The diagnosis can usually be made easily by thoroughly examining the skin lesions. They may be present on the trunk, limbs, face, neck and head, and also in the nose and throat.

If red spots, small vesicles and crusts are all present at the same time, it can be assumed that the child has chickenpox. Small ulcers in the mouth may also be seen. The extent of the rash can vary considerably. Some children only have a few spots, while others are completely covered.

TREATMENT

Treatment is aimed at relieving the itching – calamine lotion may be helpful.

If secondary infection is present, fusidic acid cream can be applied to the infected blisters (see Chapter 13).

If the chickenpox is accompanied by general symptoms of illness or fever, paracetamol is recommended. If a pregnant woman (or a woman who has just given birth) develops chickenpox, urgent specialist attention should be sought.

PREVENTION AND ADDITIONAL INFORMATION

Preventing others from becoming infected is not always worthwhile. Contact should, however, be avoided with those with a compromised immune system and pregnant women who have never had chickenpox. Pregnant contacts who have not previously had chickenpox require urgent assessment of their varicella immune status and should be managed according to the advice in *Immunisation against Infectious Disease*. Parents should try to prevent secondary infections through proper hygiene, treating the itching and disinfecting open lesions. There is a vaccine for chickenpox, but this is not yet used in the UK.

Key points

- Typically, the various stages of chickenpox (macules, papules, vesicles, pustules and crusts) are present at the same time.
- By the time they reach adulthood, 90% of people have been infected. In the rare case of infection in adults, the general symptoms are more pronounced.
- Pregnant contacts who have not previously had chickenpox require urgent assessment of their varicella immune status and should be managed according to the advice in *Immunisation against Infectious Disease*.

Literature

Enders G, Miller E, Cradock-Watson J, Bolley J, Ridehalgh M. Consequences of varicella and herpes zoster in pregnancy: prospective study of 1739 cases. *Lancet* 1994;**343**:1547–50.

Immunisation against Infectious Disease. London: HMSO, 1996.

Swingler G, Volmink J. Chickenpox. *Clin Evidence* 2002;**8**:673–9.

Wilterdink JB. *Medische virologie* [*Medical virology*]. Houten: Bohn Stafleu Van Loghum, 1992.

20

SHINGLES/HERPES ZOSTER

DEFINITION

Herpes zoster, or shingles, is a secondary manifestation of an earlier infection with the herpes-zoster varicella virus (HZV) in a dermatome. It is characterized by a well-defined rash consisting of grouped blisters on one side of the face or body, accompanied by local neuralgia.

AETIOLOGY/PATHOGENESIS

HZV is part of a group of human herpesviruses including those that cause herpes labialis, herpes keratitis and herpes encephalitis (herpes simplex type-1), herpes genitalis (herpes simplex type-2), cytomegalovirus (CMV) infection, infectious mononucleosis (Epstein–Barr virus) and roseola infantum (human herpesvirus type-6).

The primary infection with HZV is usually experienced in childhood and manifests as chickenpox. The virus then lays dormant in the spinal ganglia. At a later age, the virus reactivates, spreads via a spinal nerve to the skin and creates the characteristic symptoms in the dermatome involved.

There is an increased risk of shingles, and of serious infection, in patients with a compromised immune system. Thus, for example, AIDS or other forms of immunosuppression should be considered if shingles occurs in young people in different dermatomes, or in an exceptionally severe form.

The major complication, postherpetic neuralgia, is characterized by intense pain in the dermatome concerned after the rash disappeared. This is present at 1 month in one-quarter of patients older than 50 years. After 3 months, this percentage drops to below 18%.

PRESENTATION

The patient will usually visit the GP with the typical rash on the skin. Often, the patient may already think it is shingles, or this may have been suggested by someone else. Pain can also prompt consultation, sometimes without a visible rash or blisters. In the case of intense unilateral pain that is otherwise unexplained, herpes zoster should be considered. Sometimes, eye symptoms, numbness of the skin or other neurological symptoms will be the reason for consulting the GP.

EPIDEMIOLOGY

UK prevalence figures have been quoted as follows:

- in early adult life: 2–3/1000
- in 60s: 5/1000
- over 80 years old: 10/1000.

Twenty per cent of adults suffer an attack at some time. The disorder can recur, but this is rare (about 2% of cases). The prevalence of post-herpetic neuralgia is 19% at 1 month, 7% at 3 months, and 3.4% at 1 year, although this varies with age.

HISTORY

The GP asks:

- when the pain began
- when the rash began
- whether a fever is present
- about the nature of the pain
- about the intensity of the initial symptoms
- in the case of symptoms around or in the eye (ophthalmic shingles or zoster ophthalmicus), about eye complications, such as pain in the eye itself, a decrease in vision or double vision
- about immunity problems.

EXAMINATION

The GP inspects the skin for (sometimes very minor) signs, and the stage of the skin lesions (redness, vesicles or crusts).

In the case of herpes zoster ophthalmicus, the eye is examined, including the cornea and eye movements. The presence of shingles on the tip of the nose increases the risk of eye abnormalities in the case of zoster ophthalmicus. The cornea must be inspected with fluorescein; dendritic ulcers primarily occur in herpes simplex infections.

Additional investigations: if there are severe herpes eruptions, blood tests such as a full blood count and human immunodeficiency virus (HIV) testing should be considered.

TREATMENT

Herpes zoster is a self-limiting disease. Providing an explanation, especially about the expected development, is generally sufficient. Local treatment is not necessary. Secondary infection is not common; necrotic spots should not be mistaken for infection.

The major complaint is pain, which is more intense in older people and if the initial symptoms were severe. Usually, the pain can be treated with standard painkillers.

Oral antiviral medications, if taken early enough (within 48 hours after the appearance of the rash) do have some effect on the development of symptoms. Treatment results in significant shortening of the duration of virus shedding; the duration of the illness and the period of pain are also reduced. Whether the modest positive effects justify the costs merits careful consideration.

Those at highest risk of problems, and especially postherpetic neuralgia, probably should be treated. So, antivirals (aciclovir, valaciclovir or famciclovir) are warranted in people over 50 years old, in the case of severe initial symptoms, or if the shingles affects the head or neck region. Immunocompromised patients may require more vigorous treatment such as intravenous aciclovir – specialist advice is required. In addition, people suffering from zoster ophthalmicus (and zoster oticus infections) require treatment and specialist assessment.

Antiviral therapy does not prevent postherpetic pain, but it is likely to reduce it, especially in the elderly (aged 80 years and over). It has been shown that antidepressants (such as amitriptyline) reduce the severity and duration of the pain. Start with amitriptyline 25 mg per day, and increase this to 75 mg per day if necessary.

PREVENTION AND ADDITIONAL INFORMATION

Herpes zoster cannot be prevented. The infection can be contagious for people who have never had chickenpox (in which case they are at risk of developing chickenpox, not shingles).

Key points

- The presence of shingles on the tip of the nose increases the risk of eye abnormalities.

- In the case of intense unilateral pain that is otherwise unexplained, herpes zoster should considered.

- Necrotic spots should not be mistaken for infection.

- Those at highest risk of problems – and especially postherpetic neuralgia – probably should be treated with antiviral agents.

- Immunocompromised patients may require more vigorous treatment, such as intravenous aciclovir – specialist advice is required in this situation.

Literature

Lancaster T, Silagy C, Gray S. Primary care management of acute herpes zoster: a systematic review of evidence from randomized controlled trials. *Br J Gen Pract* 1995;**45**:39-45.

Opstelten W, Eekhof JAH, Knuistingh Neven A, Verheij ThJM. Herpes zoster. Kleine kwalen [Minor ailments. Herpes zoster]. *Huisarts Wet* 2003;**46**:101–4.

21

PRURITUS IN THE ELDERLY

DEFINITION

Pruritus in the elderly (sometimes called 'senile pruritus') describes itching in older people, for which no cause can usually be found. The term 'xerosis' is used to describe dry, lightly flaky skin, which is often found in this situation.

AETIOLOGY/PATHOGENESIS

Little is known about the pathogenesis of this problem. It is probably influenced by both exogenous and endogenous factors. Exogenous factors include warm and dry air – so central heating may be a factor – and excessive use of soap and hot water. Of the endogenous factors, changes in the skin of the elderly seems to play a role. These changes include a reduced hydration of the skin surface, a decreased protective lipid layer and the slower repair of the stratum corneum. In addition, it is possible that changes in the specific itch-sensitive nerve fibres, which are sensitive to mediators such as histamine and heat, contribute to the itching. It also seems that a change in the synthesis and clearance of neuropeptides in the skin plays a part.

The frequency and the severity of xerosis increases with age; it is often accompanied by pruritus. Sometimes, the dry skin can eventually develop into a type of eczema generally seen only in the elderly: eczema craquelé. Dry skin, however, is not necessarily the cause of the pruritus – it should only be regarded as such if there is no other apparent cause.

Many patients who visit their GP with itching have skin rashes. The rash, and therefore the underlying cause, is sometimes difficult to recognize – in the elderly in particular, presentation can be atypical.

There are a number of underlying illnesses that can cause itching: examples include Hodgkin's and other malignancies (e.g. leukaemia), uraemia, liver diseases, diabetes and other metabolic disorders (e.g. hyperthyroidism, hypothyroidism), psychological disorders, anaemia, polycythaemia and drug reactions. In such cases the skin may appear normal or may just reveal scratch marks.

PRESENTATION

The patient visits the GP because of troublesome itching, present over the entire body. The patient's sleep is often disrupted.

EPIDEMIOLOGY

Pruritus is a common and often persistent complaint in the elderly. Based on an epidemiological study in general practice in The Netherlands, the Continuous Morbidity Registration 1971–1992, an average of more than two new cases of itching without a cause are recorded per 1000 patients per year. The incidence is age related. Older men in particular (older than 75 years) seem to be bothered by this complaint.

HISTORY

The GP asks:

- about the duration of the complaint
- about washing and the use of soap
- about treatments tried by the patient
- about the presence of other symptoms, such as weight loss, thirst, general malaise, medications (as pointers to potential underlying problems).

EXAMINATION

In pruritus of the elderly, no skin abnormalities are found other than the presence of dry skin or scratch marks. Eczema craquelé may be present.

Further investigation is aimed at detecting underlying causes. A full blood count, urea and electrolytes, liver function tests, blood sugar and thyroid function tests are all appropriate.

TREATMENT

Treatment is often difficult. There are no studies on the effectiveness of local therapy. The following recommendations are therefore based on consensus and experience. Clearly, any underlying cause should be managed as appropriate. In practice, however, no cause is usually found, and the GP will prescribe symptomatic treatment depending on the severity of the complaint.

GPs often prescribe local emollients, even if there is no dry skin. There is a huge range of options – GPs are guided by previous experience, patient preference and response. Commonly used examples include aqueous cream, emulsifying ointment and unguentum M. A thin layer of these treatments should be applied to the skin once or twice daily. The ideal time to do this is immediately after bathing. However, these remedies often only provide short-term results. If desired, corticosteroids may also be added, which may have an additive, itch-relieving effect. The use of a mild topical corticosteroid, such as hydrocortisone 1% cream, is often sufficient.

Furthermore, oral remedies such as antihistamines, may be used. A double-blind, placebo-controlled study of the use of antihistamine has been described. This study showed a good improvement in itching. However, the dosage of antihistamines in the elderly is difficult due to its side-effects, such as urine retention, restlessness and an influence on psychomotor function. Also, the improvement may be the result of sedation, so a sedating antihistamine is likely to be most effective. The use of topical antihistamines is not recommended in view of the risk of sensitization.

The use of systemic corticosteroids for pruritus in the elderly is controversial.

PREVENTION AND ADDITIONAL INFORMATION

General recommendations, such as avoiding excessive soap, hot water and the application of alcohol, can help considerably. Also, attention should be paid to overly dry air in the environment, as may be the case with central heating.

Key points

- Dry skin is not necessarily the cause of pruritus in the elderly – it should only be regarded as such if there is no other apparent cause.

- Older men in particular (older than 75 years) seem to be bothered by this complaint.

- Treatment is often difficult – general recommendations, such as avoiding excessive use of soap or hot water and the application of alcohol, can help considerably.

- Local emollients and/or topical steroids may relieve the symptoms.

Literature

Beckers RCY, Vermeer BJ, Boom BW. Jeuk bij interne aandoeningen; pathogenese en behandeling [Itching due to internal disorders; pathogenesis and treatment]. *Ned Tijdschr Geneeskd* 1994;**138**:1269–72.

De Wit RFE. Huidafwijkingen bij ouderen [Skin abnormalities in the elderly]. In: Van Vloten WA, et al. (eds). *Dermatologie en Venerologie* [*Dermatology and Venereology*]. Utrecht: Bunge 1996.

Thaipisuttikul Y. Pruritic skin diseases in elderly. *J Dermatol* 1998;**25**:153–7.

Van Everdingen JJE, et al. Pruritus. In: *Dermatovenereologie voor de eerste lijn* [*Dermatovenereology for the first line*]. Houten/Antwerpen: Bohn Stafleu Van Loghum, 1991, pp. 79–83.

22

INFECTIOUS MONONUCLEOSIS/ GLANDULAR FEVER

DEFINITION

Infectious mononucleosis (glandular fever) is an infectious disease that is caused by the Epstein–Barr virus (EBV), one of the human herpesviruses.

AETIOLOGY/PATHOGENESIS

EBV infects, and replicates in, B lymphocytes. A blood film shows a moderate leucocytosis and a shift in the direction of lymphocytes and monocytes (mononucleosis). The symptoms are usually mild in young children, and consequently often go unnoticed. In adolescents, 85% of cases have a fever, sore throat and swollen glands as prominent symptoms. After the infection, the virus is present for the rest of the patient's life, and is secreted in varying degrees in the saliva. Complications are very rare. They include: rupture of the spleen, haemolytic anaemia, Guillain–Barré syndrome and pericarditis.

EBV is found throughout the world. Almost all adults carry the virus. At any given point in time, the virus can be cultured from the saliva of approximately 20% of healthy EBV carriers. It is not clear how the disease is transmitted. The commonly used label 'kissing disease' could be accurate, because the virus can be transmitted in the saliva. The incubation period is usually 4–6 weeks. Shorter incubation periods have been documented, so the incubation period probably depends on the infecting dose.

PRESENTATION

The classic case is a young adult with a fever, sore throat (which may be severe), and swollen, painful glands. However, these classic symptoms may be less marked in some cases. Other symptoms and signs that suggest infectious mononucleosis include: oedema around the eyes, a rash, jaundice, abdominal pain, arthralgia and fatigue. Because the illness is linked to general malaise, patients sometimes present this as their main complaint. However, no clear connection has been found with chronic fatigue syndrome.

The sore throat is caused by pharyngitis and tonsillitis. This is difficult to distinguish from other throat infections, such as streptococcal infection. In the case of infectious mononucleosis, the sore throat is often asymmetrical. In exceptional cases, signs of hepatosplenomegaly and jaundice can predominate.

EPIDEMIOLOGY

Little is known about how the disease is transmitted, although infectious mononucleosis is more frequently seen in closed communities of young people, such as boarding schools and barracks. Because infection in young children is often mild or asymptomatic, many cases in this age group are not brought to the attention of the GP. The total incidence is one per 1000 persons per year. Cases presenting to the GP are most common in the 15- to 25-year-old age group. Because the virus stays in the body for the rest of the patient's life, recurrence is not possible. For patients with normal immunity, reactivations, as can occur with the herpes-zoster virus (HZV), do not happen. There are no clear seasonal influences.

HISTORY

The history should be oriented towards the relevant symptoms described above. Specifically, the GP asks:

- about the symptoms noticed by the patient, such as fever and sore throat, and how long they have been present.
- about other relevant symptoms, which might point to an alternative diagnosis (very rarely, acute lymphatic leukaemia or blood dyscrasias resulting from medication side-effects can present in the same way).

EXAMINATION

Young people with infectious mononucleosis do not usually seem very ill, despite often having a high fever and severe pharyngitis.

The throat should be inspected. A distinction should be made between the swelling of the pharynx in infectious mononucleosis and the start of a peritonsillar abscess. The cervical glands are palpated. Glands in the front of the neck can be very large and swollen. Enlarged glands in the back of the neck more likely indicate infectious mononucleosis than bacterial pharyngitis. Other lymph gland areas, in the axillae and groins, are also palpated. The size of the liver and the spleen is determined by percussion and palpation. Some hepatosplenomegaly is nearly always present.

If a patient has the classic symptoms of infectious mononucleosis, additional laboratory tests may add little. Should it be necessary to confirm or rule out the diagnosis, tests can be done to identify specific antibodies against EBV. In the acute phase, both immunoglobulin M (IgM) and IgG are elevated. If the acute phase has passed, then only IgG antibodies are present. The degree of abnormality of the liver function tests has no prognostic value – they are caused not by hepatitis, but by congestion with lymphocytes. In the white cell differential, a relatively large number of atypical lymphocytes are found. However, these findings are not specific to infectious mononucleosis.

TREATMENT

There is no treatment for infectious mononucleosis available or necessary. The illness is self-limiting and patients almost always fully recover. Only in exceptional cases is the duration of the disease prolonged: no more than 1–2% of patients suffer from months of fatigue. Besides, this picture of post-viral fatigue is common to many virus infections. The GP will provide an explanation about the diagnosis and reassure the patient about the expected course of the illness. This reassurance is very important because many patients have a distorted view of infectious mononucleosis. Repeated serological tests are unnecessary.

A sore throat of this sort sometimes leads to requests for a prescription for antibiotics. In response, the GP should explain that penicillins, especially ampicillin and amoxicillin, can cause a severe rash in patients with infectious mononucleosis, which can make them very unwell. Sore throat and fever can usually be treated symptomatically with paracetamol.

Patients will adapt their activities to their subjective symptoms; measures such as bed rest and dietary changes (e.g. a low-fat diet) are not necessary. Patients can take whatever measures they feel are needed. However, in the case of splenomegaly, it is recommended that the patient avoid contact sports.

PREVENTION AND ADDITIONAL INFORMATION

Because a large majority of people carry EBV, recommendations to prevent transmission are pointless. Less than 5% of patients are aware of recent contact with a person infected with infectious mononucleosis. Any information given should be based on the evidence and aimed at changing the negative ideas that many patients have about the course of this illness.

Key points

- The symptoms are usually mild in young children, and consequently often go unnoticed. In adolescents, 85% of cases present with a fever, sore throat and swollen glands.

- Ampicillin and amoxicillin should not be prescribed in the patient with a severe sore throat. If the diagnosis turns out to be infectious mononucleosis, the patient will suffer a rash as a result.

- No clear connection has been found with chronic fatigue syndrome. Only in exceptional cases is the duration of the disease prolonged: no more than 1–2% of patients suffer from months of fatigue.

Literature

Kinderknecht JJ. Infectious mononucleosis and the spleen. *Curr Sports Med Rep* 2002;**1**(2):116–20.

Macsween KF, Crawford DH. Epstein–Barr virus – recent advances. *Lancet: Infect Dis* 2003;**3**(3):131–40.

Ohga S, Nomura A, Takada H, Hara T. Immunological aspects of Epstein–Barr virus infection. *Crit Rev Oncol Hematol* 2002;44(3):203–15.

Peter J, Ray CG. Infectious mononucleosis. *Pediatr Rev* 1998;**19**:276–9.

Swanink CMA, et al. Epstein–Barr virus (EBV) and the chronic fatigue syndrome: normal virus load in blood and normal immunological reactivity in the EBV regression assay. *Clin Infect Dis* 1995;**20**:1390–2.

Van den Bosch WJHM. Herpesvirusinfectie in de huisartspraktijk [Herpesvirus infection in general practice]. *Tijdschr Huisartsgeneeskd* 1997;**14**:114–24.

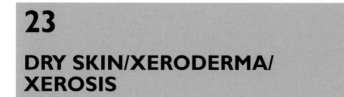

23

DRY SKIN/XERODERMA/ XEROSIS

DEFINITION

Dry skin, also known as xeroderma or xerosis, refers to a persistent, generalized feeling of dryness and roughness of the skin. There may be associated fine scaling and sometimes redness and itching. Small cracks may also be present.

AETIOLOGY/PATHOGENESIS

The horny layer of the skin is hydrated by moisture secreted from the subepidermal blood vessels. Through keratinization and fatty cell degeneration (with lipid formation) of epidermal cells, a layer is created that prevents dehydration and provides elasticity. On the surface of the skin, there is a thin layer of sebum, a fatty mixture of substances that forms an emulsion. One of the functions of sebum is to prevent the rapid evaporation of epidermal moisture. This prevents the skin from dehydrating.

Xeroderma can occur as a result of a disruption of the formation of the horny layer and decreased sebum production – such as in old age. The drying out of the skin can be aggravated by washing away lipids and sebum through the use of excessive soap, and through long baths or showers in hot water. The relative degree of moisture in the environment also affects the moisture level of the horny layer of the skin. During the winter, with dry weather and central heating, there is a relatively low humidity, so the skin loses more moisture due to evaporation.

Finally, there are certain skin disorders that are accompanied by dry, flaky skin, such as eczema, psoriasis and ichthyosis.

PRESENTATION

The patient complains about dry, rough skin, which is sometimes flaky and itchy. Cracks may also be present.

EPIDEMIOLOGY

There are few epidemiological data. In younger people, the complaint is often associated with a skin disorder, such as eczema. In older people, the cause is more often primary xeroderma (see Chapter 21).

HISTORY

The GP asks:

- whether the patient is bothered by itching, redness or cracking
- when the symptoms started, how they progressed (continuous or periodic) and whether there are seasonal variations
- about the patient's washing, showering and bathing habits, what products are used, and whether the patient must wash his hands frequently for work
- whether the patient is atopic or affected by psoriasis
- whether ichthyosis occurs in the family.

EXAMINATION

The physical examination is limited to inspecting the skin. Particular attention is paid to the hands, lower legs and back. Xeroderma is less pronounced in the skin folds and on the wrists and the face.

Are the effects of scratching present, along with flakiness and fissures (primarily on the hands and feet)? In the case of other signs of inflammation, such as light erythema and lichenification, eczema should be considered. No further investigation is necessary

TREATMENT

Treatment is aimed at repairing the protective emulsion in and on the skin. This can be accomplished by regularly applying an emollient, such as unguentum M or aqueous cream, to the skin. The success of the treatment depends closely on the frequency of application. A greasy cream or an ointment must be applied to the hands after handwashing (patients should always carry this with them). Oil can also be added to the bathwater. Dry hands with cracks can be treated in the same way.

PREVENTION AND ADDITIONAL INFORMATION

Patients should avoid long baths and showers, which cause the skin to dry out. Very hot water and vigorous drying are also bad for the skin. Frequent use of soap, bubble bath and shampoo should be discouraged; these damage the composition of the sebum. The use of a non-alkaline soap is preferred. A proper level of humidity in the patient's house can reduce symptoms.

Key points

- Remember the possibility of other skin conditions that can produce similar symptoms, such as eczema, psoriasis and ichthyosis.

- Xeroderma is less pronounced in the skin folds and on the wrists and the face.

- The success of the treatment depends closely on the frequency of application of emollients.

Literature

Loden M. Role of topical emollients and moisturizers in the treatment of dry skin barrier disorders. *Am J Clin Dermatol* 2003;**4**(11):771–88.

Norman RA. Xerosis and pruritus in the elderly: recognition and management. *Dermatol Ther* 2003;**16**(3):254–9.

24

EXCESSIVE SWEATING/ HYPERHIDROSIS

DEFINITION

Hyperhidrosis is excessive sweating, which causes problems either due to the abnormal amount of moisture, or the unpleasant odour. A distinction can be made between hyperhidrosis palmarum (palms), plantaris (feet), axillaris (armpits) and totalis (whole body).

AETIOLOGY/PATHOGENESIS

Sweat glands, with the exception of the apocrine sweat glands in the underarms and the mammary areolae, are eccrine. Hyperhidrosis can therefore either be eccrine or apocrine. The odour is also different: sweaty feet smell different to excessively sweaty underarms. Both types of sweat are odourless at the moment the sweat is secreted; skin bacteria convert it into aromatic short-chain fatty acids.

There are large individual differences in the degree of physiological perspiration due to heat, exertion, infectious disorders and menopause. The same is true about how perspiration is perceived: what one person views as normal, another may find excessive (in terms of moisture or smell).

Idiopathic local hyperhidrosis refers to unexplained excess sweating of the palms, underarms and feet. Generalized perspiration occurs in anxiety, thyrotoxicosis, hypoglycaemia, shock, tuberculosis, malignancies (e.g. Hodgkin's disease), alcoholism and as a side-effect of certain medicines (e.g. tricyclic antidepressants). Other endocrine disorders, such as phaeochromocytoma and hyperpituitarism, are very rare, but are included here as 'classic' causes of hyperhidrosis.

Finally, we include here the psychological, exclusively subjectively experienced, 'hyperhidrosis', which is an expression of one of the variants of an anxiety disorder, although it should be borne in mind that 'true' hyperhidrosis may be caused, or aggravated by, anxiety.

Unpleasant body odour, such as 'fish odour syndrome', without the presence of hyperhidrosis can be the result of a metabolic disorder (see Chapter 64).

PRESENTATION

A patient may attend because he is bothered by the sweating or the odour. The patient may also be sent by someone else. The sweat-stained areas of the clothes, discoloration of garments or damage to sensitive and soft areas of the skin (soles of the feet) can also be a reason for attending. The patient may also report problems holding on to objects, such as cutlery, glassware, pens or tools.

EPIDEMIOLOGY

GPs will only see the 'tip of the iceberg' – many patients will consult pharmacists, skin therapists or beauticians, and with success. Based on Dutch figures, it is estimated that the average GP sees about five new patients a year with this disorder. Hyperhidrosis probably occurs in 0.6–1.0% of the population.

HISTORY

The history can generally be short; the patient will volunteer most of the relevant information. The GP asks:

- about the extent and type of problem (sweat and/or odour)
- about the conditions under which the problem occurs
- about the amount of sweat and the places where it is troublesome
- about measures already taken
- about medication and alcohol use
- about symptoms of any possible underlying causes
- about whether other people notice the problem (to rule out an anxiety disorder).

EXAMINATION

A focused visual – and nasal – examination of the clothing (underarm areas, socks) and the relevant body parts may be useful to give an objective measure of the problem. The feet must be checked for fungal infection, and the underarms for intertrigo/dermatitis. If an underlying problem is suspected, the examination is expanded as necessary, and relevant investigations undertaken. However, this will rarely be necessary.

TREATMENT

Often, the most important hygiene measures have already been taken. These include regular washing, thorough rinsing of soap residue and thorough drying. Other important recommendations include frequently changing clothes, wearing wool and cotton clothing and socks (no added synthetic fibres), wearing shoes made entirely of leather, walking in bare feet as much as possible, and, in some cases, shaving the underarm hair.

There are various remedies available for treating hyperhidrosis. However, most of these have not been proven to be effective. Of the local remedies available, aluminium salts are the most effective (especially aluminium chloride hexahydrate). The effectiveness of oral remedies (e.g. clonidine), which are frequently used, has not been established. In serious cases, the patient can be referred to a dermatologist. More aggressive therapies, such as systemic treatment with anticholinergics, iontophoresis, sympathectomy, cryotherapy, subcutaneous removal of (apocrine) sweat glands and skin transplants, are only necessary in exceptional cases. Psychotherapy (including conditioning) may be indicated in the case of purely psychological, subjective perspiration.

PREVENTION AND ADDITIONAL INFORMATION

Young people find it very reassuring to know that the disorder will almost always disappear eventually. A comparison can be made with blushing, which is also a big problem, but which usually decreases in adolescence. An explanation about the physiology and useful function of perspiration can remove part of the stigma: sweating is not 'dirty'.

Key points

- Of the local remedies available, aluminium salts are the most effective (especially aluminium chloride hexahydrate).
- Young people find it very reassuring to know that the disorder will almost always disappear eventually.
- Anxiety may be the cause or the effect of the problem.
- Underlying pathology may rarely cause excess sweating (e.g. phaeochromocytoma, thyrotoxicosis).

Literature

De Ru VJ, Van Spronsen R. Onaangename lichaamsgeuren: hyperhidrosis [Unpleasant body odours: hyperhidrosis]. *Ned Tijdschr Geneeskd* 1986;**130**:862–64.

Leung AK, Chan PY, Choi MC. Hyperhidrosis. *Int J Dermatol* 1999;**38**(8):561–7.

25

GROWING PAINS

DEFINITION

'Growing pains' is the term used to describe the situation in which children complain about deep pain in both legs, usually at the end of the day and during the night. These pains occur intermittently; there are no apparent abnormalities.

AETIOLOGY/PATHOGENESIS

Although the symptom is experienced during periods of growth, growing pains probably have nothing to do with physical growth. This is because growing pains are usually not localized to the growth plates, and they do not occur specifically during growth spurts. The true cause is unknown. There have been many explanations put forward, such as that the pain is due to fatigue, improper posture or a psychosomatic disorder. There is no evidence to back up these ideas. In terms of a differential diagnosis, the following must be considered:

- Benign hypermobility syndrome: pains present in children with hypermobility – the pain occurs at the end of the day, but is localized to the joints and does not disrupt sleep.
- Chondromalacia patellae: pain around the patella, especially when walking up stairs; there is local pain during the examination.
- Intermittent night leg cramps: pain after considerable exertion during the day; the parents can clearly feel the cramped muscles (see also Chapter 105).
- Psychosomatic disorders, such as conversion, fear, tension, neglect: normal findings and normal exercise tolerance might suggest a psychosocial basis for the pains.
- Osteoid osteoma: pain at the end of the day or during the night, nagging, usually on one side; can only be excluded by a bone scan.

- Osteomyelitis: early recognition of this rare disorder is very important; serious and often localized pain accompanied by a fever can point to this diagnosis.

PRESENTATION

The parents usually ask whether the child has some significant medical problem or simply has growing pains. They explain that the child wakes up at night from pain in both legs; this occurs several times a week and may occur for several months. The problem may come and go. The pain is usually located deep in the muscles of both calves or thighs, and almost never in the arms.

EPIDEMIOLOGY

Growing pains occur in approximately 10% of children, usually those aged 4–10 years, and more often in girls than boys.

HISTORY

In the history, the questions are aimed at distinguishing between growing pains and a more serious disorder. The GP asks:

- whether the pains occur at the end of the day and at night
- whether the symptoms are constant or intermittent
- whether the pains occur in both legs
- whether there is joint pain
- whether the child has general symptoms of illness, especially fever
- whether the child is limited in his exertion.

EXAMINATION

No abnormalities are found in the physical examination. If the pains are unilateral or if the child can clearly indicate the site, a significant disorder should be suspected. Physical abnormalities, temperature differences or pain during the examination point to a diagnosis other than growing pains.

If the history does not suggest a more serious disorder and the physical examination is normal, additional investigations, such as blood tests and X-rays, are not necessary.

TREATMENT

The GP provides the parents with an explanation, reassurance and recommendations. It has been shown that rubbing the painful muscles and doing stretching exercises can help reduce the pain. According to those who view the problem as purely psychosomatic, this improvement can be attributed to the extra attention the child receives.

PREVENTION AND ADDITIONAL INFORMATION

It is advisable to reassure the child and the parents. In addition, the GP should also explain that growing pains are well recognized and harmless and that they will disappear 'by themselves' in 1–2 years. It is also important to indicate when other investigations might be necessary.

Key points

- Growing pains are intermittent pains felt in the legs of children usually aged 4–10 years, typically at night, for which no pathological cause can be found.
- They probably have nothing to do with physical growth.
- Unilateral, constant, well-localized and/or joint pain suggest an alternative diagnosis.
- They disappear spontaneously within a year or two.

Literature

Barten WCM, Streefkerk JG. Kleine kwalen in de huisartsgeneeskunde; groeipijn bij kinderen [Minor ailments in general practice; growing pains in children]. *Ned Tijdschr Geneeskd* 1994;**138**:1062–5.

Halliwell P, Monsell F. Growing pains: a diagnosis of exclusion. *Practitioner* 2001; **245**(1624):620–3.

Manners P. Are growing pains a myth? *Aust Fam Physician* 1999;**28**:124–7.

26

HOT FLUSHES

DEFINITION

Hot flushes are sudden feelings of heat and perspiration, usually accompanied by an increasing reddening of the face, neck and front of the upper body. A hot flush lasts an average of 1–3 minutes, with large individual differences. The patient experiences the feeling of heat approximately 30–45 seconds before the hot flush is actually apparent.

The objective signs consist of sweating, an acute rise in skin temperature (especially in the fingers), peripheral vasodilatation, an increase in heart rate and a drop in skin resistance. Hot flushes are the most characteristic symptom of the menopause in women.

AETIOLOGY/PATHOGENESIS

During a hot flush, the body tries to release 'excess' body heat, without there being good reason for this. Essentially, a normal physiological control mechanism is activated by an incorrect 'setting' of the thermoregulatory centre in the hypothalamus. Hot flushes can therefore be considered as a neuroendocrine phenomenon. The most plausible explanation is that a large drop in the oestrogen level results in changes in the neuroendocrine processes in the hypothalamus–pituitary axis, such as the production of gonadotrophin-releasing hormone. However, what exactly happens at this level is not entirely clear. The disruption in thermoregulation makes the body 'mistakenly' experience itself as too hot. Peripheral vasodilatation follows in an attempt to 'release' the heat. Because of perspiration, the skin conductivity increases and the temperature of the skin rises by 1°C in the face and an average of 5°C in the fingers. As a result of the heat loss, the temperature of the entire body drops, so a woman feels cold and shivery after the hot flush has ended.

PRESENTATION

A woman with hot flushes attends her GP because the complaint can
be a significant nuisance and because nocturnal hot flushes (night
sweats) can disrupt sleep. The intensity and frequency of flushes
varies among individual women and over time. Most women are
unhappy about turning red in the presence of others, especially in
combination with heavy perspiration. The patient generally wants to
have her suspicion confirmed that this complaint is due to the
menopause. In addition, she may want information about these
symptoms, their prognosis and what can be done about them.

EPIDEMIOLOGY

The frequency of flushes increases from the premenopause to the
first year of the postmenopause, by which time nearly 80% of women
are affected. The number of hot flushes per day varies, but in general,
during the menopause, only 20% of women have more than six hot
flushes per day and approximately the same percentage are
awakened at least once a night by flushes. Hot temperatures and
tension increase the number of hot flushes. Women in the
premenopause may also complain of hot flushes, even if they
menstruate quite regularly. Furthermore, women who have
undergone a hysterectomy – even without removal of the ovaries –
suffer more often from hot flushes and sweating than other women.
The frequency of hot flushes gradually decreases over time; however,
5% of women are still seriously troubled by this symptom 10 years
after their last period. Although not all women will consult about this
problem, a GP will see five to ten women with these symptoms each
year.

HISTORY

The main goal of the history is to determine the severity and nature
of the problem. The GP asks:

- about the consequences for the woman's daily activities
- about a disrupted sleep pattern
- about other (pre)menopausal complaints, such as irregular and/or
  heavy menstruation, vaginal dryness or discharge, incontinence

- about psychological symptoms, such as fatigue, agitation, depression, irritability and loss of self-confidence – these problems are more common in women with hot flushes: the more severe the hot flushes, the more symptoms (especially the first two).

Other relevant factors include:

- The social background of the patient and the significance the menopause might have in her life. This phase is related to growing older, no longer needing to care for children and the increased infirmity or loss of her parents.
- The way in which the woman is used to dealing with and tolerating symptoms.
- Issues around treatment – ask about the woman's ideas and desire for treatment, as well as possible contraindications.
- Differential diagnosis – the GP must consider disorders with similar symptoms, such as depression and anxiety, hyperthyroidism and, rarely, carcinoid and phaeochromocytoma (see also Chapter 24).

EXAMINATION

No specific or supplementary examination is needed if hot flushes alone are being experienced. If there are also symptoms involving the urogenital tract, a gynaecological examination is appropriate. The blood pressure must be taken before prescribing clonidine or oestrogens. However, for this symptom, further investigations are usually unnecessary.

TREATMENT

Before proposing a treatment, the wishes of the patient should be considered; most women already have experience of, or an opinion about, taking the pill or other hormones. Many do not want medication; an explanation about hot flushes and their prognosis may be sufficient. It is important to discuss the advantages and disadvantages of treatment.

There are three groups of medicines that have a positive effect on hot flushes and sweating (the vasomotor complaints of menopause): oestrogens, clonidine and progestogens.

If hot flushes are the most prominent complaint, or if there are other symptoms of oestrogen deficiency, oestrogens are the first choice. These are combined with progestogens at least once every 3 months for 12 days, due to an increased risk of endometrial carcinoma with unopposed oestrogens. This is, of course, not applicable for women whose uterus has been removed. The patient should be warned to expect withdrawal bleeding. There are no indications that short-term use (up to 5 years) of oestrogens significantly increases the risk of breast cancer.

If oestrogens are contraindicated (e.g. because of a history of breast cancer, liver disorders or thromboembolism) treatment with progestogens alone is an alternative. Hot flushes in men with metastatic prostate carcinoma after chemical or surgical castration also decrease if treated with progestogens. This treatment has the possible drawback of changing the lipid profile unfavourably. In addition, the relationship between progestogens and breast cancer is the subject of debate.

The follow-up consultation after the initiation of oestrogen treatment assesses the patient's subjective response and possible side-effects, such as nausea, mastalgia, weight gain and a possible change in blood pressure. Vaginal blood loss resulting from hormone replacement therapy during the postmenopause is a nuisance – but remember that erratic bleeding can also indicate a malignancy. Treatment is stopped after 6–12 months to determine whether the hot flushes remain.

If, for any reason, hormonal treatment is not desired, clonidine may be considered. Clonidine does also slightly lower the blood pressure, which may be of benefit in some cases. Patients may also experience dizziness, a slight sedative effect, and gastrointestinal disturbances. An effect can be expected after 2 weeks.

PREVENTION AND ADDITIONAL INFORMATION

Most women know what hot flushes are and that they occur in connection with menopause. There are no known measures to prevent these symptoms and, also, it cannot be predicted who will experience severe hot flushes or for how long.

In terms of informing the patient, it is helpful to temper the sometimes exaggerated expectations that can be generated by the media about the need for and success of treatment. A hysterectomy increases the risk of menopausal symptoms. For this, and other reasons as well, it is important to approach such an operation with caution.

Key points

- Hot flushes are the most characteristic symptom of the menopause in women.

- The frequency of flushes increases from the premenopause to the first year of the postmenopause, by which time nearly 80% of women are affected.

- The frequency of hot flushes gradually decreases over time; however, 5% of women still have problems 10 years after their last period.

- It is helpful to temper the sometimes exaggerated expectations that can be generated by the media about the need for and the success of treatment.

Literature

Freedman MA. Quality of life and menopause: the role of estrogen. *J Womens Health (Larchmt)* 2002;11(8):703–18.

Joffe H, Soares CN, Cohen LS. Assessment and treatment of hot flushes and menopausal mood disturbance. *Psychiatr Clin North Am* 2003;**26**(3): 563–80.

O'Bryant SE, Palav A, McCaffrey RJ. A review of symptoms commonly associated with menopause: implications for clinical neuropsychologists and other health care providers. *Neuropsychol Rev* 2003;**13**(3):145–52.

27

ORTHOSTATIC PROTEINURIA/ POSTURAL PROTEINURIA

DEFINITION

Orthostatic or postural proteinuria is characterized by protein in the urine while walking or standing (with no protein in the urine when the patient is recumbent). It can be present continuously or intermittently. The total protein loss in the urine does not usually amount to more than 2 g per 24 hours.

AETIOLOGY/PATHOGENESIS

The pathophysiological mechanism of orthostatic proteinuria is unclear. The amount of protein present in the urine depends on both glomerular filtration and reabsorption in the tubules. The glomerular filtrate normally contains 30 mg albumin per 100 ml. The proximal tubules reabsorb most of this, to the extent that only 150 mg albumin is present in the urine each day. According to most researchers, the cause lies in venous stasis of blood in the legs while walking and standing, which reduces blood flow through the kidneys. In some people, the resulting activation of the renin–angiotensin system and the increased glomerular filtration can lead to an increase in the passage of albumin through the glomeruli. Reabsorption by the tubules is apparently insufficient to 'recapture' all this excess albumin.

PRESENTATION

Orthostatic albuminuria is usually discovered by accident, such as during a medical examination.

EPIDEMIOLOGY

Epidemiological data vary in the literature, probably because the phenomenon is usually only detected if specifically looked for. In children and teenagers, the prevalence is 2–8%. In young adults, the prevalence is around 2%. Orthostatic proteinuria occurs much less frequently in adults over 30 years old. The prognosis is very good, because it does not appear to be a pathological process. A 20-year follow-up study revealed that patients with orthostatic proteinuria did not have a greater chance of developing renal disorders and/or hypertension than did the general population.

HISTORY

The GP asks:

- about the presence of oedema, high blood pressure or recurrent urinary tract infections
- whether the patient or his family has had kidney diseases in the past
- whether the patient experiences polyuria or polydipsia (diabetes)
- about weight gain (oedema).

EXAMINATION

Physical examination includes measurement of blood pressure and checking the renal areas for tenderness. Laboratory tests involve repeat urinalysis for protein (three times weekly between each test) to rule out non-recurring transitory albuminuria resulting from fever, exertion, cold, stress, etc. The protein level of an early morning urine sample is compared with that in a sample collected several hours later. To collect a suitable sample of morning urine, the patient should urinate 2 hours after going to bed – then the first morning urine is genuinely produced while the patient is recumbent. This sample should not show an increased protein level. The 24-hour protein excretion urine and the serum creatinine are also measured. Urine should also be sent for microscopy to look for erythrocytes and casts.

TREATMENT

If tests suggest orthostatic proteinuria, with normal microscopy and less than 2 g protein loss per day, then a follow-up consultation 2 years later is recommended. At this time, the protein level in the morning urine and a random sample is compared, the blood pressure taken, possibly the serum creatinine levels measured and the urine re-examined microscopically. If no abnormalities are found, further follow-up checks are not necessary.

Referral to a nephrologist is necessary in the following circumstances: more than 2 g protein loss per day, abnormal urine microscopy, or increased serum creatinine levels.

PREVENTION AND ADDITIONAL INFORMATION

Providing an explanation about the good prognosis of the disorder is important.

Key points

- Orthostatic or postural proteinuria is characterized by protein in the urine while walking or standing (with no protein in the urine when the patient is recumbent).

- The total protein loss in the urine is usually less than 2 g per 24 hours.

- Orthostatic proteinuria occurs much less frequently in adults over 30 years old.

- The prognosis is good. If initial assessment confirms orthostatic proteinuria, then review is recommended after 2 years. If all is well, no further follow-up is required.

- Referral to a nephrologist is necessary if there is more than 2 g protein loss per day, urine microscopy is abnormal, or serum creatinine levels are raised.

Literature

Sanders MH, Streefkerk JG. Diagnostiek en beleid bij orthostatische albuminurie [Diagnosis and treatment of orthostatic albuminuria]. *Modern Med* 1993;**17**:885–9.

Striegel J, Michael AT, Chavers BM. Asymptomatic proteinuria; benign disorder or harbinger of disease? *Postgrad Med* 1988;**83**:287–94.

28

ORTHOSTATIC HYPOTENSION

DEFINITION

Orthostatic hypotension is defined as an abnormal drop in blood pressure in a standing position. Because there is a slight physiological drop in blood pressure immediately after standing, minimum values are usually included in the definition. These figures vary in the literature. Those used most often are: a drop in the systolic blood pressure of more than 25 mmHg and in the diastolic blood pressure of more than 10 mmHg, for longer than 1 minute.

It is quite possible that someone with 'orthostatic hypotension', according to this definition, will have no symptoms, whereas someone else experiencing smaller drops in blood pressure will have symptoms. So a more practical definition is a drop in blood pressure that occurs on standing – usually immediately after standing up – causing symptoms, such as dizziness and near fainting, which can be attributed to decreased circulation to certain organs (especially the brain).

AETIOLOGY/PATHOGENESIS

A complex system of regulatory mechanisms enables the human body to assume a standing position without too many blood pressure fluctuations. The most important mechanism involves the baroreceptors (which are found, for example, in the wall of the aorta), which quickly register blood-pressure changes and cause sympathetic activation. There are a number of other regulatory mechanisms. These can fail for a number of reasons, including medication, hypovolaemia and dysfunction of the autonomic nervous system. There are also situations in which greater demands are made on the regulatory system, such as chronic hypotension.

Various medicines can result in orthostatic hypotension. These include all antihypertensives, many psychopharmacological drugs (especially antidepressants and antipsychotics) and vasodilators. There are many causes of hypovolaemia, such as dehydration due to diarrhoea and poor fluid intake, and chronic diuretic use. Relative hypovolaemia can also play a role when blood pools in the lower body – such as in extensive varicose veins or in the last trimester of pregnancy. In patients with neuropathy, such as diabetics and alcoholics, and in other rare neurological diseases, there may be damage to the autonomic nervous system. Arteriosclerosis can lead to cerebrovascular insufficiency and to improperly functioning autoregulation. This is particularly important in the elderly, and certainly when other risk factors are present. In the case of (relative) hypotension, a small (orthostatic) drop in blood pressure can lead to deficiencies in cerebral autoregulation, which can give rise to symptoms.

PRESENTATION

Patients complain of dizziness or 'seeing black' when standing. They may also have a history of repeatedly fainting or almost fainting under the same circumstances.

EPIDEMIOLOGY

This problem apparently occurs in 10–33% of the elderly. However, it also occurs in young people, especially during puberty and adolescence. The presence of diabetes mellitus or hypertension may also increase the risk of orthostatic hypotension.

HISTORY

The GP asks:

- whether the patient feels 'light in the head' or 'sees black'
- if there is a relationship between these symptoms and assuming a standing position
- about other possible causes of dizziness and fainting.

Vestibular dizziness must be distinguished from dizziness due to orthostatic hypotension. A feeling of dizziness from vertigo (the illusion of spinning or movement) points to a vestibular cause, while a feeling of lightness in the head or 'seeing black' when standing up is indicative of orthostatic hypotension. In the case of psychological dizziness, there is no relationship with 'standing up'.

EXAMINATION

Take the blood pressure while the patient is laying down and then after he has been standing for 1 minute. A drop in systolic blood pressure of more than 25 mmHg certainly warrants the formal diagnosis of orthostatic hypotension, but smaller or no differences do not rule out that diagnosis – the degree of hypotension can vary from day to day and hour to hour.

TREATMENT

First of all, drug side-effects should be considered. The benefit of any treatment causing this problem must be weighed up against the severity and risk of the hypotension. Explanation, reassurance and advice will often make the patient feel better. Simple recommendations may be helpful. Standing with crossed legs or on the toes or squatting on the haunches decreases the chance of orthostasis.

If the blood pressure is low in the lying down/sitting position, dietary advice or medication to increase the blood pressure can be considered, although this is only rarely required. A high salt intake can raise the blood pressure, as can liquorice. Wearing good-quality elastic hosiery may also help.

In the case of serious forms of hypotension, further investigation and treatment by a specialist is appropriate.

PREVENTION AND ADDITIONAL INFORMATION

If medications are used to treat hypertension and psychological disorders in the elderly, the risk of orthostatic hypotension should always be considered. Antihypertensive treatment for older people is started according to the adage 'start low, go slow'. A low dose of a thiazide diuretic is often adequate. If a patient with heart failure has an angiotensin-converting enzyme (ACE) inhibitor added to his diuretic therapy, it is recommended that the first dose of the ACE inhibitor be kept low, and that the patient take this in bed before sleeping. The dose can gradually be increased to the desired amount.

People with orthostatic hypotension should stand up slowly, and, if symptoms arise, they should sit down again with the head between the knees. After a few moments, they can then slowly try to stand up again.

Key points

- A common definition of orthostatic hypotension is a drop in systolic pressure of more than 25 mmHg and of diastolic pressure of more than 10 mmHg for longer than 1 minute on standing. A more practical definition is any drop in blood pressure on standing which causes symptoms.
- The problem needs to be distinguished from vertigo, in which there is an illusion of movement.
- Orthostatic hypotension is common in the elderly.
- The problem often represents a medication side-effect.

Literature

Freeman R. Treatment of orthostatic hypotension. *Semin Neurol* 2003;**23**(4): 435–42.

Hale WA, Chambliss ML. Should primary care patients be screened for orthostatic hypotension? *J Fam Pract* 1999;**48**:547–52.

Leenders JWM, Hoefnagels WHL, Thien T. Orthostatische hypotensie bij bejaarden [Orthostatic hypotension in the elderly]. *Ned Tijdschr Geneeskd* 1990;**134**:1252–4.

Wieling W, Smit AAJ, Van Lieshout JJ. Lichaamshoudingen die de orthostatische tolerantie verbeteren [Body postures that improve orthostatic tolerance]. *Ned Tijdschr Geneeskd* 1996;**140**:1394–7.

29

TRAVEL SICKNESS/MOTION SICKNESS

DEFINITION

Travel sickness (motion sickness) is characterized by symptoms and signs that arise when people experience movement they are not accustomed to. These symptoms and signs include: sighing, yawning, apathy, sleepiness, lack of interest, hyperventilation, pallor, perspiration, flatulence, gagging, vomiting and finally (complete) exhaustion.

AETIOLOGY/PATHOGENESIS

There is currently no clear picture of why motion sickness occurs. The most common explanation is based on the 'sensory conflict' theory. This is based on the fact that all of an individual's lifetime sensory experiences are stored in the brain. New movement patterns are compared with previously constructed and stored information. If the semicircular canals, the otoliths (vestibular mechanoreceptors), the retina and the proprioreceptors of the locomotor apparatus provide conflicting (i.e. novel) information about position and movement, the body responds with the symptoms described above. According to this theory, infants and very young children should not develop motion sickness, as very little information about movement patterns has been stored in their brains. Children aged 2–12 years experience motion sickness the most often, and after this, the incidence decreases gradually. Motion sickness is not common in adults over 50 years old. After a person becomes accustomed to a certain movement pattern, the symptoms soon disappear.

Everyone with a functionally intact balance organ can experience motion sickness, if the stimulus is strong enough and lasts long enough. For example, experienced seamen can easily develop motion sickness if they are exposed to a movement pattern unknown to them. The individual sensitivity varies strongly and is negatively influenced by alcohol and fatigue. Prior knowledge about an expected movement pattern and limiting head movement can reduce the chance of suffering the problem. Pilots and car drivers therefore rarely experience motion sickness during a trip.

Certain off-putting visual images and unpleasant odours can cause an identical set of symptoms.

PRESENTATION

The patient will report that he suffered from the typical symptoms during a car trip, boat ride or flight. However, not all of the symptoms need be experienced. The patient is likely to ask the GP about how these symptoms can be prevented in future.

EPIDEMIOLOGY

There are few reliable data about the epidemiology of motion sickness. In the general population, 70% are slightly sensitive, 25% sensitive and 5% very sensitive to changes in movement. Because of fewer journeys by sea, the improved road network, improved suspension of cars and the higher flying altitude of larger aircraft, motion sickness probably occurs less often than in the past. In military aviation and space travel, where people are exposed to extreme movements, motion sickness remains a major problem.

HISTORY

The GP asks:

- what symptoms are experienced
- under what circumstances the symptoms occur
- about the severity of the symptoms
- if the patient has had this problem before and, if so, under what circumstances
- whether the symptoms (gradually) went away after the patient was no longer exposed to the movement pattern.

EXAMINATION

The history is so characteristic that examination is not necessary.

TREATMENT

When a person is actually experiencing motion sickness, the only rational action is, if possible, to ensure that the patient is no longer exposed to the movement pattern. For people who regularly suffer from motion sickness in their work (pilots, astronauts), adaptation will take place over time and the severity of the symptoms will decrease.

Concentrating on an object that moves along with the moving vehicle, such as the bottom of a car or boat, can ease the symptoms.

PREVENTION AND ADDITIONAL INFORMATION

Explaining the mechanisms that cause motion sickness and providing information about what measures can be taken help to a degree.

Travel sickness can be treated with the following medications:

- Cinnarizine 30 mg, 2 hours before departure; if necessary, 15 mg every 8 hours
- Cyclizine 50 mg, 1–2 hours before departure; if necessary, repeat every 4–6 hours
- If antihistamines do not have a satisfactory effect and if long-lasting treatment is desired, scopolamine patches can be used. A scopolamine patch of 1 mg is placed on a dry, non-hairy spot behind the ear, 5–6 hours before departure. If necessary, it can be replaced after 72 hours. The patches can have many side-effects and are therefore not suitable for use in children less than 10 years old.

Key points

- The precise cause of motion sickness remains uncertain.
- Children aged 2–12 years experience motion sickness the most often; after this age, the incidence decreases gradually.
- Concentrating on an object that moves along with the moving vehicle, such as the bottom of a car or boat, can ease the symptoms. Various medications can also be tried.

Literature

Cheung BS, Herkin R, Hofer KD. Failure of cetirizine and fexofenadine to prevent motion sickness. *Ann Pharmacother* 2003;**37**:173–7.

Nicholson AN, Stone BM, Turner C, Mills SL. Central effects of cinnarizine: restricted use in aircrew. *Aviat Space Environ Med* 2002;**73**:570–4.

Oosterveld WJ. Capita selecta: bewegingsziekte [Capita selecta: motion sickness]. *Ned Tijdschr Geneesk* 1989;**133**:2430–3.

Pyykko I, Schalen L, Jantti V. Transdermally administered scopolamine vs dimenhydrinate. I. Effect on nausea and vertigo in experimentally induced motion sickness. *Acta Otolaryngol* 1985;**99**(5–6):588-96.

Ruckenstein MJ, Harrison RV. Motion sickness. Helping patients tolerate the ups and downs. *Postgrad Med* 1991;**89**(6):139–44.

Van Marion WF, Bongaerts MC, Christiaanse JC, Hofkamp HG, Van Ouwerkerk W. Influence of transdermal scopolamine on motion sickness during 7 days' exposure to heavy seas. *Clin Pharmacol Ther* 1985;**38**(3):301–5.

30

EXCESSIVE CRYING IN INFANTS/INFANTILE COLIC

DEFINITION

Excessive crying in infants, or infantile colic, is defined as excessive crying that occurs in 'attacks' in a healthy, properly growing infant – usually beginning in the first few weeks of life. These attacks tend to occur in the early evening when, without any clear reason, the child begins to cry inconsolably, bends the knees and pulls the legs up towards the abdomen, seems to be in pain, and may pass wind. An arbitrary definition to distinguish excessive crying from normal crying is the 'rule of three': crying/whimpering for at least 3 hours a day, at least 3 days a week, for a minimum of 3 weeks. Other terms used to refer to this problem include 'intestinal cramps' and 'inconsolable crying'. It is better to avoid these terms, and the commonly used 'infantile colic'; the key point is to distinguish between primary and secondary excessive crying. In 'primary excessive crying' no cause is found.

AETIOLOGY/PATHOGENESIS

Excessive crying in infants is not a single syndrome, but a symptom (a final common pathway) of various disorders. Some excessive crying has somatic causes, and some has psychosocial causes. Cow's milk intolerance, gastro-oesophageal reflux and abnormal intestinal motility are possible somatic explanations. The possible roles of colonic distension (due to swallowed air via an incorrect feeding technique, or an increase in gas formation as a result of fermentation of excess lactose), the type of feeding (breast- or bottle-feeding) or brain damage as a result of a traumatic birth have not been proven. Possible psychosocial causes include stress resulting from problems during the mother's pregnancy (hyperemesis gravidarum, pelvic pain, psychological problems) and the manner in which the child is cared for.

PRESENTATION

It is unclear how many parents of infants who cry excessively actually seek help. Parents usually attend because the persistent and recurring nature of the problem has exhausted them, and because they fear something might be wrong with their child.

EPIDEMIOLOGY

This problem results in one in six families seeking medical help. Incidence and prevalence figures differ significantly from study to study. The best prospective studies report prevalances in the range 5–19%. Gender, socio-economic status and the birth order of the child do not influence the incidence of the problem. There are suggestions that the phenomenon of excessive crying in infants does not occur in non-western cultures.

HISTORY

The GP asks:

- how many hours per day the infant cries
- how long the problem has been going on
- about other symptoms (inconsolable crying, problems with defaecation, bloated abdomen, flatulence, vomiting)
- about any connection between the feeding times and when the symptoms occur
- what action the parents have already taken
- about whether the parents are worried or scared.

EXAMINATION

If presented acutely, the examination is oriented towards excluding any clear cause for the crying. Otherwise, a general physical examination is unlikely to reveal any problem, but may help reassure the parents, although the presence of signs of atopy may be a useful clue. A simple urinalysis may be performed.

TREATMENT

If no abnormalities are revealed, general advice and reassurance should be given. Simple advice about care of the child might include: the infant should be exposed as little as possible to all kinds of stimuli; continually picking up and carrying around the child should be avoided; a regular pattern should be established; the parents should get adequate rest (e.g. by having someone else care for the child temporarily).

One option is a trial of treatment for 2 weeks with a hypoallergenic formula, although the evidence base for this is limited. A whey hydrolysate can be used for this purpose. If the child has a cow's milk intolerance, the crying will stop within a few days. To confirm the diagnosis, a provocation test with the original formula is conducted. If successful, the treatment with hypoallergenic formula should be continued until the child is 1 year old.

To rule out rare cases of excessive crying due to reflux oesophagitis, a trial of treatment can be carried out that involves thickening the formula with carob powder. If the test treatment with thickened formula is successful, it should be continued for several months.

The management of excessive crying often requires a number of consultations. Parents appreciate guidance and reassurance in this difficult phase.

Insufficient evidence exists to recommend other treatments, although many have been tried. Insufficient evidence exists to recommend other treatments, although many have been tried.

PREVENTION AND ADDITIONAL INFORMATION

In the case of primary excessive crying, the emphasis should be placed on the harmless character (in medical terms) of the symptom and the favourable prognosis: by 4 months, most infants' crying has dropped to a normal level. It is not possible to prevent excessive crying in infants.

Key points

- An arbitrary definition to distinguish excessive crying from normal crying is the 'rule of three': crying/whimpering for at least 3 hours a day, at least 3 days a week, for a minimum of 3 weeks.

- Parents usually attend because they are exhausted, and because they fear something might be significantly wrong with their child.

- If presented acutely, the examination is oriented towards excluding any clear cause for the crying.

- One option is a trial of treatment for 2 weeks with a hypoallergenic formula, although the evidence base for this is limited.

- By 4 months, most infants' crying has dropped to a normal level.

Literature

Hill DJ, Hosking CS. Infantile colic and food hypersensitivity. *J Pediatr Gastroenterol Nutr* 2000;**30**(Suppl):S67–76.

Gupta SK. Is colic a gastrointestinal disorder? *Curr Opin Pediatr* 2002;**14**(5): 588–92.

Lucassen PLBJ, Assendelft WJ, Gubbels JW, Van Eijk JT, Van Geldrop WJ, Knuistingh Neven A. Effectiveness of treatments for infantile colic: systematic review. *BMJ* 1998;**316**(7144):1563–9.

Lucassen PL, Assendelft WJ, van Eijk JT, Gubbels JW, Douwes AC, van Geldrop WJ. Systematic review of the occurrence of infantile colic in the community. *Arch Dis Child* 2001;**84**(5):398–403.

Vomberg PP, Eckhardt PG, Büller HA. Excessief huilen bij baby's; een literatuuroverzicht en praktische aanbevelingen [Excessive crying in babies; a literature overview and practical recommendations]. *Ned Tijdschr Geneesk* 1995;**139**:119–22.

31

NIGHT TERRORS AND NIGHTMARES (IN CHILDREN)

DEFINITION

Night terrors and nightmares are nightly sleep disturbances that usually occur in childhood. In a night terror, the child is incompletely aroused from deep, slow-wave sleep. The child is not completely awake, and seems confused. He may make random movements with his arms and legs, does not respond when spoken to, and does not remember anything about the episode the next day. These attacks rarely last longer than 15 minutes.

Nightmares are frightening dreams that wake the child from sleep, and which are not accompanied by motor agitation. The child is woken by the dream and can still remember it.

AETIOLOGY/PATHOGENESIS

Night terrors occur due to a sudden arousal from deep (non-REM sleep), generally at the beginning of the night. An episode usually begins with a loud, penetrating scream, followed immediately by random movements of the arms and legs, and sometimes the entire body, with the tendency to sit bolt upright in bed. Characteristically, the child will have an intensely frightened facial expression (with bulging, wide-open eyes), and sometimes heavy perspiration with rapid heartbeat and breathing. After a few minutes, the severity of the symptoms decreases, but the child remains confused for several minutes before falling asleep again. There is a familial predisposition, possibly in combination with sleepwalking and nocturnal enuresis. Upper respiratory disorders that disrupt sleep can aggravate the problem.

Nightmares are very frightening dreams that wake the patient from REM sleep, usually in the second half of the night. These are almost always long and complex dreams that become increasingly threatening towards the end. In contrast to night terrors, they are not accompanied by mental confusion, disorientation and pronounced motor agitation; the autonomic symptoms are also less pronounced. After waking, the patient is still aware of the frightening dream, which makes falling asleep again difficult. Children in particular sometimes have difficulty distinguishing the dream from reality.

Adults seldom suffer from sleep terrors and nightmares. These disorders may be triggered by an irregular sleeping pattern, tension, stress or medication use. If the clinical picture is not typical, additional tests may be necessary to check for epilepsy or other sleep disorders.

PRESENTATION

The parents usually explain that the child wakes up confused and acts strangely, or that the child regularly has frightening dreams.

EPIDEMIOLOGY

Night terrors occur in approximately 3% of children, peaking at around 6 years of age. They usually disappear before the age of 14, and are very rare in adults. Night terrors seem to occur slightly more often in males.

Nightmares occur in around 20–50% of children between the ages of 3 and 6 years. They usually begin gradually at the age of 2–3 years, and disappear when the child is 12 or 13. However, a small subgroup continues to experience nightmares through adulthood. They occur two to four times as often in women than men.

HISTORY

The GP asks:

- when the problem started
- whether the episodes occur at the beginning or more towards the end of the night
- whether the patient is conscious of the night-time agitation

- whether the parent can describe exactly what happened when the child woke up
- whether the problem is accompanied by motor or other symptoms
- whether the child falls asleep again easily after the episode.

EXAMINATION

Physical examination is non-contributory.

TREATMENT

For both sleep terrors and nightmares, the treatment is limited mainly to explaining to the child and parents the benign character of the episodes and the favourable prognosis. In addition, the GP should explain the importance of following a bedtime sleep routine, maintaining a regular sleeping pattern and eliminating factors that might trigger the problem.

In the case of sleep terrors, forcibly stopping the child's movements and waking the child is not recommended, as this may aggravate the disturbance. A small study reported in the *BMJ* showed that waking the child about 15 minutes before the anticipated onset of the night terror – or when autonomic arousal is first noted – for 1 week seems to produce a long-term cure.

With nightmares, the treatment consists primarily of explaining the nature and prognosis of the problem and avoiding factors that induce them. If the child experiences extreme fear, a behavioral approach can be useful. This may occasionally require referral to the community paediatric or psychology services, especially if there seem to be underlying emotional problems.

In serious cases in adults that cause significant insomnia, antidepressants or benzodiazepines may be tried for a short period of time. However, such treatment must be used very conservatively, because of the possibility of symptoms recurring, perhaps more severely, once the medication is stopped.

If the symptoms, due to their duration, frequency and the patient's age, are atypical, the patient should be referred for further tests (such as polygraphic testing with video monitoring) to check for epilepsy or other sleep disorders.

PREVENTION AND ADDITIONAL INFORMATION

A proper sleep routine (going to bed on time), a regular sleeping pattern and eliminating triggers are all essential for a good night's sleep. It is sensible not to let children watch an exciting or frightening television programme before going to bed.

Key points

- In a night terror, the child is not completely awake, and seems confused. He may make random movements with his arms and legs, does not respond when spoken to, and does not remember anything about the episode the next day. These attacks rarely last longer than 15 minutes. They peak at around 6 years of age and usually disappear before the age of 14.

- Nightmares are frightening dreams that wake the child from sleep, and which are not accompanied by motor agitation. The child is woken by the dream and can still remember it. They occur in around 20–50% of children between the ages of 3 and 6 years. They usually disappear by the time the child is 12 or 13.

- Night terrors tend to occur at the beginning of the night. Nightmares usually occur in the second half of the night.

- In night terrors, waking the child about 15 minutes before the anticipated onset of the event, or when autonomic arousal is first noted, for 1 week may produce a long-term cure.

Literature

Lask B. Novel and non toxic treatment for night terrors. *BMJ* 1988;**297**;592.

Thiedke CC. Sleep disorders and sleep problems in childhood. *Am Fam Physician* 2001;**63**(2):277–84.

Wills L, Garcia J. Parasomnias: epidemiology and management. *CNS Drugs* 2002;**16**(12):803–10.

32

DIFFUSE HAIR LOSS AND MALE-PATTERN (ANDROGENIC) ALOPECIA

DEFINITION

Diffuse hair loss is widespread rather than localized loss of hair on the head.

AETIOLOGY/PATHOGENESIS

Hair growth has three phases: the anagen phase (active growth), the catagen phase (intermediate phase between active growth and cessation of growth) and the telogen phase (resting stage). Anagen is the longest phase, with up to 90% of follicles in it at any one time. On the head, the life cycle of a hair is 2–6 years.

There are many causes of diffuse hair loss, including chronic illnesses (malignancies, leukaemia, renal insufficiency), deficiencies (iron, folic acid), medication (e.g. cytotoxic agents) and hormonal changes (pregnancy, hypo/hyperthyroidism, diabetes mellitus). The latter can cause the anagen phase to end prematurely. As a result, a larger number of hairs than normal end up in the telogen phase synchronously. Three months later, after the telogen phase, these (telogen) hairs all fall out at the same time (telogen effluvium). This type of hair loss is generally mild – a person rarely loses more than 50% of their hair. If the cause can be eliminated, normal hair growth can be expected within 6 months.

Alternatively, the cell division activity of the hair matrix can temporarily be stopped entirely (anagen arrest) – as is the case with cytotoxic agents or radiotherapy. In this situation, nearly all the hair (80–90%) falls out within 1–3 weeks (anagen effluvium). The hairs that fall out are in the anagen phase. Once the precipitating factor has been resolved, the hair follicles resume their activity. Complete recovery of hair growth, however, takes a long time (months to years).

A recently described disorder (loose anagen hair syndrome) occurs almost exclusively in children, who usually have short hair that can be easily and painlessly pulled out. The pulled-out hairs are in the anagen phase. There are no cures for this. In most cases, the thickness, density and length of the hair increase spontaneously at the start of adolescence.

Abnormalities in the hair shaft are usually a result of improper hair care; rarely, they are congenital. The hair breaks off at the weakest point of the hair shaft. Aggressive cosmetic applications (perms, hair straighteners) and strong sunlight weaken the hair, so excessive exposure to these aggravating factors should be avoided. If no external cause is found, it is appropriate to refer the patient to a dermatologist to rule out a (rare) congenital disorder of the hair shaft.

Male-pattern baldness involves genetically determined, increased sensitivity of the hair follicles to androgenous steroids. Testosterone and its metabolites promote atrophy of the hair follicle. The growth phase of a hair is consequently shortened, while the hair growth cycle is accelerated, resulting in a situation where the hair follicles are 'used up' prematurely. In men, the front hairline recedes and there is visible hair loss on and around the crown and on the temples. The balding areas converge and the familiar 'horseshoe' strip of hair remains. In women with this disorder, the hair follicles are probably extra sensitive to testosterone. There may be a connection with seborrhoea, especially in women.

PRESENTATION

Hair loss as a complaint must always be taken seriously. Some patients exaggerate the loss of hair to achieve this. It is very important to determine the patient's motivation for consulting the GP – dissatisfaction, fear, a need for information, or treatment?

For humans, hair is not essential. However, hair is significant in an aesthetic and social sense. The effect of hair loss and baldness (or the threat thereof) can have a considerable influence on a person's personality and psychosocial well-being. Furthermore, diffuse hair loss can be a symptom of a systemic disorder.

EPIDEMIOLOGY

There are no specific incidence data on the various forms of hair loss. The prevalence of male-pattern baldness in men more or less parallels the 'age decade': 30% in men aged 20–29 years, 40% in men aged 30–39 years, and so on.

HISTORY

The GP asks:

- whether the problem is increasing baldness or increasing hair loss
- whether it runs in the family
- whether the patient has a chronic illness or is on medication
- whether there are other symptoms that indicate an endocrine disorder (hypothyroidism, hyperthyroidism, diabetes mellitus).

Increasing baldness usually involves a natural process (such as male-pattern baldness in men), while increasing hair loss indicates a more acute and unnatural process (telogen or anagen effluvium).

EXAMINATION

Local examination is usually sufficient. In the early stages, it is sometimes difficult to see the hair loss; approximately 50% of the normal number of hairs on the head can fall out before the hair clearly becomes thinner. The structure and form of the hair and the hair-loss pattern are examined. The scalp is inspected for skin abnormalities, such as flaking, infection, scarring and the presence or absence of follicles.

A rough objective measure is the 'pull test'. Four days after hair washing, hold 30–40 hairs between the thumb and index finger, and pull firmly, letting the hair glide through the fingers. Normally, no more than six hairs may be pulled out. A negative pull test, however, does not rule out abnormal hair loss.

In order to differentiate between the forms of diffuse hair loss, it is useful to determine whether the hairs fall out with the root (in the telogen phase) or are broken off (in the anagen phase). The hairs pulled out with the pull test can be examined for this purpose. The general examination is guided by the patient's history and the findings on scalp examination. It may involve checking the body hair and the thyroid status, looking for the presence of hirsutism and acne (alopecia in women), and examining for malnutrition, anaemia and malignancies. Because many systemic illnesses affect both the hair and the nails, the latter should also be inspected.

Additional tests are rarely necessary. Laboratory investigations, such as thyroid function tests, are only arranged if the patient's history or examination suggests an underlying disorder.

TREATMENT

Diffuse hair loss. Treatment for diffuse hair loss is not necessary in most cases. Even if the cause is clear, treatment is often not possible. In telogen and anagen effluvium, treatment consists, where possible, of eliminating the causative agent – and, in telogen effluvium, the good prognosis should be emphasized.

Male-pattern hair loss. No completely satisfactory therapy is available for androgenic alopecia. The GP should provide realistic information about the chances of success offered by medication. The effectiveness of local remedies (e.g. minoxidil) is disappointing. Finasteride (also used for benign prostate hypertrophy) results in a significant increase in hair growth in 65% of men. But when medication is stopped, the beneficial effect disappears within 6–12 months.

Other alternatives include the use of wigs, or, in exceptional cases, referring the patient for reconstructive surgery (reduction of the bald area by plastic surgery, skin transplants or hair transplants). These treatments are expensive and are not available on the National Health Service.

PREVENTION AND ADDITIONAL INFORMATION

In addition to providing information about the cause of the hair loss and the relatively poor chance of successful treatment with medication, it is essential to address the psychosocial aspects of hair loss. Young men with alopecia androgenica should be encouraged to accept their hair loss as a normal, natural process. Proper information provision by the GP has a good chance of preventing people from seeking salvation in the often expensive and ineffective 'miracle cures' propagated in the media.

Key points

- Increasing baldness usually involves a natural process (e.g. male-pattern baldness in men), while increasing hair loss indicates a more acute and unnatural process (telogen or anagen effluvium).

- Approximately 50% of the normal number of hairs on the head can fall out before the hair clearly becomes thinner.

- The effect of hair loss and baldness (or the threat thereof) can have a considerable influence on a person's personality and psychosocial well-being.

- In telogen effluvium, patients can be reassured that the prognosis is good.

Literature

Ellis JA, Sinclair R, Harrap SB. Androgenetic alopecia: pathogenesis and potential for therapy. *Expert Rev Mol Med* 2002;**19**:1–11.

Sinclair R. Fortnightly review: male pattern androgenetic alopecia. *BMJ* 1998;**317**:865–9.

33

ALOPECIA AREATA AND OTHER FORMS OF PATCHY HAIR LOSS

DEFINITION

Alopecia areata is a disorder in which hair loss occurs in a circumscribed area, usually on the scalp, but occasionally also in the beard area or eyebrows. If the scalp looks abnormal, then other forms of patchy hair loss should be considered.

AETIOLOGY/PATHOGENESIS

Hair growth has three phases: the anagen phase (active growth), the catagen phase (intermediate phase between active growth and cessation of growth) and the telogen phase (resting stage). Anagen is the longest phase, with up to 90% of follicles in it at any one time. On the head, the life cycle of a hair is 2–6 years.

In alopecia areata, the hair follicles in the affected areas cycle into the catagen phase and then the telogen phase more rapidly than normal. There are many theories as to the cause. Some believe it is due to a disruption in the circulation of the scalp, while others think it may be an autoimmune problem. Other relevant factors include: genetic influences, hormonal influences (thyroid disorders, pregnancy) and 'increased ectodermal activity', which refers to the combination of alopecia areata with cataract, atopia and nail changes. Stress can be a trigger.

Stress can also make people nervously pull out their hair. This trichotillomania can cause large bald spots. Certain scalp disorders, such as psoriasis and tinea capitis, can also cause a clinical picture similar to alopecia areata. Long-term light pressure on the head, such as caused by a hat or cap, or long-term pulling on the hair, such as from a tight ponytail or plait, can cause persistent alopecia.

PRESENTATION

Patients consult their GP because they are worried about a bald spot that has suddenly appeared. They are usually afraid that they will soon be completely bald.

EPIDEMIOLOGY

In Great Britain, 2% of consultations in dermatology outpatient clinics apparently involve alopecia areata; the figure in The Netherlands is 1%. The disorder occurs most often in people between 20 and 40 years old, and equally often in men and women.

HISTORY

The GP asks:

- how long the bald spot has been present
- about the presence of an atopic constitution
- about repeated nervous pulling out of hair (trichotillomania)
- if the patient has a history of psoriasis or other skin disease
- about local flakiness (this can indicate a fungal infection).

EXAMINATION

Alopecia areata appears as a circumscribed bald spot, usually on the scalp, and sometimes in the beard area or eyebrows. If there is no intradermal inflammation present, the skin on the bald spot generally looks normal. There is no atrophy of the hair follicles and the follicle openings are therefore visible to the naked eye. Different bald spots can appear at the same time or consecutively. If the spots encroach on the hairline, this can result in a jagged pattern. Hairs at the edge of an affected area often take the form of an exclamation mark: they are narrow at the base and the short distal part is wide. Thirty per cent of patients also suffer from nail abnormalities, such as pitting, ridges and increased brittleness. During the examination, it is important to look for signs of mycosis, psoriasis or other skin disease.

TREATMENT

In the majority of cases, hair growth resumes in several months, regardless of treatment. Many therapies have been described. Most of these are based on a vasodilative or an immunosuppressive effect. None have been proven effective.

The results of locally applied minoxidil are disappointing. Local injections of corticosteroids are championed by several authors, but this is not supported by the literature. Because of the potentially serious side-effects of this treatment, there is no real indication for its use.

Some patients do not respond to any kind of treatment, and their hair may not regrow. The disorder can be a huge psychological burden, to the extent that counselling is necessary. These patients may benefit from a wig.

PREVENTION AND ADDITIONAL INFORMATION

It is not possible to prevent alopecia areata. The patient can be told that the condition generally has a good prognosis. It usually completely disappears after a time, without treatment. If the disorder is present in patients with an atopic constitution or with an endocrine disorder, the prognosis is less positive. This is also the case when the hairline is affected. The presence of the disorder in places other than the scalp points to a more severe and long-term prognosis, with a significant chance of alopecia totalis.

Key points

- In alopecia areata, the scalp usually looks normal – if it does not, another diagnosis should be considered.

- In the majority of cases of alopecia areata, hair growth resumes in several months, regardless of treatment.

- Poor prognostic features include associated atopy or endocrine disorders, disease affecting the hairline, and alopecia in areas other than the scalp.

Literature

Fiedler VC. Alopecia areata. A review of therapy, efficacy, safety, and mechanism. *Arch Dermatol* 1992;**128**:1519–29.

Fiedler VC, Alaiti S. Treatment of alopecia areata. *Dermatol Clin* 1996;**14**: 733–7.

Freyschmidt-Paul P, Happle R, McElwee KJ, Hoffmann R. Alopecia areata: treatment of today and tomorrow. *J Invest Dermatol Symp Proc* 2003;**8**(1): 12–7.

Price VH. Therapy of alopecia areata: on the cusp and in the future. *J Invest Dermatol Symp Proc* 2003;**8**(2):207–11.

Van Duijn HJ, Mulder Dzn JD. Kleine kwalen in de huisartsgeneeskunde; alopecia areata [Minor ailments in general practice; alopecia areata]. *Ned Tijdschr Geneeskd* 1987;**131**:1856–7.

34
DANDRUFF

DEFINITION

Dandruff, or pityriasis capitis, is a dry flaking of the scalp. It is primarily a cosmetic complaint, although it can be accompanied by itching.

It is sometimes difficult to distinguish from seborrhoeic eczema, a chronically recurring skin disorder, which may affect the scalp. This is characterized by erythematous lesions (the inflammatory component) with greasy yellow flakiness in areas with active sebaceous glands (see Chapter 35). Besides the scalp, the typical areas affected are the eyebrows, the nasolabial folds and the beard area.

Because the distinction between dandruff and seborrhoeic eczema is not always clear, in the literature dandruff is considered by some authors as a less serious form of seborrhoeic eczema (with flaking, but no inflammation). Generally, however, these problems are viewed as separate entities. This chapter focuses exclusively on dandruff rather than seborrhoeic eczema.

AETIOLOGY/PATHOGENESIS

In keratinized simple squamous epithelium, cells continuously divide in the epidermis and new keratinocytes are formed. These keratinocytes gradually move to the exterior, to become the 'horn cells'. These are eventually shed, and stick together in particles that are usually smaller than 0.2 mm. In the case of dandruff, the particles are larger due to increased adhesion and increased production of the horn cells.

An important role is played by the yeast *Pityrosporum ovale* (and, to a lesser degree, *P. orbiculare*) in the pathogenesis of dandruff. This causes the flakiness: more *Pityrosporum* spores are found in people with dandruff than in people without it. Individual sensitivity is also relevant: *Pityrosporum* is frequently present, but not everyone develops dandruff. In this sense, the situation is similar to pityriasis versicolor (see Chapter 14). Conditions favourable for the growth of the yeast, such as moisture or occlusion, can exacerbate dandruff.

PRESENTATION

The main complaint is dandruff, recognized by the patient as such, and posing a cosmetic problem. It is sometimes accompanied by itching. The patient's hairdresser may also have recommended consulting the GP.

EPIDEMIOLOGY

There are no known figures on the occurrence of dandruff, but it is clearly very common.

HISTORY

The history may be short. The GP asks:

- about how the symptoms have developed
- about whether there are other symptoms in addition to the dandruff/flakiness (such as itching, redness or crusts on the scalp)
- about signs of a secondary infection (e.g. from scratching)
- whether similar problems are present on other parts of the body and whether there are signs of other skin disorders, such as psoriasis or seborrhoeic eczema.

EXAMINATION

The examination focuses on inspecting the scalp. Is the flaking present on the entire scalp or only part of it? Also, check for the presence of redness or crusts. Based on the history, the rest of the skin is checked for abnormalities. Other skin disorders, such as seborrhoeic dermatitis or psoriasis, can also cause excessive flaking. Additional investigations are unnecessary.

TREATMENT

Dandruff can be satisfactorily treated with shampoo containing zinc pyrithione. If this does not have the desired effect, ketoconazole, coal tar and selenium sulphide are other options.

PREVENTION AND ADDITIONAL INFORMATION

Dandruff cannot be 'cured', but it can be effectively suppressed with regular thorough washing with one of the shampoos described above. Covering the head with a hat, cap or helmet can make the dandruff worse.

Key points

- It can be difficult to distinguish dandruff from seborrhoeic eczema.
- The yeast *Pityrosporum ovale* plays an important role in dandruff.
- Dandruff cannot be cured, but a variety of shampoos will ease the problem.

Literature

Anon. Scales in the balance: dandruff reconsidered [editorial]. *Lancet* 1985;**ii**:703–4.

Janniger CK, Schwartz RA. Seborrheic dermatitis. *Am Fam Physician* 1995;**52**:149–55.

Pierard-Franchimont C, Hermanns JF, Degreef H, Pierard GE. From axioms to new insights into dandruff. *Dermatology* 2000;**200**(2):93–8.

Polano MK. Hoofdroos [Dandruff]. *Ned Tijdschr Geneeskd* 1986;**130**:2340–2.

35

SEBORRHOEIC ECZEMA OF THE SCALP/CRADLE CAP

DEFINITION

Seborrhoeic eczema, also known as seborrhoeic dermatitis, is a chronically recurring skin disorder characterized by erythema with greasy, yellow crusts in areas with active sebaceous glands. Besides the scalp, the typical sites are: the nasolabial folds, other body folds, the beard area, eyebrows, eyelashes, the outer ear and ear canals, and the postauricular, presternal and interscapular areas. In young children, seborrhoeic eczema is often called 'cradle cap'. It begins in the first few weeks after birth and usually resolves rapidly. In flakiness of the scalp, the main distinguishing feature from dandruff (see Chapter 34) is that seborrhoeic eczema clearly involves an inflammatory component that manifests as erythema.

AETIOLOGY/PATHOGENESIS

The name of this disorder indicates a relationship with the sebaceous glands, but it is not simply the result of seborrhoea (an abnormally high sebum production): people with seborrhoea are not more likely to suffer from seborrhoeic eczema. However, there does seem to be a link with sebum production:

- Seborrhoeic eczema occurs more often in men than in women (men have a higher sebum production – this increases during puberty under the influence of male sex hormones).
- An artificial reduction of the, often normal, level of sebum production in people with seborrhoeic eczema results in a reduction of symptoms.

The main exogenous factor is the yeast *Pityrosporum ovale*, which plays a role in the inflammation – sebum may promote the growth of this yeast. Other factors that can influence the course of the disorder are both external (clothing, local irritation due to soap or cosmetics, climate) and internal (stress, diet).

PRESENTATION

The main complaints are itching, greasy, yellow flakes and redness on the scalp, sometimes with similar lesions on other sites. The flakes may be fine, but they can also take the form of large greasy crusts at the hairline. The symptoms vary over time, but they do not usually disappear completely.

EPIDEMIOLOGY

Available data reveal an incidence of six patients per year in the average general practice. The actual incidence is probably much higher, because many people do not visit their GP but self-treat.

HISTORY

The GP asks:

- whether there are only flakes, or whether itching and redness are also present
- about the progression of the condition over time
- about the presence of similar abnormalities on other parts of the body.

EXAMINATION

The physical examination consists first of inspecting the scalp. Attention should be paid to whether the flakiness is present on the entire scalp or only at the hairline, and to whether redness, crusts and signs of secondary impetiginization are present. The skin on the rest of the body is assessed for the presence of flakes, as well as on the face for crusts (eyebrows, eyelashes, around the mouth), behind the ears or in the ear canal (seborrhoeic eczema can cause otitis externa), in the body folds and on the sternum and between the shoulder blades. Additional investigations do not help in making the diagnosis.

TREATMENT

The GP first explains that seborrhoeic eczema is a life-long disorder, which will never completely disappear. There are, however, various remedies that reduce the symptoms. Zinc pyrithione, selenium sulphide, ketoconazole, sulphur and tar are active against *P. ovale*. Salicylic acid and resorcinol dissolve the flakes, so these can be washed out of the hair. Corticosteroids reduce the inflammation and the itching. For mild forms of this disorder, twice weekly treatment with a shampoo containing zinc pyrithione is sufficient. Selenium sulphide in a shampoo is also effective, but it also makes the hair somewhat greasy.

For more serious problems with the scalp, cocois should be used. Topical steroids (class III) are also helpful, as is ketoconazole shampoo. The corticosteroid can usually be stopped after 1 week; use of ketoconazole is continued until the symptoms have disappeared. As a maintenance treatment, applying the ketoconazole gel twice monthly after washing is recommended.

In women with severe seborrhoeic eczema accompanied by excessive sebum production, systemic cyproterone acetate (as Dianette) can be tried to see if it has an effect.

In children, the disorder usually disappears before the child's first birthday. Thick crusts on a baby's scalp can be removed by soaking them with baby oil for 20–30 minutes every day. The hairy area of the scalp is then washed with zinc pyrithione shampoo.

PREVENTION AND ADDITIONAL INFORMATION

Yeasts flourish in a warm, moist and closed environment, which means that covering the head should be avoided. Exposure to the sun and other ultraviolet radiation reduces the symptoms.

Key points

- The typical sites for seborrhoeic eczema are the scalp, the nasolabial folds, other body folds, the beard area, eyebrows, eyelashes, outer ear and ear canals, and the postauricular, presternal and interscapular areas.

- Seborrhoeic eczema involves an inflammatory component that manifests as erythema. This helps distinguish it from simple dandruff.

- It is important that patients understand that seborrhoeic eczema is a life-long disorder, which will never completely disappear.

Literature

Gupta AK, Bluhm R. Seborrhoeic dermatitis. *J Eur Acad Dermatol Venereol* 2004;**18**(1):13–26.

Johnson BA, Nunley JR. Treatment of seborrheic dermatitis. *Am Fam Physician* 2000;**61**:2703–10.

36
EARLOBE INFLAMMATION

DEFINITION

Earlobe inflammation is typically exudative, accompanied by redness, itching, oedema, blisters and crusts. The clinical picture primarily has the characteristics of a dermatitis.

AETIOLOGY/PATHOGENESIS

Earlobes can become inflamed by wearing pierced or clip earrings. A distinction can be made between two forms: acute and chronic. The acute, often infectious, form can occur after perforation of the earlobe, such as after ear piercing. Rare complications, such as keloid scars, staphylococcal sepsis, hepatitis, cysts and haematomas, are described in the specialist literature. If the cartilage of the ear is pierced, there is a risk of perichondritis. Due to the risks of infection, many jewellers nowadays use sterile sets with hypoallergenic metals to make a hole in the earlobe or auricular cartilage.

The chronic, usually allergic, form is often the result of a nickel allergy. This is a type IV (late) lymphocyte-mediated allergy. Earrings can therefore be the cause of extensive allergic skin disorders on the entire body. The reverse can also occur: sensitization due to jewellery containing nickel worn on other body parts can cause a local reaction if the patient wears 'cheap' earrings. Combinations of allergy and (secondary) infection are very common.

PRESENTATION

The patient usually consults the GP to ask whether the inflammation means the earrings need to be removed. In some cases, the patient may have already removed the earrings, and simply request something to combat the inflammation. Pain, itching, swelling behind the ear, the inflammation spreading behind the ear and fever can also be reasons for consulting the GP.

EPIDEMIOLOGY

A comprehensive study revealed that, when asked, 34% of women with pierced ears experienced chronic local complications such as redness, swelling or infection. Contact hypersensitivity to nickel is ten times more common in women than in men. It appears that 15% of girls aged 8–15 years with pierced ears already have a sensitivity to nickel. The main cause of this is probably wearing jewellery containing nickel.

HISTORY

The history is usually short. The GP asks:

- how the disorder has developed
- about other symptoms or signs of contact allergies
- about the extent of the reaction
- about what action the patient has already taken
- whether the patient is willing not to wear earrings
- about hygiene measures.

EXAMINATION

A local examination is usually sufficient. Inspecting the skin of the earlobe and the outer ear is required to exclude impetiginization or erysipelas (see Chapter 13). If the hole is located in the cartilage of the earlobe, perichondritis may be present. The pre- and post-auricular glands should be palpated.

A more extensive examination is carried out if allergy or atopy is suspected. The skin is inspected elsewhere, especially the popliteal and antecubital fossae, and the fingers, to check for signs of eczema. Signs of nickel allergy are found mainly on the wrists, throat and neck. Allergy tests are rarely necessary.

TREATMENT

If there is pain, redness, pus or swelling, the earring needs to be removed. A piece of cotton wool saturated with alcohol applied to the inflamed area, and possibly stuck to the earlobe with a plaster, will provide relief. Alternatives are povidone iodine or chlorhexidine. If the inflammation is due to an allergy, the allergen needs to be eliminated or avoided. Remember, too, that the problem may be caused by jewellery worn on other areas of the body.

If necessary, an antibiotic ointment may be applied (e.g. fusidic acid ointment). Erysipelas is treated with oral antibiotics (e.g. phenoxy-methylpenicillin or flucloxacillin). Perichondritis requires similar treatment. Occasionally, systemic treatment of (generalized) allergic reactions (severe itching, rash) with antihistamines is necessary.

PREVENTION AND ADDITIONAL INFORMATION

After the ear is pierced, the hole must be cleaned twice daily with an antiseptic liquid until it is epithelialized. To decrease the pressure on the contact points in the ear lobe, it is advisable to twist the earring in the hole several times a day for the first 4 weeks. Piercing holes in the cartilage of the ear, and wearing pierced or clip earrings if a person is sensitive to nickel or chrome, are not recommended.

Key points

- Ear lobes become inflamed because of infection or allergy, or both.
- If the cartilage of the ear is pierced, there is a risk of perichondritis.
- Contact hypersensitivity to nickel is ten times more common in women than in men.

Literature

Steigleder GK. *Dermatologie und Venereologie fur Ärzte und Studenten mit 122 Prüfungsfragen* [Dermatology and venereology for doctors and students with 122 examination questions]. Stuttgart: Thieme, 1987.

Van Vloten WA, et al. (eds). *Dermatologie en venereologie* [Dermatology and venereology]. Utrecht: Bunge, 1996.

37

EAR WAX BLOCKAGE/ CERUMEN IMPACTION

DEFINITION

Cerumen, or ear wax, is the physiological secretion of ceruminous glands located in the outer third of the external auditory canal. It becomes a problem if a plug of wax blocks the external auditory canal, causing deafness or a sensation of blockage.

AETIOLOGY/PATHOGENESIS

The secretory part of the ceruminous glands is surrounded by myoepithelial cells. These respond to physical and chemical stimuli by contracting. This causes cerumen to be secreted, which initially consists of white watery drops. As a result of oxidation, the cerumen turns into the familiar brown, semi-liquid 'wax'. The amount varies per individual, as does the colour. Also, each ear can produce different amounts of cerumen.

After it dries out on the skin of the external auditory canal, the cerumen is dispersed and eventually disappears. This process can be disrupted if there is significant flaking (dry eczema) or considerable sebum production (seborrhoea). In these situations, cerumen accumulates and mixes with the skin flakes, dust, etc. The resulting cerumen plug slowly dries out, increases in size from deposits, and blocks the ear canal partly or completely.

During showering or swimming, a cerumen plug can absorb water, swell up, and cause an acute total blockage of the ear canal. The frequent use of cotton buds, earplugs, and so on (physical stimuli) promotes the production of cerumen, pushes the cerumen inwards, and removes the protective keratin layer of the skin, which may trigger otitis externa.

Cerumen is usually not present in the affected ear canal if a patient has acute otitis media, because of the temperature rise – so, in a patient with earache, the presence of cerumen makes acute otitis media unlikely.

PRESENTATION

The patient complains of a full feeling or abnormal noises in the ear, itching, dizziness and loss of hearing, which may occur acutely after showering or swimming. A hard cerumen plug can sometimes cause pain and may occasionally cause a troublesome tickly cough.

EPIDEMIOLOGY

In general practice, the diagnosis is made 32–38 times per 1000 people per year, slightly more often in women, and appears to have been increasing in frequency in recent years. These incidence figures also include relapses.

The diagnosis is made more often as people age. In the group aged 5–14 years there are 20 new cases per 1000 people per year; in the group aged 75 years and above, there are almost four times as many.

HISTORY

The GP asks:

- about symptoms such as a full feeling in the ear, ringing or other noises in the ear, deafness or a tickly cough
- about discharge from the ear, ear pain and itching
- how the symptoms developed (gradual or acute)
- whether the symptoms occurred after showering or swimming
- whether the patient uses cotton buds in the ear, or puts (sharp) objects (e.g. matchsticks) in the ear
- whether there are predisposing factors, such as eczema or dermatitis
- whether the ear drum may be perforated (this will influence treatment).

EXAMINATION

In an area with proper lighting, gently pull the outer ear up and posteriorly, stretching the external auditory canal and making the opening visible. This is sometimes sufficient to see the plug with the naked eye. Otherwise, examination involves otoscopy.

This first focuses on the cerumen and whether there is a blockage. Is this located deep in the canal, or closer to the external auditory meatus? If the cerumen plug does not block the ear completely, the visible part of the ear drum is inspected. Is the ear drum perforated? The wall of the external auditory canal is also inspected. Is otitis externa present? Are there other causes of blockage, such as a foreign body or furuncle?

After the cerumen plug has been removed, the GP can determine whether the patient is (still) suffering from hearing loss, if necessary.

TREATMENT

Hard cerumen plugs that block the distal part of the external auditory canal should preferably be removed mechanically, using a cerumen hook (or loop) for this purpose.

In practice, these plugs are usually removed by means of irrigation, as are the deeper cerumen plugs. The syringe, containing approximately 100 ml of water, must be firmly held in the hand and work smoothly (it must glide easily). It should be fitted with a pointed extension, and be easy to clean.

Warm tap water is used to avoid irritating the auditory canal and the eardrum. The syringe must not contain any air. The ear should be irrigated from various angles, with gentle, brief spurts.

If the syringe has been emptied three times (approximately 100 ml each time) and the plug has not come loose, the GP or nurse should ask the patient to wait 15–30 minutes. Often, the warm water will loosen the plug.

If, after two attempts at removal, there is still no result, the patient is asked to continue treatment at home using oil. This involves the patient putting drops of some type of oil (olive, sunflower, almond, baby or salad oil) in the ear: three drops, twice daily, for a maximum of 3 days. A new attempt to remove the plug after this is nearly always successful.

After the cerumen has been successfully removed, the outer ear should be inspected by means of otoscopy to make sure that all the cerumen has been cleared.

If it is known or suspected that the ear drum is perforated, the wax must be suctioned out after the plug has been soaked with oil – this is likely to require referral to the local ear, nose and throat department (see also Chapter 38).

PREVENTION AND ADDITIONAL INFORMATION

If a cause is present (eczema or dermatitis; use of ear plugs) it should be managed as appropriate. The GP should also explain that cerumen production is a physiologically useful phenomenon, and that the ear canal continually cleans itself. The use of cotton buds or other objects to clean the external auditory canal is not recommended.

Key points

- Ear wax tends to be most troublesome in patients who suffer eczema or seborrhoea.

- In a patient with earache, the presence of cerumen makes acute otitis media unlikely.

- If it is known or suspected that the ear drum is perforated, removal of wax will probably require referral to the local ear, nose and throat department.

- The use of cotton buds or other objects to clean the external auditory canal is not recommended.

Literature
Eekhof JAH, De Bock GH, Le Cessie S, Springer MP. A quasi-randomised controlled trial with water as a quick dispersant for persistent earwax in general practice. *Br J Gen Practice* 2001;**51**(469):635–7.

Eland PF, Van Geldrop WJ, Mokkink HGA. Cerumen en otitis media acuta in de huisartspraktijk [Cerumen and otitis media acuta in general pratice]. *Huisarts Wet* 1995;**38**(7):302–3.

Sharp JF, Wilson JA, Ross L, Barr-Hamilton RM. Ear wax removal: a survey of current practice. *BMJ* 1990;**301**:1251–338.

38

FOREIGN BODY IN THE EAR

DEFINITION

This chapter deals with foreign bodies in the exterior auditory canal that cannot be removed without the help of a device or instrument.

AETIOLOGY/PATHOGENESIS

Classic objects include beads, paper, food, peanuts, and so on, which children may put into every possible body orifice while playing. Cotton buds are occasionally even pushed into the ear, and form a foreign body deep in the ear canal. Broken-off matches and intact needles sometimes end up in the ear in a similar way. Finally, insects are also included here, as they can end up in the ear canal and are not able to crawl or fly out by themselves.

PRESENTATION

Either on purpose or by accident, an object ends up in the ear and cannot be removed. Children sometimes have an earache and ear discharge due to the inflammation that is caused by the object present in the ear canal. Sometimes, the foreign body affects the child's hearing.

EPIDEMIOLOGY

On average, a GP sees one patient a year with this problem.

HISTORY

The history is usually very short: the patient will usually confess that he has put something in his ear. The GP asks:

- about the nature of the object

- how long the object has been in the ear.

In the case of children and the mentally disabled, the history can be less clear, and the foreign body may have been present in the ear for a long time before presentation (see also Chapter 37).

EXAMINATION

Careful inspection of the auditory canal with an otoscope, or indirect lighting with a forehead mirror, is necessary. When there is significant swelling, drops of adrenaline 0.1% or xylometazoline solution 0.1% can be put in the ear. If the examination itself is painful, a few drops of lidocaine solution 1% may be put in the ear canal beforehand.

TREATMENT

The best method involves removing the object by suction. This works only for round objects and with an instrument that provides continuous suction. In most cases, this will require referral to the local ear, nose and throat department. Another method involves removing the foreign body by positioning a hook or loop behind it and pulling it out of the ear canal.

A third method involves irrigating the ear. However, this risks pushing the object further into the ear canal. This method can cause considerable pain particularly if there is not enough room to irrigate around the foreign body, and it is pushed against the eardrum. It is therefore helpful to put a few drops of lidocaine solution 1%, possibly with adrenaline 1%, into the ear canal and to wait a few minutes before beginning irrigation. Make sure that, when irrigating, the water is pointed beside the object, and not straight at it.

It is risky to attempt to remove the foreign body with a pair of tweezers. If this method is chosen, small surgical tweezers with sharp points are recommended. This should only be tried if it is possible to 'grab' the object – tweezers can grab a soggy brown bean, but not a bead.

After removing any foreign body, it is important to inspect the tympanic membrane for signs of damage.

PREVENTION AND ADDITIONAL INFORMATION

When children are at the age when they put things in various body orifices, they should not be allowed to play with beads, marbles, peanuts, etc.

Key points

- In the case of children and the mentally disabled, the history can be unclear, and the foreign body may have been present in the ear for a long time before presentation.

- Foreign bodies may be removed by suction (the best method), with a hook or loop, or by irrigation.

- It is risky to attempt to remove the foreign body with a pair of tweezers.

- After removing any foreign body, it is important to inspect the tympanic membrane for signs of damage.

Literature

Huizing EH, Snow GB (eds). *Leerboek keel-, neus- en oorheelkunde* [*Textbook for throat, nose and ear medicine*]. Houten: Bohn Stafleu Van Loghum, 1993.

Vereecken A, Verheij ThJM. Kleine kwalen in de huisartspraktijk. Het corpus alienum in het oor [Minor ailments in general practice. The corpus alienum in the ear]. *Tijdschr huisartsgeneesk* 1998;**15**:199–202.

39

EAR PAIN DURING AIR TRAVEL

DEFINITION

Ear pain that results from air travel (barotitis media, barotrauma) is due to an acute or chronic traumatic inflammation of the middle ear, a result of an air pressure difference between the outside air and the middle ear.

AETIOLOGY/PATHOGENESIS

Aeroplanes do have a pressurized cabin, but the air pressure maintained during the flight is around 600 mmHg: this is the natural air pressure at an altitude of 2000 m, and is therefore much lower than the pressure on the ground. As a result, relative excess pressure is exerted on the closed middle ear. The anatomy of the eustachian tube enables it to function as a valve. If there is excess pressure in the tympanic cavity, the necessary amount of air is usually let out easily, which restores the pressure balance. During landing, the opposite should occur. However, the pharyngeal part of the eustachian tube, functioning as a valve, has more difficulty in letting air into the middle ear. Therefore, forced movements (swallowing, yawning, moving the jaw, Valsalva manoeuvre) are needed to actively open the eustachian tube.

If the local mucous membrane is swollen, due to infection (e.g. influenza) or an allergy (e.g. hay fever), it is even more difficult for air to flow into the middle ear through the eustachian tube (difficulties may also be encountered with the outflow of air). The resulting relative lower pressure in the middle ear causes the pain. This is why an overly rapid landing or insufficient swallowing and similar manoeuvres during landing can also cause pain even with a eustachian tube that is functioning normally.

Long-term lower pressure in the middle ear causes secondary congestion of blood in the retracted eardrum and the mucous membranes of the middle ear. Haemorrhagic transudate can develop as a result, followed ultimately by traumatic eardrum perforation.

Air pressure changes are made very gradually in commercial air travel, to reduce as much as possible the risk of barotrauma.

PRESENTATION

The patient usually attends immediately after the barotrauma. The history is one of ear pain during a flight; there may also be nausea, tinnitus, loss of hearing or dizziness. The patient may also present for advice for a future flight, wanting to know if there is a chance that this unpleasant (and painful) experience will recur.

EPIDEMIOLOGY

Outside military air travel, there are no reliable data about this problem. Upper respiratory infections are very common, as are hay fever and allergic rhinitis. Because barotrauma is linked with these ailments, it might be expected to occur relatively frequently. In commercial air travel, however, the pressure changes are minimal and gradual. Consequently, the frequency of barotrauma is probably lower than might be anticipated. In military air travel, pilots are exposed to extreme changes in pressure. Of a group of 50,000 US pilots, 8500 (17%) suffered from barotrauma in a high-pressure cabin.

HISTORY

The GP asks:

- about the patient's acute symptoms, such as pain, 'pressure' in the ear, dizziness or difficulties with hearing
- whether one or both ears are affected
- whether the patient had a cold, runny nose, flu, fever or blocked ears prior to the air travel
- whether there was fluid or blood in or from the ear (or ears)
- about the patient's current symptoms
- what the patient did during the flight while the symptoms were present, such as yawning, swallowing, moving the jaw or plugging the nose and breathing out to push air into the eustachian tubes.

EXAMINATION

The GP examines the outer ear to see if blood or fluid is present in the external auditory canal. Otoscopy is used to assess the eardrum. It is important to check for colour, perforation, retraction, blood vessel injection, blood or exudate in the middle ear. Audiometry can be carried out as an additional test, but only for difficulties with hearing that have been present for longer than approximately 2 months.

TREATMENT

If barotrauma has occurred, the treatment is, in principle, expectant. Inflamed ear drums and ear drum perforation almost always heal spontaneously, although this may take weeks. Transudate in the middle ear, with a retracted eardrum, will also usually settle spontaneously in 3–10 weeks. Decongestant nose drops are unhelpful. If problems persist, the patient should be referred to a specialist.

PREVENTION AND ADDITIONAL INFORMATION

Patients with an upper respiratory infection (cold, flu) or allergic rhinitis should preferably not fly. People who fly professionally (pilots, cabin attendants, etc.) are not considered fit to carry out their duties if they are suffering these problems. It has not been demonstrated that decongestant nose drops are able to keep the eustachian tubes open, although they are often used to prevent barotrauma. Systemic treatment of allergic disorders can, however, have a favourable effect on the eustachian tubes. While landing, it is important to swallow, yawn or move the jaw frequently. If this does not help, the Valsalva manoeuvre can be carried out. The patient pinches the nose shut, breathes in deeply through the mouth, presses forcefully, and swallows while pressing. This can be repeated every minute during landing.

Key points

- Ear pain that results from air travel (barotitis media, barotrauma) is due to an acute or chronic traumatic inflammation of the middle ear, as a result of an air pressure difference between the outside air and the middle ear.
- Infection or allergy make it more difficult for the patient to equalize pressures.
- Resolution of barotrauma may take weeks; decongestants are unhelpful.

Literature

Dehart RL (ed). *Fundamentals of aerospace medicine*. Philadelphia: Lea & Febiger, 1985.

Phaff Ch, Van de Beek J, Hendriks JT. *Het onderzoek van oor, gehoor en evenwichtsorgaan* [*Study of the ear, hearing and balance organ*]. Utrecht: Bunge, 1995.

Silman S, Arick D. Efficacy of a modified politzer apparatus in management of eustachian tube dysfunction in adults. *J Am Acad Audiol* 1999;**10**(9): 496–501.

Westerman ST, Fine MB, Gilbert L. Aerotitis: cause, prevention, and treatment. *J Am Ostheopath Assoc* 1990;**90**:926–8.

40

FOREIGN BODY IN THE NOSE

DEFINITION

A wide range of foreign objects can end up in the nose. This chapter covers how these objects can be removed when then they do not fall out spontaneously.

AETIOLOGY/PATHOGENESIS

The classic objects are beads, pieces of paper, small toys, peanuts, and so on, that children sometimes put in a variety of body orifices while playing. The nose is a favourite hiding place. This problem also very occasionally presents in adults.

PRESENTATION

The patient may simply present with an object present in the nose after unsuccessful attempts at removing it. Children and adults may attend with a foul discharge from one nostril and may not mention, or may have forgotten, the foreign body. If a child has put an object in both nostrils, a blocked nose may be the main complaint. Bad breath is also sometimes caused by a foreign body in the nose.

EPIDEMIOLOGY

There are no known epidemiological data, but every GP encounters this from time to time.

HISTORY

This is usually short (unless presenting with a unilateral discharge caused by a forgotten, or unmentioned, foreign body): the patient has put something in the nose and is no longer able to remove it. The GP asks:

- how long the object has been in the nose
- what kind of object it is (e.g. a bean (which could swell up) or a glass bead (relatively neutral)).

The child's parent may suspect a blocked nose due to allergy or the common cold, or fear that there is something remaining in the nose after an object has already been removed.

EXAMINATION

Carefully inspect both nostrils. If necessary, drops of xylometazoline 0.1% can be put in the nose first, if there is much swelling; wait 5 minutes before continuing. Ensure there is proper lighting with the nose speculum on the otoscope (direct rhinoscopy) or with a forehead mirror (indirect).

TREATMENT

Of course, care should be taken to ensure the object is not pushed deeper into the nose. In general, the GP should have a very low threshold for referral to the ear, nose and throat (ENT) department to avoid possible aspiration.

A foreign body always causes the mucous membranes to swell up. Therefore, if attempts at removal are appropriate, put two or three drops of xylometazoline 0.1% in each nostril before beginning.

The foreign body can be removed by suction. A hook device can also be used to remove the object. Be careful if using tweezers, because they can damage the mucous membranes of the nose. Use a pair of small surgical tweezers with sharp points if necessary, and make sure the foreign object is soft or rough enough to be grabbed by the tweezers. However, if a foreign body presents any real difficulty during attempts at removal, it is sensible to refer to an ENT specialist for possible treatment under general anaesthetic.

PREVENTION AND ADDITIONAL INFORMATION

When children are at the age when they put things in various body orifices, they should not be allowed to play with beads, marbles, peanuts, etc.

Key points

- Children and adults may attend with a foul discharge from one nostril and may not mention, or may have forgotten, the foreign body.
- The GP should have a very low threshold for referral to the ENT department to avoid possible aspiration.
- Be careful if using tweezers, because they can damage the mucous membranes of the nose.

Literature

Huizing EH, Snow GB (eds). *Leerboek keel-, neus- en oorheelkunde* [*Textbook for throat, nose and ear medicine*]. Houten: Bohn Stafleu Van Loghum, 1993.

41
NOSEBLEED/EPISTAXIS

DEFINITION

Epistaxis is bleeding from the nasal cavity.

AETIOLOGY/PATHOGENESIS

There are two types of nosebleed: those in which the cause is in the nose itself (local cause), and those due to a disorder elsewhere in the body (systemic cause).

The first group mainly consists of spontaneous bleeding from Little's area on the nasal septum. This area has a network of small blood vessels, originating from branches of the internal and external carotid arteries. Here, the nasal mucous membrane often lies directly on top of the cartilage, without a protective layer of muscle or connective tissue. When damage occurs, such as via infection, dehydration or nose picking, bleeding can easily result. However, because a clear cause cannot always be determined, this is sometimes referred to as an 'idiopathic nosebleed'. Other local causes include a foreign body, trauma and a tumour/polyp in the nose or the paranasal sinuses.

Systemic causes include infectious illnesses, which can lead to a nosebleed as a result of hyperaemia of the nasal mucous membrane. Allergic rhinitis can have a similar effect. The use of some medications, especially warfarin and salicylates, can increase the risk of epistaxis. Alcohol use also influences blood coagulation and creates a higher risk of epistaxis. Hypertension can occasionally cause posterior nosebleeds, especially if arteriosclerotic blood vessels are present, such as in older people. Less frequent systemic causes include bleeding due to thrombocytopenia and other bleeding tendencies.

PRESENTATION

Nosebleeds are often minor, and so medical attention is not always sought. The alarm is raised only if the patient cannot stop the bleeding or if the nosebleed recurs. The GP must be aware that the bleeding can occasionally be very serious, especially in the elderly.

EPIDEMIOLOGY

A GP with an average practice sees approximately 5–7 patients per year with this problem (acute or recurring). In addition, he will provide telephone advice several times on how to stop an acute nosebleed. Nosebleeds are most common in children and the elderly: one study found that 9% of children aged 11–14 years had frequent episodes of epistaxis. In children, the nosebleeds occur almost without exception from Little's area. In the elderly, they tend to originate more posteriorly and can cause significant problems.

HISTORY

If the bleeding has not yet stopped, the GP needs to know what action the patient has already taken. The GP asks:

- what body position the patient has assumed
- whether the patient has blown clots out of the nose
- whether the patient squeezed the nose and, if so, for how long.

Any further history will be aimed at detecting possible causes. The GP asks:

- whether nose picking was the cause, if there is another cause, or if the bleeding started spontaneously
- whether this was the first episode or the nosebleeds are recurring – if the latter, the frequency and severity
- whether the patient is suffering from a cold
- whether the patient has an irritated nose passage due to, for example, an allergy
- whether there is a history of trauma
- whether there is a foreign body in the nose
- whether the patient is on any medication
- whether the patient is hypertensive.

EXAMINATION

In the case of recurrent epistaxis, the nasal septum and nasal cavity
are inspected. The following may be found: a superficial blood vessel,
an erosion, a foreign body or, rarely, a tumour.

If there has been severe loss of blood, the blood pressure and pulse
are checked. In the case of long-term blood loss and frequently
recurring nosebleeds, the haemoglobin level is measured. If
indicated, a clotting screen can be useful, particularly if the patient is
on anticoagulants, or there is a suspicion of thrombocytopenia.

TREATMENT

The following instructions are given for an acute nosebleed (this can
usually take place over the telephone). The patient must sit down
and lean slightly forwards, so that any blood that runs down the
back of the nose and throat cavity can be spat out. The patient should
then blow the nose well to remove any clots. Next, the nostril on the
side of the bleeding should be pinched shut for at least 10 minutes. It
is important to time this by the clock, because there is a tendency to
stop too quickly. If the bleeding is successfully stopped, the nose
must be left alone for 2 days: the patient should not blow or pick the
nose.

In serious cases, the nose can be packed with gauze, which can be
coated with Vaseline to prevent additional damage. The gauze should
be packed horizontally; insert this in the nose, layer by layer, moving
from the base to up inside the nose. Note: the packing is often started
in too cranial a direction. The gauze can be removed after 2 days.
Many GPs would tend to refer patients to casualty for packing.

If the bleeding originated from the posterior part of the nose, this
may well continue, even after pinching the nose shut and packing
the nose with gauze. Such patients require urgent referral to an ear,
nose and throat specialist.

Any underlying systemic cause suspected (hypertension,
anticoagulants, etc.), should be dealt with as appropriate.

In the case of recurrent nosebleeds, there is some evidence that
antibiotic cream (chlorhexidine/neomycin) reduces episodes
compared with no treatment. Some people find the smell and taste of

these creams unpleasant. Cautery is also often used; it is painful, despite the use of local anaesthesia.

PREVENTION AND ADDITIONAL INFORMATION

Preventing nosebleeds is difficult. It is always helpful to advise the patient not to pick his nose; the use of decongestant nose drops during a cold can be useful for those with a tendency towards nosebleeds. However, be sure to warn the patient about the deleterious effect of chronic use of this type of nose drops.

Many patients do not use the correct technique to stop a nosebleed: they lean their head back, put cotton wool in the nose, press a cold key to the neck without pinching the nose shut, and so on. Ask about this, give other instructions, and clearly explain how to stop the bleeding.

Key points

- There are two types of nosebleed: those in which the cause is in the nose itself (local cause), and those due to a disorder elsewhere in the body (systemic cause).

- Epistaxis can occasionally be very serious, especially in the elderly.

- In recurrent nosebleeds, antibiotic cream (chlorhexidine/neomycin) may reduce the number of episodes. Cautery is an alternative.

- Many patients do not use the correct technique to stop a nosebleed.

Literature
Alvi A, Joyner-Triplett N. Acute epistaxis. How to spot the source and stop the flow. *Postgrad Med* 1996;**99**(5):83–90.

Burton MJ, Doree CJ. Interventions for recurrent idiopathic epistaxis (nosebleeds) in children. *Cochrane Database Syst Rev* 2004;**1**:CD004461.

Huizing EH, Snow GB (eds). *Leerboek keel-, neus- en oorheelkunde* [*Textbook for throat, nose and ear medicine*]. Houten: Bohn Stafleu Van Loghum, 1993.

Josephson GD, Godley FA, Stierna P. Practical management of epistaxis. *Med Clin North Am* 1991;**75**(6):1311–20.

McGarry G. Recurrent idiopathic epistaxis (nosebleeds). *Clin Evid* 2002;**7**:349–51.

McGarry G Nosebleeds in children. *Clin Evid* 2003;**10**:437–40.

Tan LK, Calhoun KH. Epistaxis. *Med Clin North Am* 1999;**83**(1):43–56.

42

COLDS IN YOUNG CHILDREN/ CORYZA

DEFINITION

The common cold (coryza) in a child results in clear or purulent nasal discharge, possibly accompanied by a blocked nose or sneezing. Other symptoms may also be present, such as fever, coughing, sore throat and general malaise.

AETIOLOGY/PATHOGENESIS

The common cold is caused by a variety of viruses, the rhinovirus being by far the most common. Other viruses that can be implicated include: adenovirus, (para)influenza virus, enterovirus, echovirus, respiratory syncytial virus (RSV) and coxsackievirus. RSV can also cause bronchiolitis or pneumonia in young children; in older children, this is limited to an upper respiratory infection. Generally, the common cold disappears by itself in a few days to several weeks. In exceptional cases, it can cause complications, such as otitis media, acute sinusitis or a lower respiratory infection. RSV in particular has a higher risk of causing serious problems in infants and children with risk factors (e.g. an immune disorder).

The virus particles are transmitted mainly by air and physical contact: coughing and touching. Children who go to a day nursery, a playgroup or school, and their younger siblings at home run the risk of being infected.

Chronic adenoidal hypertrophy should be considered in children who appear to suffer from a cold for months at a time. A foreign body can also cause a blocked nose on one side (see Chapter 40).

PRESENTATION

The reasons for visiting the GP are varied. It is important to understand the reason for consulting, so that management can be tailored accordingly. In many cases, the parents feel that their child has had a cold for longer, or is suffering colds more frequently, than they would expect. The child may suffer from sneezing, a blocked nose or coughing, which result in sleep or eating problems. An infant will often cry more and have more difficulty with feeding than normal, and be irritable. The parent does not usually consult the GP just for a runny nose, but rather because the child is listless and complains of a headache or stomach ache, for example. Other causes then need to be considered.

EPIDEMIOLOGY

Colds are most common in childhood. A young child will suffer a cold, on average, six times a year. By encountering these infections, the child is able to gradually build up its immunity. The incidence rises sharply in the autumn and winter; however, most patients do not visit their GP.

HISTORY

The GP asks (particularly in recurrent or persistent problems):

- about the duration of the symptoms
- about other symptoms, such as fever, cough, headache or malaise
- about the amount of nasal discharge (the colour of the discharge does not indicate anything about the possible cause)
- about the child's appetite, growth and development (if relevant)
- about a possible relationship with other factors, such as environmental factors or illness in the surrounding environment
- whether anyone smokes around the child – the harmful effect of smoking should be strongly emphasized
- about earache (pulling at the ear) or a sore throat
- about whether the child breathes with its mouth open or snores during the night, even if the child does not have a cold

- whether the parent has already taken action or given the child something for the cold.

EXAMINATION

The examination focuses mainly on ruling out complications or alternative diagnoses, such as otitis media, bronchitis or tonsillitis. Colds themselves do not require any physical examination. The GP considers how the child looks: healthy or sick. In a young child, the lungs are examined first. This provides important information and is the least threatening. Usually, no abnormalities are found. Any wheezing is noted; this information may be useful at a later date if asthma is suspected. If the child complains of a stomach ache, the abdomen should be examined for the sake of completeness. When inspecting the ears, the GP should examine the eardrums for any dullness or redness, which might indicate serous or infective otitis media. Palpable lymph glands in the neck are normal in young children. Finally, the throat is inspected.

Examining the nose is only useful if a foreign body is suspected, or if the symptoms have persisted for a long time (more than 6 weeks). The patient should blow the nose before inspection; in a young child, the nose may be cleaned out using suction. Placing a mirror under the nose will enable the GP to see if the patient is breathing through both nostrils (condensation will form). General inspection of the nose is possible by pushing upwards on the tip of the nose and using a small light. A nasal speculum may be used in older children.

TREATMENT

Based on the history, examination and previous history, the GP can assess whether there is any evidence of, or risk of, complications. In the uncomplicated situation, the treatment focuses on responding to parents' concerns and promoting their ability to manage the situation (self-help measures, such as steaming in the bathroom, and over-the-counter medication). Symptomatic treatment may also be given, or advised: saline nose drops in babies, nasal decongestants for short-term use, or painkillers if necessary. The preference is not to give the child anything for the cough. Antibiotics are never necessary for a simple cold. If there is a high chance of complications (e.g. an otitis-prone child) a follow-up consultation may be offered, particularly if the child becomes symptomatic.

PREVENTION AND ADDITIONAL INFORMATION

It is important to explain that the cold will go away by itself and that the recurrent pattern is normal. An explanation about the build up of immunity is also helpful. If possible and appropriate, the GP can explain that consultation for an uncomplicated cold is not actually necessary. The GP can also provide information about how to deal with such infections: keeping the child at home or in bed is not warranted. It is not possible to prevent colds. Some recommendations that can be given, however, include washing the hands more frequently, and touching the nose and face less. There is no reason for the child's activities to be limited: lots of exercise, fresh air and healthy food improve resistance to infections.

Key points

- A young child will suffer a cold, on average, six times a year.
- Chronic adenoidal hypertrophy should be considered in children who appear to suffer from a cold for months at a time. A foreign body can also cause a blocked nose on one side.
- The examination focuses mainly on ruling out complications or alternative diagnoses, such as otitis media, bronchitis or tonsillitis.
- Palpable lymph glands in the neck are normal in young children.

Literature

Heikkinen T, Jarvinen A. The common cold. *Lancet* 2003;**361**(9351):51–9.

Jacobs VEJ, Numans ME. Vitamine C bij verkoudheid: ratio of religie? [Vitamin C for colds: reason or religion?]. *Huisarts Wet* 1998;**41**:524–7.

Jones M. Childhood coughs and colds. *J Fam Health Care* 2002;**12**:39–41.

Semmekrot BA. Hoestmedicatie bij kinderen [Cough medication in children]. *Geneesmiddelenbulletin* 2000;**34**:127–34.

Turner RB. Epidemiology, pathogenesis, and treatment of the common cold. *Ann Allergy Asthma Immunol* 1997;**78**(6):531–9.

Zaat JOM, Van der Most K. Over snotteren, snuiten, stomen en druppelen [About sniffling, blowing the nose, steaming and giving drops]. *Huisarts Wet* 1997;**40**:471–80.

43

FOREIGN BODY IN THE EYE

DEFINITION

A foreign body in the eye, for the purposes of this chapter, includes an object or an irritating substance in the conjunctival sac or on the cornea, or, in rare cases, in the eyeball itself.

AETIOLOGY/PATHOGENESIS

A foreign body in the eye usually occurs when working with materials for work or a hobby – particularly in the metal industry (steel splinters and iron filings), construction (splinters, sawdust) and when working with chemicals. Dust, dirt and sand can end up in the eyes due to strong wind, sports and play.

PRESENTATION

Patients with this problem may experience pain, but more often a sensation of irritation or photophobia, accompanied by a watering, red eye. They may recall a feeling of something hitting their eye. If the corneal epithelium is damaged by a finger or twig, pain is the prominent symptom. In contrast, a perforation is often not very painful.

EPIDEMIOLOGY

Incidence figures vary considerably. One large study gave an incidence of 3.9 per 1000 patients per year. Approximately 3.5% of people with an ocular foreign body are referred to an ophthalmologist by their GP.

HISTORY

The GP asks:

- about the nature of the foreign body
- how it ended up in the eye
- how long ago it happened
- whether the patient is suffering from irritation or a burning sensation in the eye
- whether there is a change in the patient's eyesight.

The aim is to estimate the risk of corneal damage or perforation.

EXAMINATION

In addition to inspecting the eye, it is important that vision is checked, as almost all intraocular lesions are accompanied by a loss of visual acuity. If the patient's vision is normal, serious damage to the cornea or the lens is less likely.

The eye is inspected using a strong light source directed diagonally at the eye. If blepharospasm makes examination difficult, a local anaesthetic can be used.

In the case of chemical burns, the eye should first be rinsed thoroughly. Be sure to remember the area under the eyelids. The eye is then inspected and checked for signs of possible perforation: asymmetrical or otherwise abnormal pupils, iris prolapse, lens cloudiness or subconjunctival bleeding. Remember that a perforation may not be visible to the naked eye. To locate the foreign body, first the bottom and then the top eyelids are turned inside out: close the eye, place a cotton bud against the eyelid, grab the eyelid from under the bud and pull the hairs upwards. Finally, the cornea is meticulously inspected and checked for possible damage. If in doubt, use blue light after applying fluorescein.

TREATMENT

If no foreign body is found and there are no other abnormalities, it is appropriate to wait and see; the symptoms will usually resolve after a good night's sleep.

A foreign body under the eyelid which scratches the cornea during blinking can be removed with a moist cotton bud after everting the eyelid. Local anaesthetic drops may be applied before starting.

A foreign body in the cornea must be removed to prevent infection. A damp cotton bud can be used after the application of local anaesthetic. If this does not work, the tip of a needle may be used – cautiously, and with the tip as near horizontal as possible to avoid the risk of perforation.

If the foreign body cannot be removed easily, the patient should be referred to an ophthalmologist.

If the cornea has been damaged, an antibiotic eye ointment is applied – a single application is usually sufficient. The patient must return after 24 hours for reassessment. The epithelium that quickly grows over the damaged area protects the cornea against infection. This usually heals in approximately 24 hours. Eye pads do not seem to accelerate the healing.

Patients with ongoing symptoms need regular reassessment and may well require referral.

In the case of thermal or chemical injuries, the eye should be irrigated for a long time with running tap water or an eye bath. Any particles that have stuck to the eye must be removed. If the cornea is clear and there are no signs of conjunctival necrosis, an antibacterial ointment is applied and follow-up advised as above. Patients with superficial trauma and superficial chemical burns without conjunctival redness only need to return for a follow-up consultation if, despite proper treatment, the symptoms have not subsided after 3 days.

Infection of a corneal abrasion causes a white necrotic area around the lesion and, possibly, a greyish-white exudate. Such infections can lead to ulceration, panophthalmitis and, finally, the loss of the eye. So, if infection is a possibility, referral to an ophthalmologist is absolutely vital.

The patient should be referred if there is a serious injury due to perforation, if damage to the cornea has not healed after 3 days, if a chemical burn is accompanied by cloudiness of the cornea, and if an infection of a corneal erosion is suspected.

PREVENTION AND ADDITIONAL INFORMATION

An accurate history will reveal how the problem occurred. On this basis, the GP may be able to suggest how future incidents can be prevented. Wearing safety glasses is one of the most important preventive measures if the injury occurred during work or hobby activities.

Key points

- If the patient's vision is normal, serious damage to the cornea or the lens is less likely.

- If no foreign body is found and there are no other abnormalities, it is appropriate to wait and see.

- A foreign body in the cornea must be removed to prevent infection. If it cannot be removed easily, the patient should be referred to an ophthalmologist.

- The patient should be referred if there is a serious injury due to perforation, if damage to the cornea has not healed after 3 days, if a chemical burn is accompanied by cloudiness of the cornea, and if an infection of a corneal erosion is suspected.

Literature

Baggen J. *Oogheelkunde in de huisartspraktijk* [*Ophthalmology in general practice*]. Dissertation. Amsterdam: Thesis Publishers, 1990.

Blom GH, Cleveringa JP, Louisse AC, De Bruin W, Gooskens P, Wiersma TJ. NHG-standaard: het rode oog [NHG standard: the red eye]. *Huisarts Wet* 1996;**39**:225–38.

Hubert MFG. Efficacy of eyepad in corneal healing after corneal foreign body removal. *Lancet* 1991;**337**:643.

Mester V, Kuhn F. Intraocular foreign bodies. *Ophthalmol Clin North Am* 2002;**15**(2):235–42.

Owens JK, Scibilia J, Hezoucky N. Corneal foreign bodies – first aid, treatment, and outcomes. Skills review for an occupational health setting. *AAOHN J* 2001;**49**(5):226–30.

Shields SR. Managing eye disease in primary care. Part 2. How to recognize and treat common eye problems. *Postgrad Med* 2000;**108**(5):83–6, 91–6.

Van de Beek G, Dekkers NWHM, Schiffelers H. *Oogheelkunde* [*Ophthalmology*]. Lege artis. Utrecht: Bunge, 1991.

44

CONJUNCTIVITIS

DEFINITION

Conjunctivitis is a painless inflammation of the conjunctiva of one or both eyes, characterized by redness of the white part of the eye and usually accompanied by burning, a foreign-body sensation, or itching. There is a discharge with a watery to purulent consistency, and the vision is not affected. Conjunctivitis usually settles spontaneously within 1–2 weeks, and complications are rare.

AETIOLOGY/PATHOGENESIS

The conjunctiva is the mucous membrane that lines the inside of the eyelids and which continues via the fornix (turning fold), onto the eyeball to the transition to the cornea, the corneal limbus. In 70% of cases, conjunctivitis is infectious and usually viral. In the remaining 30%, the inflammation is caused by allergy or a tear-duct disorder.

Bacterial conjunctivitis in adults is caused primarily by staphylococci (70%). In younger people, *Haemophilus influenzae* (21%) and streptococci (16%) are causes, but *Staphylococcus* remains responsible for 35% of the infections. In newborns, *Neisseria gonorrhoea* and *Chlamydia* can cause (kerato)conjunctivitis, but both are uncommon. In infants with persistent or recurring eye infections, the GP should consider the possibility of an improperly functioning nasolacrimal duct (see Chapter 48).

Viral conjunctivitis is usually caused by adenoviruses. There are two main types: pharyngoconjunctival fever with pharyngitis, enlarged preauricular glands, and conjunctivitis; and keratoconjunctivitis epidemica, which has the same characteristics, and in which subepithelial cornea infiltrates can develop, with a risk of visual damage. In adenovirus infections, the plica and caruncule are usually swollen and hyperaemic quite early on, and in the fornix the eyelid shows glassy sago-like granular follicles due to local lymphocyte accumulation. Conjunctivitis due to the herpes simplex virus (HSV) is notorious; this may be accompanied by vesicular blepharitis on the margins of the eyelids. Keratoconjunctivitis is frequently seen in recurring infections, with dendritic ulcers as possible complications, which can lead to visual impairment if not treated properly. Enteroviruses and cold viruses can cause a conjunctivitis with purulent discharge, which is difficult to distinguish from a bacterial infection. More uncommon viral causes of (kerato)conjunctivitis are mumps, measles, influenza and herpes-zoster.

In allergic conjunctivitis, a distinction is made between atopic conjunctivitis and conjunctivitis due to a contact allergy. Atopic conjunctivitis is usually seasonal, and is accompanied by very itchy eyes, excessive watering and nasal symptoms, with photophobia and chemosis in extreme cases. Most cases involve an atopic constitution with oversensitivity to pollen, allergens of an animal nature or food ingredients. Conjunctivitis due to a contact allergy is based on a sensitization to substances that are placed directly in the eye, such as eye drops, cosmetics and contact-lens solution; the accompanying redness is most prominent in the fornices. Eczematous changes in the skin around the eye can also develop.

Conjunctivitis sicca is caused by qualitative and quantitative changes in tears. This disorder occurs almost exclusively in older patients, or as part of the so-called 'sicca syndrome' in Sjögren's syndrome, Besnier–Boeck disease or rheumatoid arthritis. The patient complains of dry, burning eyes with mild conjunctival redness; some keratitis may also be present.

An exceptional form of conjunctivitis can result from blepharitis (see also Chapter 45). In this case, there is usually seborrhoeic dermatitis, with a chronic staphylococcal infection of the margins of the eyelids; the conjunctivitis is probably caused by bacterial endotoxins. If blisters are present on the margins of the eyelids, HSV conjunctivitis must be considered.

PRESENTATION

Patients present with symptoms of burning, red eyes, and often the feeling of a foreign body. They may also complain about an unpleasant discharge and eyelids that are 'glued' shut in the morning. Blurred vision may be mentioned, but this disappears after blinking the eyes repeatedly or removing the discharge.

EPIDEMIOLOGY

GPs see conjunctivitis at a rate of about 6–8 per 1000 consultations. This means the average GP will see one or two cases a week. It occurs in all age categories and is not gender related. However, the aetiology, and therefore also the treatment, are age-related.

If it occurs in newborns, the GP must consider an infection due to *N. gonorrhoeae* or *Chlamydia*, and in infants a tear-duct dysfunction. Children generally suffer from viral conjunctivitis as a component of an adenovirus infection with lymphadenopathy. In older children and young adults, allergic conjunctivitis occurs more frequently, due to hay fever. In the elderly, tear-production disorders often play a role in the aetiology.

HISTORY

The GP asks about 'alarm' symptoms, which might indicate a problem more serious than conjunctivitis:

- pain should be distinguished from itching and a foreign body sensation – true eye pain points to an alternative diagnosis
- photophobia is usually accompanied by eye pain and indicates an irritated iris or cornea
- decreased vision is a sign of media cloudiness or problems at the level of the retina or optic nerve.

Next, depending on the symptoms presented, the GP may ask about the following:

- the duration and progression of the symptoms
- whether one or both eyes are affected
- the nature and colour of any discharge or excessive watering
- a foreign-body sensation
- itching or symptoms that are part of an atopic syndrome, such as sneezing, runny nose, shortness of breath, wheezing or eczema
- the use of contact lenses
- any preceding trauma

- the presence of chronic illnesses
- medication use; use of eye drops, cosmetics and contact-lens solution.

EXAMINATION

The GP examines the following areas of the affected eye: eyelids, discharge, cornea, extent of redness and the anterior chamber of the eye. The extent of the examination will reflect the degree of certainty, or otherwise, derived from the history

The eyelids may be red and/or swollen. Look for vesicles or pustules, foreign bodies on the inside of the eyelids, follicles, whether the eyelids are positioned correctly (ectropion or entropion) and whether the eyelids can be closed normally.

Purulent discharge indicates probable bacterial infection. If serous discharge is present, a viral infection is likely. Allergic and irritative conjunctivitis are accompanied by watery exudate and usually excessive watering (epiphora). The lack of discharge or watering points to tear-gland disorders as a part of a sicca syndrome.

Redness can indicate inflammation or bleeding, and vary from superficial to deep, pericorneal or peripheral (conjunctival) redness. The superficial redness of the eye in conjunctivitis occurs due to hyperaemia of the superficial subconjunctival blood vessels. The (brick red) colour is most prominent in the fornix and decreases in intensity towards the cornea. Superficial redness must be distinguished from deep redness, which has more of a purple colour. In the case of inflammation of the iris, the ciliary body, the sclera or the cornea, deep redness occurs in a more central or pericorneal position – these features do not suggest conjunctivitis.

The cornea is inspected with illumination, allowing the GP to examine the clarity and shininess of the cornea, looking for erosions and foreign bodies. Epithelial defects can be revealed with the use of fluorescein and blue light.

The anterior chamber of the eye is inspected for the presence of pus (hypopyon) and blood (hyphaema). The colour of the iris, and the size, light reaction and the left–right differences of the pupils are also assessed.

If the red eye is accompanied by alarm symptoms (see above) additional tests are carried out to differentiate further or rule out disorders of the deeper structures of the eye. Discussion of this is beyond the scope of this chapter and is likely to involve specialist referral.

TREATMENT

The treatment depends on the type of conjunctivitis. In general, contact lenses should not be worn, at least until the problem has resolved. If there is considerable discharge, the eye can be cleaned with tap water.

Bacterial conjunctivitis usually clears up without treatment within a week. If the symptoms are troublesome or if a great deal of suppurating discharge is present, the use of antibiotic eye drops (e.g. chloramphenicol 0.5% or fusidic acid 1% eye drops) is advised.

In the case of viral conjunctivitis, the patient should wait for the symptoms to clear up spontaneously; symptoms may persist for 2 weeks. Referral to an ophthalmologist is indicated for keratoconjunctivitis with corneal infiltrate. Herpes-simplex conjunctivitis is treated with aciclovir eye ointment five times daily, until a week after the symptoms have disappeared. A follow-up consultation every 3 days is desirable to assess the spread of the infection to the cornea, using fluorescein. In the case of keratitis, referral to an ophthalmologist is indicated.

Allergic conjunctivitis caused by atopia is treated with sodium cromoglycate, one to two drops, four times daily or, if rapid results are desired, with an antihistamine, such as levocabastine, one drop, two to four times daily. For severe symptoms, prednisolone 0.5% eye drops can be prescribed for several days, one drop three times daily, with a follow-up consultation after 3 days.

Conjunctivitis symptoms caused by a contact allergy can be reduced with cromoglycate eyedrops (one or two drops 4–6 times daily) or antihistamine eyedrops (one drop 2–4 times daily).

For conjunctivitis sicca, a trial of treatment is given with hypromellose drops hourly. If the results are not satisfactory and/or frequent use is a problem, an artificial-tear gel can be tried. Insufficient improvement or an increase in symptoms despite local treatment justifies referral to the ophthalmologist.

Conjunctivitis in the case of blepharitis is treated by cleaning the margins of the eyelids twice daily with diluted baby shampoo, and using fusidic acid to the lids, avoiding contact with the eyes, two to four times daily for a week to eliminate any staphylococcal reservoirs (see also Chapter 45).

If hyperacute conjunctivitis occurs in an infant less than 10 days old, infection with *N. gonorrhoeae* is likely. This requires an emergency referral to the ophthalmologist for rapid parenteral and local treatment with antibiotics, to prevent corneal perforation. *Chlamydia* should also be considered in this situation.

In the case of chronic conjunctivitis (an infection present for longer than 2 weeks, treatment not effective, doubt about the cause), the patient should be referred to an ophthalmologist.

PREVENTION AND ADDITIONAL INFORMATION

Infectious conjunctivitis is contagious; the shared use of flannels, handkerchiefs/tissues, towels, etc. should be avoided. Conjunctivitis due to a contact allergy can generally be prevented by using, for example, hypoallergenic contact-lens solution and/or cosmetics. The patient should be advised to return for a follow-up consultation if the symptoms are not any better after 3 days despite appropriate treatment. If, in the meantime, pain and/or photophobia increase or the visual acuity decreases, the patient should immediately contact the GP.

Key points

- In conjunctivitis, the vision is not significantly affected.
- In newborns, *N. gonorrhoea* and *Chlamydia* can cause (kerato) conjunctivitis.
- In infants with persistent or recurring eye infections, the GP should consider the possibility of an improperly functioning nasolacrimal duct.
- If blisters are present on the margins of the eyelids, HSV conjunctivitis must be considered.
- True eye pain, photophobia and/or decreased vision point to an alternative diagnosis.
- Purulent discharge indicates probable bacterial infection. If serous discharge is present, a viral infection is likely. Allergic and irritative conjunctivitis are accompanied by watery exudate and, usually, excessive watering (epiphora).
- In inflammation of the iris, the ciliary body, the sclera or the cornea, deep redness occurs in a more central or pericorneal position – these features do not suggest conjunctivitis.
- In the case of chronic conjunctivitis (an infection present for longer than 2 weeks, treatment not effective, doubt about the cause), the patient should be referred to an ophthalmologist.

Literature

Bertolini J, Pelucio M. The red eye. *Emerg Med Clin North Am* 1995;**13**(3): 561–79.

Brodovsky SC, Snibson GR. Corneal and conjunctival infections. *Curr Opin Ophthalmol* 1997;**8**(4):2–7.

Coote MA. Sticky eye, tricky diagnosis. *Aust Fam Physician* 2002;**31**(3):225–31.

Friedlaender MH. A review of the causes and treatment of bacterial and allergic conjunctivitis. *Clin Ther* 1995;**17**(5):800–10.

Polak BCP. Antimicrobiële middelen bij ooginfecties [Antimicrobial remedies for eye infections]. *Ned Tijdschr Geneesk* 1988;**132**:1731–4.

Redactioneel. Nieuwe geneesmiddelen: levocabastine [New medicines: levocabastine]. *Geneesmiddelenbulletin* 1992;**26**:13.

Syed NA, Hyndiuk RA. Infectious conjunctivitis. *Infect Dis Clin North Am* 1992;**6**(4):789–805.

Vafidis G. When is red eye not just conjunctivitis? *Practitioner* 2002; **246**(1636):469–71, 474–5, 478–81.

Weber CM, Eichenbaum JW. Acute red eye. Differentiating viral conjunctivitis from other, less common causes. *Postgrad Med* 1997;**101**(5):185–6.

45

BLEPHARITIS

DEFINITION

Blepharitis is an inflammation, usually chronic, of the eyelid margins
of both eyes.

AETIOLOGY/PATHOGENESIS

Two factors contribute to the development of blepharitis. The first
is pre-existing skin disorders: seborrhoeic eczema is present in
many cases, and rosacea, atopic eczema and psoriasis sometimes
have a role. The second involves infectious processes – in most
cases, a bacterial infection. The cause is often a *Staphylococcus*,
in particular *Staphylococcus aureus*, followed by *Staphylococcus
epidermidis*. The infection occurs in the follicles of the eyelashes
and the accompanying sebaceous and sweat glands. A viral
infection (e.g. herpes simplex), a fungal infection (e.g. *Candida*) or
a parasite infestation (e.g. the mite *Demodex folliculorum*) may
sometimes be present.

A combination of seborrhoeic and infectious blepharitis is often seen.
Blepharitis is always characterized by flaky skin between the
eyelashes, which is greasy and crusts over if seborrhoea is present.
This helps to create and maintain the inflammation. In infectious
blepharitis, the inflammation is more severe and is also accompanied
by small ulcers and crusts.

Complications arise mainly in the infectious form of blepharitis.
Bacterial toxins can cause mild conjunctivitis and even keratitis. The
eyelashes can fall out or become malpositioned, which can in turn
lead to corneal damage. Styes and chalazions occur more frequently
if infectious blepharitis is present.

Blepharitis is characterized by chronicity and can be an extraordinarily
stubborn problem.

PRESENTATION

The patient attends with eyelid margins that are irritated, burning or painful, and often complains about the cosmetic effect (red-ringed eyes).

EPIDEMIOLOGY

The GP diagnoses two to three new cases per 1000 patients per year. The disorder is present in people of all ages, and the frequency is about the same in both men and women.

HISTORY

The GP asks:

- about the development and duration of the symptoms
- about the presence of itching, burning, redness, excessive watering and photophobia.

Often, the patient has had symptoms for years, the most prominent being itching, burning, a sensation of grit in the eyes, pain and redness of the eyelid margins. The symptoms are most prominent in the morning upon waking. Once in a while, excessive watering or photophobia may be present.

EXAMINATION

The eyelid margins are red and slightly swollen. Small flakes (dry or greasy) can be seen between the eyelashes. The lashes are crusted together to a certain extent in the morning. It may be necessary to remove flakes and crusts to check for ulcers on the eyelid margin. It may also be apparent that eyelashes have fallen out or grow in a misdirected way. Pay particular attention to eyelashes pointing inwards, as these can irritate the cornea. Check whether a chalazion or stye is present (see Chapters 46 and 47). Watch out for signs of conjunctivitis or keratitis. Particularly on the lower third of the cornea, pinpoint lesions (infiltrates or small ulcers) may be visible. Superficial corneal defects can be best detected with the use of fluorescein. Finally, the forehead, eyebrows, scalp and face should be inspected for signs of seborrhoeic eczema or any other relevant skin disorder.

If there are clear signs of infection (prominent inflammation or ulcers) a swab of the eyelid margin for culture and sensitivity can be considered, but this is rarely necessary.

TREATMENT

The GP should always begin by instructing the patient to clean the eyelid margins. A cotton bud or mascara brush is dipped in baby shampoo diluted with warm water (1:1), and carefully used to wash away all flakes and crusts while the eyelids are shut. The eyelids are then rinsed with lukewarm water. This must be done every morning, and possibly also before going to bed. Artificial tears can offer relief if the patient complains of burning. If bathing alone does not solve the problem, or there are clear signs of infection (especially in the case of ulcers), an antibiotic ointment such as fusidic acid should be applied to the eyelid margins at night, and possibly also in the morning. This treatment may be necessary for several months. If seborrhoeic eczema is found, the recommended treatment is hydrocortisone cream 1%. Referral to an ophthalmologist is indicated in resistant cases.

PREVENTION AND ADDITIONAL INFORMATION

For a mild case of blepharitis, daily washing can prevent secondary infections. Also, the patient must avoid touching the eyelids as much as possible to avoid the risk of contamination with staphylococci. It is a good idea to point out the recurring nature of this ailment. Patients should avoid cosmetics, smoke and dust as much as possible.

Key points

- Two factors contribute to the development of blepharitis: pre-existing skin disorders, such as seborrhoeic eczema, and infectious processes.

- Blepharitis is characterized by chronicity and can be an extraordinarily stubborn problem.

- Treatment involves instruction about eyelid bathing; antibiotic ointment may be necessary.

Literature

Carter SR. Eyelid disorders: diagnosis and management. *Am Fam Physician* 1998;**57**:2695–702.

McCulley JP, Shine WE. Changing concepts in the diagnosis and management of blepharitis. *Cornea* 2000;**19**(5):650–8.

McCulley JP, Shine WE. Eyelid disorders: the meibomian gland, blepharitis, and contact lenses. *Eye Contact Lens* 2003;**29**(1 Suppl):S93–5.

Smith RE, Flowers CW Jr. Chronic blepharitis: a review. *CLAO J* 1995;**21**(3): 200–7.

46

CHALAZION/MEIBOMIAN CYST

DEFINITION

A chalazion is a well-defined small swelling on the upper or lower eyelid caused by a chronic inflammation of the meibomian gland.

AETIOLOGY/PATHOGENESIS

The meibomian glands are found in the dense connective tissue in the middle of the eyelid. The duct of a meibomian gland can become blocked, so secretions accumulate; these secretions are composed primarily of lipids. This creates a sterile inflammation reaction in the form of a granuloma. The cause is usually unknown, but the duct can sometimes become blocked due to blepharitis, rosacea or vitamin A deficiency (in developing countries).

Several chalazia may be present at the same time. Rarely, a large chalazion can lead to astigmatism due to pressure on the cornea, which results in blurred vision. Also, the visual field may be limited by an eyelid with a large chalazion.

Secondary infection is possible, and a chalazion can occasionally perforate, usually on the inside of the eyelid. If this happens, jelly-like papillae may be present for quite a while (chalazion luxurians). Small chalazia may disappear spontaneously.

PRESENTATION

The patient attends with a painless lump in an eyelid, which can cause worry or visual problems. The patient may also find the swelling cosmetically unattractive.

EPIDEMIOLOGY

A GP sees about one new chalazion per 1000 patients per year. Most do not resolve spontaneously. After excision, there is a reasonable chance that a new chalazion will develop.

HISTORY

The GP asks:

- how long the swelling has been present in the eyelid
- if it has grown in size
- whether it hurts
- if it affects the vision.

EXAMINATION

During the examination, a swelling is visible in the upper or lower eyelid slightly removed from the margin. The diameter of the lump can vary from several millimetres to a maximum of about 1 cm. The lump can be easily palpated, feels firm and the skin covering it can be moved easily. If the eyelid is everted, a bump can be seen, which is velvety red at an early stage and later bluish-grey.

A chalazion is often confused with a stye: a small abscess of a sweat or sebaceous gland on the skin side of the eyelid. A stye characteristically causes pain, redness on the skin side of the eyelid, a lump that is located more on the eyelid margin, and the development of a pus head in the skin. A chalazion should also be distinguished from a basal cell carcinoma: this can also cause a well-delineated lump, but is located in the skin of the eyelid.

If an apparent chalazion recurs in the same spot, supplementary histological tests are indicated to rule out a sebaceous gland carcinoma or a malignant tumour of the meibomian gland or its duct.

TREATMENT

The consensus is that most chalazia should be surgically removed. For small chalazia that do not cause symptoms, a 'wait and see' treatment is reasonable, in view of their harmless nature and the possibility of spontaneous regression. Carefully massaging the area several times a day and also applying hot compresses and/or taking a hot shower can speed up this process. Excision is indicated if there are cosmetic worries, visual problems or secondary infections. Surgical removal is usually performed by an ophthalmologist. This operation may also be carried out by a GP with the proper skills and correct tools.

In the surgical removal of a chalazion, the eyelid is everted and the tissue around the chalazion is infiltrated with lidocaine. The chalazion is fixed in a chalazion clamp and an incision with a small knife is made in the jelly-like mass, perpendicular to the eyelid margin. The chalazion is then carefully curetted with a sharp scoop. The incision does not need to be sutured. The patient is given a piece of gauze to hold on the eyelid for a while, along with a prescription for antibiotic ointment, for 5–7 days.

A review of the literature reveals that a corticosteroid injection in the chalazion is just as effective as surgery. The GP can easily perform this procedure. First, administer local anaesthesia. Then evert the eyelid and inject a small amount (0.1–0.2 ml) of local steroid. Repeated injections are not necessary.

PREVENTION AND ADDITIONAL INFORMATION

There are no known preventive measures. When the GP explains the problem to the patient, emphasis should be placed on the harmless nature of the chalazion. If, in the future, the patient finds another eyelid swelling, the GP should again be consulted to rule out the remote possibility of any malignant causes.

Key points

- A chalazion is often confused with a stye: the latter characteristically causes pain, redness on the skin side of the eyelid, a lump that is located more on the eyelid margin, and has a head.

- Small chalazia may disappear spontaneously.

- A corticosteroid injection into the chalazion is just as effective as surgery.

- If an apparent chalazion recurs in the same spot, histological tests are necessary to rule out rare abnormalities such as a sebaceous gland carcinoma or a malignant tumour of the meibomian gland or its duct.

Literature

Baijens ATJM, Giesen PHJ. Behandeling van het chalazion door middel van corticosteroïdinjecties. Een literatuuronderzoek [Treatment of the chalazion by means of corticosteroid injections. A literature survey]. *Huisarts Wet* 1997;**40**(13):644–8.

Bron AJ, Benjamin L, Snibson GR. Meibomian gland disease. Classification and grading of lid changes. *Eye* 1991;**5**:395–411.

McCulley JP, Shine WE. Eyelid disorders: the meibomian gland, blepharitis, and contact lenses. *Eye Contact Lens* 2003;**29**(1 Suppl):S93–s5.

Paranjpe DR, Foulks GN. Therapy for meibomian gland disease. *Ophthalmol Clin North Am* 2003;**16**(1):37–42.

Van Bijsterveld OP, Van Es JC. *Oogheelkundige problemen [Ophthalmological problems]*. Utrecht: Bunge, 1983.

47
STYE/HORDEOLUM

DEFINITION

A stye, or hordeolum, is an abscess-like acute infection in an eyelid. Anatomically, a distinction can be made between a hordeolum externum and hordeolum internum. The first involves a sweat gland or a sebaceous gland on the skin side of the eyelid, while the second involves a meibomian gland, located under the tarsal conjunctiva. A hordeolum internum can develop from a chalazion, and vice versa (see Chapter 46).

AETIOLOGY/PATHOGENESIS

A staphylococcal infection is nearly always present, and a small abscess with a pus head forms. The infection is self-limiting to the extent that the abscess usually spontaneously perforates, and then heals.

In patients with poor health, styes can occur as part of the more extensive clinical picture. Such a situation is beyond the scope of this book.

PRESENTATION

The patient usually experiences pain, and is distressed by the look of the red, swollen eyelid.

EPIDEMIOLOGY

The disorder occurs with the same frequency in all age categories, but more women than men are affected. People who are prone to staphylococcal infections develop styes more frequently. The supposed relationship with diabetes is rarely present. In many cases, a stye develops due to chronic blepharitis (see Chapter 45). Detailed epidemiological data are lacking, but GPs see this problem fairly frequently – although the vast majority are probably managed by patients themselves.

HISTORY

The GP asks:

- how long the stye has been present
- if the patient often experiences this problem
- whether the patient often has abscesses
- whether the eyelid margins are often inflamed.

EXAMINATION

A small swelling is visible on the inside or outside of the eyelid. The lid is red and shows oedematous swelling. Pressing on the lump with a cotton bud is painful – in contrast to a chalazion. There may also be a pus head present.

Taking a culture of the pus is not useful, because it will not affect management. Pay particular attention to signs of blepharitis.

TREATMENT

In general, it is recommended that the patient holds warm, moist compresses on the eye for half an hour at a time. The idea is that this will help the stye come to a head more quickly. If the abscess spontaneously perforates, the pain will be relieved, and the eyelid will heal within a few days. If the spontaneous perforation takes longer than 48 hours and the patient is bothered by the stye, an incision made with a needle can offer relief. The incision is made in the yellow pus head, always in a vertical direction, perpendicular to the row of eyelashes.

If pus is present, antibiotic ointment can be applied to the eye.

PREVENTION AND ADDITIONAL INFORMATION

Blepharitis forms a breeding ground for staphylococci (see Chapter 45). In this case, effective blepharitis treatment is the best way to prevent styes.

Key points

- Recurrent or multiple styes may be caused by underlying poor health or by associated blepharitis.
- Unlike chalazia, styes are tender to the touch.
- Styes are usually self-limiting.
- If pus is present, antibiotic ointment is indicated.

Literature

Axenfeld Th, Pau H (eds). *Lehrbuch der augenheilkunde* [*Textbook of ophthalmology*]. Stuttgart: Fischer, 1992.

Giesen PHJ, Van de Lisdonk EH. De diagnostiek en behandeling van het hordeolum in de huisartspraktijk [Diagnosis and treatment of the hordeolum in general practice]. Report of a conference on general practice. *Huisarts Wet* 1995;**38**:348–50.

Lederman C, Miller M. Hordeola and chalazia. *Pediatr Rev* 1999;**20**(8):283–4.

Miller SJH. *Parsons's diseases of the eye*. Edinburgh: Churchill Livingstone, 1990.

Raskin EM, Speaker MG, Laibson PR. Blepharitis. *Infect Dis Clin North Am* 1992;**6**(4):777–87.

48

BLOCKED TEAR DUCT IN CHILDREN

DEFINITION

A blocked tear duct is a congenital disorder in infants that leads to drainage problems of the tear fluid.

AETIOLOGY/PATHOGENESIS

Tears, which clean the exterior eye and protect it from drying out, drain through the two lacrimal canals. In the upper and lower lid, approximately 5 mm from the medial corner of the eye, a small spot the size of a pinprick is visible. This is the tear point, or punctum lacrimale, the opening of each of the two canals. Both end in the tear sac, which in turn drains into the nasal cavity just under the inferior concha via a bony passageway (the nasolacrimal duct). The nasolacrimal opening can remain blocked after birth by a thin membrane, which means tears cannot pass through. This leads to an accumulation of the tear fluid in the tear sac and, once this is filled, the tears will drain from the inferior conjunctival fornix onto the cheek. A secondary bacterial infection can occur in the tear sac, which can result in purulent discharge from the punctum lacrimale.

PRESENTATION

Infants usually develop symptoms when they are 2–3 weeks old: a watering or 'pussy' eye. Despite frequent wiping, the eye does not stay clean. The parents want to know what the problem is and how it can be treated.

EPIDEMIOLOGY

A significant number of children are born with a blocked nasolacrimal duct. Between 6% and 20% develop symptoms of sticky eye because of this in the first month of life. In most, the membrane will spontaneously rupture in the first 4–6 weeks after birth. Only in a small number (around 0.3 per 1000 patients per year) will this not occur, and symptoms will continue. Even in this group, in time the tear duct can become unblocked (sometimes with simple therapy). In very occasional cases, the obstruction is located in the punctum lacrimale or elsewhere in the drainage system.

HISTORY

The GP asks:

- when the symptoms began (if almost immediately after birth, it is congenital)
- about the presence of purulent discharge
- whether the child has a cold (possibly accompanied by conjunctivitis) or a fever.

EXAMINATION

The GP first inspects whether the disorder is present in one or both eyes. Swelling and redness in the corner of the eye indicate an infected tear sac (dacryocystitis – usually accompanied by general symptoms of illness, such as fever). If light pressure is applied to the tear sac, either only excess tear fluid, or purulent discharge (dacryocystitis) come out of the punctum lacrimale. Putting drops of fluorescein solution in the lower eyelid, then inserting a cotton bud in the nose under the inferior concha can indicate whether the solution drains to this point: if fluorescein is not present on the bud, an obstruction is present. However, fluorescein observed in the nose does not rule out a partial obstruction.

TREATMENT

If the blockage is uncomplicated and the infant only has one watering eye, an attempt can be made to resolve the problem by massaging the tear sac three times daily, starting at the punctum lacrimale and moving in an inferomedial direction.

The treatment is different in the presence of complications. If purulent discharge is present, antibiotic eye-drop therapy is necessary in addition to the above measures. Before the drops are put in the eye, the tear sac should be squeezed empty. In the case of dacryocystitis, systemic therapy with an antibiotic is necessary. The skin under the watering or pussy eye can be protected with a barrier cream.

Most affected children will achieve spontaneous resolution by 12 months of age; ophthalmologists are unlikely to undertake treatment before that age. Explain to the parents the aetiology and prognosis and the probability of spontaneous resolution. Some cases fail to resolve and require probing, but it is not possible to identify these cases early on. While waiting for resolution, the treatment is limited to simple cleaning (with tap water) of discharge from the lids. Avoid antibiotic treatment for the usual presentation of mild discharge from a white eye in the absence of true conjunctivitis. If the obstruction is still present at 12 months of age, a referral for ophthalmological assessment is necessary.

The specialist will insert a probe in the duct under general anaesthesia. If, after this procedure, the symptoms persist, a dacryocystorhinostomy can be carried out, in which a direct connection is made between the lacrimal sac and the nasal cavity.

PREVENTION AND ADDITIONAL INFORMATION

It is important to point out that the disorder will usually clear up over the course of several weeks to 6 months. Give clear instructions about how the tear sac should be massaged: three times daily in the correct direction. If necessary, the eye can be cleaned with water. However, intensive cleaning should be discouraged, as this irritates the conjunctivae.

Key points

- Infants usually develop symptoms when they are 2–3 weeks old: a watering or 'pussy' eye.

- Between 6% and 20% of children develop symptoms of sticky eye because of a blocked tear duct in the first month of life.

- Most affected children will achieve spontaneous resolution by 12 months of age.

- Avoid antibiotic treatment for the usual presentation of mild discharge from a white eye in the absence of true conjunctivitis.

Literature

Calhoun JH. Problems of the lacrimal system in children. *Pediatr Clin North Am* 1987;**34**(6):1457–65.

King RA. Common ocular problems in children: conjunctivitis and tear duct obstructions. *Pediatrician* 1990;**17**(3):142–51.

Paul TO, Shepherd R. Congenital nasolacrimal duct obstruction: natural history and the timing of optimal intervention. *J Pediatr Ophthalmol Strabismus* 1994;**31**(6):362–7.

Sakol PJ. Tearing: lacrimal obstructions. *Pa Med* 1996;**99**(S):99–104.

Verdonk HER, Gill K. Kleine kwalen in de huisartsgeneeskunde; dacryostenose bij zuigelingen [Minor ailments in general practice; dacryostenosis in infants]. *Ned Tijdschr Geneeskd* 1988;**132**:959–60.

Young JD, MacEwen CJ. Managing congenital lacrimal obstruction in general practice. *BMJ* 1997;**315**(7103):293–6.

49
FLOATERS

DEFINITION

Floaters are an optical phenomenon in which vitreous opacities are seen as strings, fluff or clouds that move with the vision in a slightly delayed manner. They are most obvious when looking at a blank or clear background, such as a blue sky or a white wall. It is not possible to fix on one of these spots, as they move out of the field of vision. Floaters can occur in one or both eyes.

AETIOLOGY/PATHOGENESIS

Most floaters are a physiological phenomenon. The vitreous body is composed of a gel, through which runs a three-dimensional network of fine collagen threads. During childhood, this is usually an optically homogenous structure. As a person ages, the vitreous gel becomes more fluid and shrinks. The posterior vitreous membrane can then slowly or suddenly come loose from the inside of the retina (posterior vitreous detachment). The shrunken vitreous body and the partially detached posterior vitreous membrane move along with eye movements: the cast shadow is perceived on the retina as a gradual or sudden occurrence of floaters. The risk of a posterior vitreous detachment increases with age – up to 50% of 50 year olds, although about 20% of these are asymptomatic. Myopic patients are at particular risk.

The posterior vitreous detachment can be accompanied by flashes of light, especially if there is traction on the retina. If a vitreous detachment is present, there is a 20% chance of a retinal tear. Untreated symptomatic retinal tears give an estimated risk of a retinal detachment of 40%. In patients with floaters and flashes of light, the risk of a retinal detachment is estimated at 15%. This percentage increases the more floaters are present. For patients experiencing only floaters, there is no significantly higher risk of a retinal tear.

If retinal detachment occurs, the patient will see a number of floaters, or a 'veil', accompanied by flashes of light and/or a loss of field of vision. Risk factors for retinal detachment include advanced age, myopia, previous cataract extraction, sharp or blunt trauma to the eye, retinal detachment in the other eye, and a family history of the same problem.

Another possible complication of posterior vitreous membrane detachment is vitreous haemorrhage. The symptoms can vary from a few, diffuse floaters to a decrease in visual acuity.

Other things that can be perceived as floaters are leukocytes (e.g. in uveitis), cholesterol crystals, asteroids (particles containing calcium and phosphorus) and amyloidosis. A foreign body on the cornea can also be perceived as a floater.

Some disorders can cause symptoms similar to floaters, such as migrainous phenomena, cataracts, a scotoma and visual hallucinations. Ophthalmic migrainous phenomena are a non-age-related, bilateral symptom of migraine. They usually begin with a light-grey spot without clear borders in the central visual field. After 10–20 minutes, this spreads to the periphery, until it covers approximately half of the visual field. This is usually followed by a unilateral headache. Cataracts generally occur after the age of 50 years. The first symptoms involve seeing stationary black spots. Double or triple vision or a decrease in visual acuity can also occur. A scotoma is a dark spot that moves with the eye, but which can be seen at a fixed point in relation to the fixation point. The cause is a pathological process in the fundus, retina and/or choroid. Visual hallucinations can vary from simple perceptions of light to very complex effects that may occur in acute confusion.

PRESENTATION

The patient may well be worried that the problem is serious. He complains of seeing moving strings, fluff or lines for several seconds, possibly accompanied by flashes of light. The complaint may have developed suddenly or might have been present for several months. The number of floaters can also vary.

EPIDEMIOLOGY

Only a small percentage of patients with floaters consult their GP. The majority (92%) of floaters disappear within 4 weeks. The prevalence of floaters increases with age and is higher in women than in men.

HISTORY

The GP will try to rule out a serious cause when taking the patient's history. The GP asks:

- about the nature of the floaters
- whether a few or many floaters are present
- whether the objects move in the direction of vision or stand still
- whether they are present in one or both eyes
- whether there are accompanying symptoms (flashes of light, reduction of field of vision, decrease in visual acuity, headache, watering or burning eyes)
- when the floaters began
- about the progression of the symptoms and whether they worsened suddenly
- about risk factors for retinal detachment (myopia, previous cataract extraction, or a preceding blunt or sharp trauma)
- about risk factors for vitreous bleeding (diabetes mellitus, ocular trauma).

EXAMINATION

Using a strong light source, the GP examines the exterior eye and the eyelids for a foreign body or signs of trauma. The vision in both eyes is assessed to rule out a decrease in visual acuity. An attempt should be made to detect any scotoma. The retina should be inspected via fundoscopy to detect a retinal tear or detachment; similarly, cataracts and vitreous distortions should be looked for.

TREATMENT

If the history and the examination do not suggest any pathology, the floaters are probably physiological. The implication is that the symptoms are harmless and often temporary, so it is important to reassure and inform the patient. However, the patient must receive clear instructions about the symptoms for which the GP should be consulted again. Symptoms suggesting complications are a sudden increase in the number of floaters, a decrease in visual acuity, field of vision loss and floaters that do not move along with the vision. If the GP suspects the patient has a retinal detachment, vitreous bleeding or a scotoma, an (emergency) referral to the ophthalmologist is appropriate.

PREVENTION AND ADDITIONAL INFORMATION

In view of the physiological nature of most floaters, prevention is not possible. However, it is important to prevent possible complications.

Key points

- The majority (92%) of floaters disappear within 4 weeks.
- In patients with floaters and flashes of light, the risk of a retinal detachment is estimated at 15%. This percentage increases the more floaters are present. However, for patients experiencing only floaters, there is no significantly higher risk of a retinal tear.
- The patient must receive clear instructions about the symptoms for which the GP should be consulted again. These include a sudden increase in the number of floaters, a decrease in visual acuity, field of vision loss and floaters that do not move along with the vision.

Literature

Alwitry A, Chen H, Wigfall S. Optometrists' examination and referral practices for patients presenting with flashes and floaters: 1. *Ophthal Physiol Opt* 2002;**22**(3):183–8.

Baggen JL. *Oogheelkunde in de huisartspraktijk [Ophthalmology in general practice]*. Dissertation. Amsterdam: Thesis Publishers, 1990.

Diamond JP. When are simple flashes and floaters ocular emergencies? *Eye* 1992;**6**:102–4.

Duguid G. Ocular flashes and floaters. *Practitioner* 1998;**242**:302–4.

Hichiki T, Trempe CL. Relationship between floaters, light flashes, or both, and complications of posterior vitreous detachment. *Am J Ophthalmol* 1994;**117**:593–8.

Sebag J. The vitreous. In: Adler FA (ed). *Adler's physiology of the eye*. St. Louis: Mosby, 1992, pp. 268–347.

Serpetopoulos CN, Korakitis RA. An optical explanation of the entoptic phenomenon of 'clouds' in posterior vitreous detachment. *Ophthal Physiol Opt* 1998;**18**(5):446–51.

Van Overdam KA, Bettink-Remeijer MW, Mulder PG, Van Meurs JC. Symptoms predictive for the later development of retinal breaks. *Arch Ophthalmol* 2001;**119**(10):1483–6.

Wilkinson C. Interventions for asymptomatic retinal breaks and lattice degeneration for preventing retinal detachment. *Cochrane Database Syst Rev* 2001;**3**:CD003170.

50

ARC EYE/WELDER'S FLASH/ SNOW BLINDNESS/ PHOTOKERATITIS

DEFINITION

Arc eye, welder's flash and snow blindness are all types of photokeratitis – an inflammation of the cornea due to overexposure to ultraviolet rays.

AETIOLOGY/PATHOGENESIS

Ultraviolet (UV) rays are a part of electromagnetic radiation. UV rays have a shorter wavelength than visible light, which means that the photons have a higher energy.

Problems resulting from overexposure to electromagnetic radiation generally occur in the tissue layers where the radiation is absorbed. The cornea and conjunctiva absorb radiation from the UVB and UVC spectra, giving rise to photokeratitis.

The injuries that can arise from this do not depend on the radiation energy per time unit, but on the total dose of radiation. The same injury can therefore occur in several seconds or several hours. In arc eye, damage can occur even if the welder works for only a few seconds without protective glasses. Snow blindness usually occurs after several hours' exposure to sunlight, in which rays are reflected off ice, snow or water. There is a higher risk of snow blindness at higher altitudes, due to the greater intensity of the rays.

PRESENTATION

Photokeratitis has a characteristic clinical picture. There is always a latent period, which can vary according to the intensity and duration of the exposure to UV rays. This period usually ranges from 6 to 12 hours, so that the first symptoms arise in the evening or at night. If the exposure is extreme, the latent period can be very short (up to 30 minutes). The damage to the cornea causes a foreign-body sensation, as if there is 'sand' in the eye; this is accompanied by extreme pain and photophobia with blepharospasm. If the patient is not familiar with these symptoms, the situation can be very alarming.

EPIDEMIOLOGY

There are no known reliable data on the occurrence of photokeratitis. To provide an impression, a random group of GPs was asked about their experience of this problem. On this basis, the incidence in a normal practice was estimated at five times a year to once in 7 years; the average was about once a year.

HISTORY

The history is characteristic. Often, the patient is fully aware of the diagnosis. The GP asks:

- whether the patient was exposed to a welding flame without eye protection, or to bright sunlight
- when the symptoms began
- if one or both eyes are affected
- whether it is possible there is a foreign body in the eye
- whether the patient wears contact lenses.

EXAMINATION

Both eyes are red and bloodshot. It is often difficult to inspect the eye because of the blepharospasm and watering. The eyelids may also be swollen and red. A single use of a local anaesthetic, such as amethocaine 0.5–1.0%, may be necessary to examine the eye properly.

In cases of doubt, to rule out a foreign body, the eye and the areas under the lids should be inspected thoroughly. The eye should also be examined with fluorescein.

If photokeratitis is present, the characteristic punctate corneal erosions will clearly fluoresce green.

TREATMENT

Once the diagnosis has been made, the treatment is aimed at alleviating the symptoms. A local anaesthetic should not be given (at least, not more than once) by the GP. The use of such treatment should be confined to the GP's surgery; it shouldn't be used at home by the patient. An anaesthetic delays the regeneration of the epithelium (spontaneous recovery takes 12–24 hours) and can in itself cause eye pain. This can lead to a vicious cycle in which the patient uses the eye drops more and more often. As a result, a more severe keratitis can develop, with the risk of eyeball perforation. In addition, a local anaesthetic renders the cornea insensitive to external stimuli.

The treatment subsequently involves a bandage, with ointment to reduce the pain. Because the effectiveness of antibiotic ointment for photokeratitis has not been demonstrated, a neutral ointment may be used with a bandage or an eye pad. Oral painkillers can be administered for the pain. Cold compresses can be helpful.

If the patient objects to having the eye covered, wearing sunglasses is recommended.

The severe pain usually resolves after 12–24 hours. After 48 hours, nearly all the symptoms should have disappeared. If the exposure was extreme, the patient may suffer from headache and minor visual disturbance for several weeks. Permanent damage is rare.

Referral to an ophthalmologist is only necessary if there is doubt about the diagnosis.

A rare chronic form of photokeratitis may occur in welders and residents of snowy areas. This involves visual disturbance, increased sensitivity to light and signs of chronic blepharoconjunctivitis; cornea ulceration may also occur.

PREVENTION AND ADDITIONAL INFORMATION

Prevention is very important for arc eye. Considerable attention is paid to this subject in the technical training programmes for welders. The GP must warn the patient about being lax about eye protection, to prevent future recurrences. For those travelling to snowy mountainous areas, wearing effective sunglasses with proper coverage is essential.

It is important for the GP to offer patients with photokeratitis reassurance and provide information about the harmlessness of the symptoms, which usually disappear by themselves.

Key points

- Arc eye is a type of photokeratitis, an inflammation of the cornea caused by overexposure to ultraviolet rays.

- The damage does not depend on the radiation energy per time unit, but on the total dose of radiation – so the same injury can occur in several seconds or several hours.

- There is always a latent period, usually 6–12 hours, before symptoms appear. Therefore, the problem usually becomes obvious in the evening or at night.

- A single use of a local anaesthetic, such as amethocaine 0.5–1.0%, may be necessary to properly examine the eye. However, an anaesthetic delays the regeneration of the epithelium and can in itself cause eye pain, so it should not be used as a remedy.

- The severe pain usually resolves after 12–24 hours. After 48 hours, nearly all the symptoms should have disappeared.

Literature

Cullen AP. Photokeratitis and other phototoxic effects on the cornea and conjunctiva. *Int J Toxicol* 2002;**21**(6):455–64.

Gerts MJJ, De Jongh TOH. Kleine kwalen in de huisartsgeneeskunde; keratitis door ultraviolette straling [Minor ailments in general practice; keratitis due to ultraviolet rays]. *Ned Tijdschr Geneeskd* 1992;**136**:685–7.

Longstreth J, De Gruijl FR, Kripke ML, Abseck S, Arnold F, Slaper HI, Velders G, Takizawa Y, Van der Leun JC. Health risks. *J Photochem Photobiol B* 1998;**46**(1–3):20–39.

Sterk CC. Acute traumata in de oogheelkunde [Acute traumas in ophthalmology]. *Ned Tijdschr Geneeskd* 1987;**131**:2246–9.

Tenkate TD. Occupational exposure to ultraviolet radiation: a health risk assessment. *Rev Environ Health* 1999;**14**(4):187–209.

51
PTERYGIUM

DEFINITION

A pterygium is a degenerative abnormality of the eye, in which the conjunctiva grows over the cornea in the nasal and/or temporal areas as a triangular, vascularized fold. The tissue grows in, and is firmly attached to, the most superficial layers of the cornea.

AETIOLOGY/PATHOGENESIS

To date, there has been no consensus on the pathogenesis of pterygia. Ultraviolet light is an aetiological factor – it is striking how the problem occurs so often in areas between the latitudes 37° north and 37° south. Other commonly cited causative factors include heat, dryness and dust, but these appear to have only a minor role. Many other contributory factors are reported in the literature, such as heredity, immunology and other environmental factors.

Wearing hard contact lenses can result in a 'pseudo-pterygium'. In an existing pterygium, hard contact lenses can result in the lens bumping against the lesion with each blink.

A growth rate of more than 1 mm/year in a pterygium is exceptional; if a patient has several pterygia, those on the temporal side will be the most recent.

A distinction can be made between three types of pterygia: progressive, stationary and atrophic. Each of these varieties can change into one of the other types. The progressive pterygium has a fleshy structure, with a redness caused by blood-vessel growth (typically horizontal in nature). This form is more common in younger people (aged 20–35 years). The stationary pterygium is thinner and less fleshy than the other types; there is more of a balance between growth and involution. Atrophic pterygium is thin and pale grey. This is more common in older people (over the age of 50 years).

PRESENTATION

Patients with pterygia attend because of eye symptoms (e.g. irritation or a burning sensation), or because they are worried about a 'bump' on the eye, and the possible implications of this for their eyesight. The patient may have been advised to attend by someone who has noticed the abnormality.

EPIDEMIOLOGY

In Europe, this problem occurs most often in areas around the Mediterranean Sea. Accurate prevalence data are sparse; most cases are probably not brought to medical attention.

HISTORY

The GP asks:

- how the problem has developed
- about the presence of symptoms, such as irritation, a burning sensation, or a foreign-body sensation, which may be present in progressive pterygia
- about visual symptoms, especially when the abnormality has been present for a long time
- about the patient's concerns, such as anxieties about malignancy or the potential effect on eyesight.

EXAMINATION

The GP inspects (using a magnifying glass, if necessary) the eyeball, eyelids and the entire cornea. The type of pterygium may be identified according to the classification and description given above. Eye movements and vision are also checked (also for astigmatism).

A number of disorders are relevant when considering the differential diagnosis. A pinguecula is a small, whitish-yellow, slightly raised swelling in the conjunctiva, usually on the nasal side of the cornea. A pinguecula usually remains small and does not lead to complications; treatment is not necessary.

A pseudo-pterygium looks very similar to a pterygium. However, a pseudo-pterygium can develop along the entire cornea. This is due to a difference in pathogenesis: a pseudo-pterygium always develops secondary to another eye disorder. It can occur if the conjunctiva comes into contact with an inflammatory process from the inside (e.g. keratitis). A pseudo-pterygium can also develop due to an external factor: for example, trauma, such as a chemical burn, or hard contact lenses. It can be distinguished from a true pterygium by the ability to insert a probe between the cornea and the conjunctival fold.

A carcinoma of the conjunctiva is rare, but as it usually develops from the limbus, it should be borne in mind if an abnormality is present at this site.

TREATMENT

Small lesions are usually not treated surgically unless they present a real threat to the vision. The GP should offer the patient explanation and reassurance. A follow-up consultation after a year may be worthwhile, or sooner if problems develop in the interim.

Pterygia are usually asymptomatic. Treatment with artificial tears, antihistamines and decongestants offer temporary relief from irritation (see Chapter 45). Vasoconstrictive medication cannot be used longer than a few days, due to the possibility of rebound. Locally administered corticosteroids only alleviate the symptoms a little and should not be used in view of the possible complications.

Surgery may be indicated if the pterygium reaches the edge of the pupil, if the growth causes astigmatism to increase, or if it grows more than 1–2 mm on the cornea. Surgery is also appropriate if the pterygium causes a mobility problem with the eyeball or there are recurring infections. The problem may also be surgically corrected for cosmetic reasons.

If the abnormality recurs after an operation (more rapid and extensive growth than the original pterygium, usually within 6 months), referral is again necessary. The figures for risk of recurrence vary in the range 5–75%.

PREVENTION AND ADDITIONAL INFORMATION

Patients should be aware that contact lenses can create a 'pseudo-pterygium' or may aggravate an existing pterygium. Protective goggles for outside work in hot, dusty environments may be of benefit.

Key points

- The differential diagnosis of pterygium includes a pinguecula, a pseudo-pterygium and, rarely, carcinoma of the conjunctiva.
- Pterygia are usually asymptomatic. Treatment with artificial tears, antihistamines and decongestants offer temporary relief from irritation.
- Surgery may be indicated if the pterygium reaches the edge of the pupil, aggravates astigmatism, grows onto the cornea, affects eye movements, causes recurrent infections or for cosmetic reasons.

Literature

Coroneo MT, Di Girolamo N, Wakefield D. The pathogenesis of pterygia. *Curr Opin Ophthalmol* 1999;**10**(4):282–8.

Di Girolamo N, Chui J, Coroneo MT, Wakefield D. Pathogenesis of pterygia: role of cytokines, growth factors, and matrix metalloproteinases. *Prog Retin Eye Res* 2004;**23**(2):195–228.

Hirst LW. The treatment of pterygium. *Surg Ophthalmol* 2003;**48**(2):145–80.

Reenalda H, Mulder JD. Kleine kwalen in de huisartsgeneeskunde; het pterygium van de conjunctiva [Minor ailments in general practice; pterygium of the conjunctiva. *Ned Tijdschr Geneeskd* 1989;**133**:1683–5.

52

SUBCONJUNCTIVAL HAEMORRHAGE

DEFINITION

A subconjunctival haemorrhage is bleeding under the conjunctiva that produces a clearly defined homogenous red patch.

AETIOLOGY/PATHOGENESIS

Subconjunctival haemorrhage results from the rupture of a conjunctival blood vessel. In most cases, no clear cause can be identified. There may be a connection with hypertension, extensive arteriosclerosis, the lifting of heavy objects and periods of severe coughing, vomiting or straining. Most subconjunctival bleeding, either occurring spontaneously or after a trauma, is only important because of its cosmetic impact. However, it may also be related to more serious disorders, such as blood dyscrasias, local blood vessel anomalies and acute infections. Subconjunctival bleeding may also be seen in contusions of the eye, perforating injuries and as part of an orbital haematoma (which is very rare and results from a cranial injury or subarachnoidal bleeding).

PRESENTATION

Patients with a spontaneous subconjunctival haematoma generally worry about the possibility of a serious disorder, due to the dramatic appearance and the sudden onset. They do not experience pain or problems with visual acuity.

EPIDEMIOLOGY

Subconjunctival bleeding usually arises spontaneously in older people, but it can also occur in people of other ages. In 1978, Hodgkin gave an incidence of 1.8 per 1000 patients per annum, and in his research Baggen (1990) found an incidence of 0.9 per 1000 patients per year.

HISTORY

The GP asks:

- about alarming symptoms, such as a decrease in visual acuity and pain
- about a perforating eye injury or other trauma
- about the use of anticoagulants.

EXAMINATION

The diagnosis is made by simple inspection. Check the vision if necessary. Depending on the situation, additional eye examination may be desirable. Check if there are signs of a perforating eye injury – but beware that a perforation is not always easily visible. Be alert, especially in children, for small penetrating wounds in the eyelid: these may be hiding a perforation injury of the eyeball. In such a case, no pressure should be put on the eyeball during the examination.

In uncomplicated subconjunctival haemorrhage, there will be a clearly delineated, clear red patch located next to, or sometimes around, the cornea. The cornea will be clear, and no cloudiness will be present in the anterior chamber of the eye. If a hyphaema (blood in the anterior chamber of the eye) is present, there must be a complication.

TREATMENT

For a spontaneous subconjunctival haemorrhage, the only treatment required is to reassure the patient: explain that the blood will disappear within 1–2 weeks, and that the patch will change colour (to green and yellow) during the recovery process, as the blood pigments are broken down. In very rare cases, a large haematoma can significantly raise the conjunctiva and cause symptoms. A small incision can allow the blood that has not coagulated to be released, which will help alleviate the situation. However, after this procedure, the patient should be referred. Referral is always indicated if a perforating eye injury is suspected. The eye is covered using an eye bandage, patch or a plastic cup.

PREVENTION AND ADDITIONAL INFORMATION

Prevention is not possible, except when it is caused by the use of anticoagulants. It is helpful to emphasize that this conjunctival bleeding is harmless and, if it occurs again, a serious disorder is unlikely.

Key points

- In most cases, no clear cause can be identified.
- Rarely, there may be a significant underlying cause, such as a blood dyscrasia or trauma.
- The haemorrhage will disappear within 1–2 weeks, with colour change (to green and yellow) during the recovery process.

Literature

Huang FC, Tseng SH, Shih MH, Chen FK. Effect of artificial tears on corneal surface regularity, contrast sensitivity, and glare disability in dry eyes. *Ophthalmology* 2002;**109**(10):1934–40.

Maclean H. *The eye in primary care*. Edinburgh: Butterworth-Heinemann, 2002.

Shields SR. Managing eye disease in primary care. Part 2. How to recognize and treat common eye problems. *Postgrad Med* 2000;**108**(5):83–6.

Wright PW, Strauss GH, Langford MP. Acute hemorrhagic conjunctivitis. *Am Fam Physician* 1992;**45**(1):173–8.

53

DRY EYE SYNDROME/ XEROPHTHALMIA

DEFINITION

Dry eye syndrome, or xerophthalmia, consists of a set of symptoms caused by insufficient tear production or insufficiently frequent blinking. Terms used in this context are: keratoconjunctivitis sicca, keratitis filiformis, sicca syndrome, Sjögren's syndrome and age-related atrophy of the tear gland. These terms refer to different causes, as well as differences in the severity of the symptoms.

AETIOLOGY/PATHOGENESIS

The cornea is dependent on tears for nourishment. Poor-quality tear fluid, insufficient tear production or non-continuous lubrication of the cornea from blinking cause metabolic disorders in the corneal tissue, which manifests as inflammation: keratitis sicca.

The main cause is inadequate lacrimal gland secretion, which is usually due to atrophy secondary to old age. Lack of tear fluid may also be associated with collagen disorders and with the side-effects of medication, such as antidepressants.

Dry eyes can also occur due to a lack of regular lubrication of the cornea from incomplete or insufficient blinking. This occurs in a number of disorders, such as facial palsy, severe ectropion, extreme exophthalmos or a lower eyelid deformed due to scarring. There is also evidence that some people without any obvious abnormalities sometimes sleep with their eyes partially open, resulting in insufficient lubrication of the cornea.

Environmental factors can play a role. The drier the air, the greater the chance of dry eyes. Central heating, air conditioning and a dry, (sub)tropical climate can cause problems.

A rare disorder in which dry eyes can occur is Sjögren's syndrome. This is an autoimmune illness involving an acute or chronic lymphocytic inflammatory reaction and the destruction of tear and/or salivary gland tissue (see Chapter 57), accompanied by joint problems. The erythrocyte sedimentation ratio (ESR) is elevated. This disease mainly affects middle-aged women.

Problems with the cornea are determined by the severity and duration of the dry eyes. Even if tear production drops only slightly or occasionally, the patient will experience symptoms, but not keratitis. If the severity increases, problems will develop that are almost always located in the lower part of the cornea.

PRESENTATION

Dry eyes rapidly produce troublesome symptoms in patients. In minor cases, patients complain of 'burning', a 'gritty feeling' or, curiously, 'watering' eyes, that lead to repeated rubbing. Only in a minority of patients is the actual complaint dry eyes. If the disorder worsens, the symptoms increase to severe pain and photophobia. Some patients suffer mainly at night, and experience eyelid movements as very painful. They do not dare to open their eyes in the morning for fear of the pain. The patient's symptoms, however, do not always correspond to the severity of the problem. For example, patients with a corneal ulcer do not always experience severe pain.

EPIDEMIOLOGY

Dry eyes are primarily seen in the elderly and more often in women. However, young people also suffer from this disorder, especially if they work in dry areas. The type of dry eyes due to abnormal blinking is rare, but this occurs in people of all ages.

HISTORY

The GP asks:

- when the symptoms started
- what kind of work the patient does and whether the symptoms seem related to this

- whether there were previous eye injuries
- about the use of medications
- about rheumatological disorders or any autoimmune illness.

EXAMINATION

The GP first inspects the eye and the surrounding structures. The vision is tested if necessary. The anterior segment of the eye is then examined (the eye may be dyed with fluorescein). If sicca syndrome is present, abnormalities are rarely seen. The most reliable 'test' probably involves prescribing artificial-tear remedies and assessing the response.

TREATMENT

Artificial tears (e.g. hypromellose drops 0.3%, one drop hourly) always resolve the symptoms and any minor complications, and are therefore a very useful therapy. The patient will have to use this treatment indefinitely. Responses to the different remedies for decreased tear secretion are very idiosyncratic, and this should be taken into account when determining the best one for a patient. If the corneal epithelium is damaged, local antibiotics (e.g. chloramphenicol) are also administered. If the dry-eye symptoms represent a side-effect of medication, the GP should consider stopping the treatment and substituting another, if possible. In more severe forms of keratitis sicca, corneal damage or ulcers, referral is recommended.

PREVENTION AND ADDITIONAL INFORMATION

Prevention is not really possible. Serious complications can be prevented by using artificial tears.

Key points

- Dry eye syndrome is the result of insufficient tear production or insufficiently frequent blinking.

- The main cause is inadequate lacrimal gland secretion, which is usually due to atrophy secondary to old age.

- Patients usually complain of 'burning', a 'gritty feeling' or, curiously, 'watering' eyes – only in a minority of patients is the actual complaint dry eyes.

Literature

Axenfeld T, Pau H (eds). *Lehrbuch der augenheilkunde* [*Textbook of ophthalmology*]. Stuttgart: Fischer, 1992.

Hara JH. The red eye: diagnosis and treatment. *Am Fam Physician* 1996;**54**(8):2423–30.

Polak BCP, Henkes HE. Droge ogen [Dry eyes]. *Ned Tijdschr Geneeskd* 1982;**126**:1025.

Rosenthal BP. Ophthalmology. Screening and treatment of age-related and pathologic vision. changes. *Geriatrics* 2001;**56**(12):27–31.

Van Haeringen NJ. Brandende en droge ogen [Burning and dry eyes]. In: Van Es JC, Mandema E, Olthuis G, et al. (eds). *Het Medisch Jaar 1991*. Houten: Bohn Stafleu Van Loghum, 1991.

54

EPIPHORA/WATERING EYES

DEFINITION

Epiphora – excessively watering eyes – usually involves troublesome watering in one or both eyes resulting from disrupted drainage of tear fluid. It is only rarely caused by increased tear production.

Problems with a non-functioning nasolacrimal duct in newborns are not covered here (see Chapter 48).

AETIOLOGY/PATHOGENESIS

Under normal circumstances, tears collect in the nasal corner of the eye. Excess tears drain through the nasolacrimal duct – helped by blinking, which has a suction effect in this area – which empties under the inferior turbinate in the nose. There are various causes of disrupted tear drainage. In facial palsy, blinking is less frequent. With an ectropion, the external opening (punctum) of the nasolacrimal duct can be turned outward and so is no longer in contact with the tears. This opening can also be disrupted by trauma (e.g. glass injuries caused by road traffic accidents) near the medial corner of the eye. Other local causes can also interfere with tear drainage, such as thick mucus in the nasolacrimal duct, mucosal folds in the corner of the eye and nasal abnormalities near the inferior turbinate.

Excessive tear secretion can be the result of chronic blepharitis due to a (staphylococcal) infection (see Chapter 45).

PRESENTATION

The patient complains of troublesome watering of the eye; he has to continually dry the face with a tissue. Some patients only experience problems in cold outside air or if it is windy. People wearing glasses complain that their lenses continually get dirty. Others complain about dry, painful skin resulting from constant wiping with a tissue.

EPIDEMIOLOGY

Little is known about the prevalence in the general population and the incidence in general practice. Research has revealed that the disorder is usually caused by puncta that do not touch the eye or a drainage system blocked by mucus, which is age-related. For this reason, older people more commonly experience this complaint.

HISTORY

The history volunteered by the patient is usually very clear. The GP asks:

- when the symptoms started
- whether there are conditions that exacerbate the symptoms
- whether there was trauma to or near the eye
- whether there are nasal abnormalities.

It should be noted that the history does not usually provide much additional or useful information.

EXAMINATION

The lower tear punctum is examined. In the correct position, it is turned 180° from the observer, and is therefore not immediately visible. It can only be seen by carefully pulling the lower eyelid downwards. If the opening of the tear punctum points (spontaneously) upwards, or worse, to the front, this is likely to be the cause of the problem.

TREATMENT

If the tear puncta are not positioned correctly or if the drainage system appears to be disrupted, referral to an ophthalmologist should be considered. Attempts to put a probe in the tear canal is definitely not recommended, as this can cause irreversible damage to the drainage system.

If watery eyes are due to hypersecretion, treating the underlying cause (e.g. chronic blepharitis) can help. If no pathological cause of hypersecretion can be established, tear secretion can be reduced by administering a local beta blocker, once or twice daily.

PREVENTION AND ADDITIONAL INFORMATION

There are no specific measures that can prevent this disorder.

Key points

- Epiphora usually involves troublesome watering in one or both eyes resulting from disrupted drainage of tear fluid.
- Some patients only experience problems in cold outside air or if it is windy.
- Hypersecretion of tears (e.g. in chronic blepharitis) is sometimes the cause.

Literature

Axenfeld T, Pau H (eds). *Lehrbuch der augenheilkunde* [*Textbook of ophthalmology*]. Stuttgart: Fischer, 1992.

Foulks GN. The evolving treatment of dry eye. *Ophthalmol Clin North Am* 2003;**6**(1):29–35.

Pflugfelder SC, Solomon A, Dursun D, Li DQ. Dry eye and delayed tear clearance: 'a call to arms'. *Adv Exp Med Biol* 2002;**506**:739–43.

55

ANGULAR CHEILITIS/ ANGULAR STOMATITIS

DEFINITION

Angular cheilitis, also known as angular stomatitis, is characterized by maceration and fissures in the corners of the mouth, sometimes accompanied by crusts and extension to the surrounding skin.

AETIOLOGY/PATHOGENESIS

The formation of folds in the corners of the mouth is the main cause of angular cheilitis. These particularly develop in people who wear dentures, especially if the dentures are ill-fitting. People with their own teeth can also suffer from abnormal folds in the corner of the mouth, because the skin loses elasticity with age. Patients predisposed to other skin disorders, such as atopic eczema, seborrhoeic eczema and psoriasis, are more likely to develop angular cheilitis. This disorder can be linked with excess salivation and, occasionally, with iron or vitamin B deficiencies. According to some researchers, infections in the mouth, throat and nose can also be a cause. Based on the literature, no clear statements can be made about the pathogenic micro-organisms. However, it is likely that infection with *Candida albicans* is often present, in addition to a secondary bacterial infection with staphylococci and possibly streptococci. The disorder can be very persistent and often recurs.

PRESENTATION

Patients with angular cheilitis visit their GP because the disorder can be very painful, may itch and is often unattractive. Because it can spread to the surrounding skin, and may be accompanied by crusts and fissures, patients are sometimes worried about the possibility of a serious skin disorder.

EPIDEMIOLOGY

There are few reliable epidemiological data about this disorder. A figure of 1.3 per 1000 patients per year has been reported, but this is probably an underestimate.

HISTORY

The GP asks:

- about the development of the symptoms
- about whether the patient wears dentures and if these fit correctly
- whether there are relevant symptoms related to the mouth, throat or nose
- about habits such as drooling, licking the corners of the mouth and sucking the thumb
- about the patient's diet (milk products, vegetables, meat, fish, unrefined grains).

EXAMINATION

The GP assesses the extent of the lesions and checks for signs of impetiginization (see Chapter 13). The dentures (if worn) may be examined to determine how well they fit and if they are cleaned regularly. Inspect the mouth and throat to check for signs of stomatitis or other infections. Also consider examining for other skin disorders.

Additional tests for *C. albicans* or bacteria are not particularly reliable and are therefore not useful; taking a culture is only indicated if a severe, progressive skin infection is present. A full blood count may be appropriate to check for possible iron or folic acid deficiencies.

TREATMENT

The edges of the mouth can be treated with an antimycotic cream (e.g. miconazole cream 2%) combined with a local disinfecting agent (e.g. chlorhexidine) twice daily. This treatment should be continued for at least 2 weeks; sometimes up to 5 weeks of treatment is necessary.

When there are clear signs of a bacterial infection, such as yellow crusts, an antibiotic cream (e.g. fusidic acid cream 2% three times daily) can be applied. If the complaint is very persistent or spreads, treatment with oral antibiotics (flucloxacillin 500 mg four times daily for 7–10 days) is indicated.

If the patient wears dentures, the following measures should be taken. Ill-fitting dentures should prompt a referral to the dentist. If the dentures fit correctly, it is recommended that the dentures are not worn for 1–2 weeks. In addition, an oral gel (e.g. miconazole) can be prescribed. The patient should keep this in the mouth as long as possible before swallowing and can also brush the dentures with the gel. Treatment should continue until the symptoms have disappeared.

Any underlying or exacerbating cause, such as infection of the mouth, throat or nose or deficiency of iron or B vitamins, should be treated as appropriate.

PREVENTION AND ADDITIONAL INFORMATION

If dentures are worn, it is helpful to point out that careful cleaning can prevent infections. Any food particles remaining on the dentures will promote the growth of *Candida*. Also, explain the relationship between ill-fitting dentures and angular cheilitis. Providing information about harmful habits, such as licking the edges of the mouth, can have a preventive effect.

Key points

- The main cause of angular cheilitis is the formation of folds in the corners of the mouth. These, in turn, are caused by ill-fitting dentures or the loss of skin elasticity with age.

- It is likely that infection with *C. albicans* is often present, in addition to a secondary bacterial infection with staphylococci and, possibly, streptococci.

- Treatment should be continued for at least 2 weeks; sometimes up to 5 weeks of treatment is necessary.

Literature

Appleton SS. Candidiasis: pathogenesis, clinical characteristics, and treatment. *J Calif Dent Assoc* 2000;**28**(12):942–8.

Feldmann CT. Kleine kwalen in de huisartsgeneeskunde: angular cheilitis [Minor ailments in general practice: angular cheilitis]. *Ned Tijdschr Geneeskd* 1989;**133**:1638–40.

Ohman SC, Jontell M. Treatment of angular cheilitis. The significance of microbial analysis, antimicrobial treatment, and interfering factors. *Acta Odontol Scand* 1988;**46**(5):267–72.

Smith AJ, Jackson MS, Bagg J. The ecology of *Staphylococcus* species in the oral cavity. *J Med Microbiol* 2001;**50**(11):940–6.

56
COLD SORES/HERPES LABIALIS

DEFINITION

Herpes labialis, commonly known as cold sores, is the manifestation of a recurring infection with the herpes-simplex virus (HSV). It is usually found on or around the lips and is characterized by a localized collection of blisters with a red base. These develop into crusts and then disappear without scarring.

AETIOLOGY/PATHOGENESIS

After a primary infection, herpesviruses lie dormant in the ganglia of the central nervous system. Various stimuli can cause their active replication, resulting in a clinical manifestation.

A distinction can be made between two types of herpes-simplex viruses: type-1 (HSV-1), which usually causes abnormalities around the mouth and which is also the cause of herpes keratitis and herpes encephalitis; and type-2 (HSV-2), which causes herpes genitalis (and herpes neonatorum). As a result of orogenital sexual contact, HSV-2 can also be responsible for herpes around the mouth, and herpes in the genital area can be caused by HSV-1. The two types cannot be accurately distinguished purely on the clinical picture.

During active infection, the virus can be isolated from the saliva. Primary transmission occurs by mouth or orogenital contact with a person excreting the virus, or via contaminated objects.

The primary infection with HSV-1 can manifest as acute gingivostomatitis in children less than about 6 years old. These children can become very ill, with symptoms such as fever, pain, general malaise, cervical lymphadenitis, excessive salivation and refusal to eat and drink. In adolescents, the primary infection can develop as ulcerating glossitis, which clears up in a period of 10–14 days. However, the majority (probably 90%) of primary infections are asymptomatic. A primary infection can also manifest on the fingers (e.g. in dentists) or on the eyes, resulting in paronychia or herpetic keratoconjunctivitis, respectively. After this primary infection, the virus probably remains present for the rest of the patient's life in the sensory ganglia of the dermatome affected – usually the trigeminal ganglion.

There are various apparent triggers that lead to recurrence, which is usually at the same site as the primary infection. These include stress, exposure to ultraviolet light, hormonal changes during the menstrual cycle and intensive rubbing of the skin (which may take place in some contact sports, hence 'herpes gladiatorum'). In approximately 5% of patients with a primary infection, the infection recurs frequently (more than six episodes a year).

The clinical picture of a recurrence can be divided into three phases. The characteristic prodromes of burning and itching usually precede the visible lesions. Redness and swelling develop next (first stage), followed by grouped blisters on a red base filled with clear fluid (second stage). These blisters are all in the same stage of development at the same time. The blisters then open and form crusts (third stage), which dry out. The lesions are present for 1–2 weeks. Occasionally, a bacterial superinfection can give rise to impetiginization.

There are recent suggestions that the virus may play a role in acute idiopathic facial paralysis (Bell's palsy).

PRESENTATION

Many patients with herpes labialis do not visit their GP, because it is well recognized that the disorder is self-limiting. The main reasons for seeking medical advice are pain, the cosmetic effects, and for questions about treatment and how recurrences can be prevented.

EPIDEMIOLOGY

Herpes labialis is a common problem. It accounts for around 1% of primary care consultations in the UK each year. Between 20% and 40% of people have suffered cold sores at some time. In The Netherlands, 50–70% of the population is a carrier of the virus; this figure may even be as high as 90%. However, not every carrier has symptoms – probably only about half of them. The disorder seems to occur one and a half times more often in women than in men; this may be related to the menstrual cycle.

HISTORY

The GP asks:

- when the symptoms began
- if blisters appeared immediately, or were preceded by pain
- about predisposing factors, such as exposure to ultraviolet light
- about any relationship with the menstrual cycle and stress.

The patient usually attends for the first time after the prodromal stage has ended, at which point antiviral treatment is ineffective. Patients may present sooner if they detect an impending recurrence.

EXAMINATION

Simple inspection of the lesions is sufficient to make the diagnosis. The GP must also check for signs of complications, such as secondary bacterial infection or eczema herpeticum. The latter is a disseminated herpes-simplex infection in a patient who already has atopic eczema. Patients with decreased immunity can also have very severe herpes infections.

Additional tests, such as viral culture, are only indicated in very exceptional cases (e.g. patients with lowered resistance).

TREATMENT

Various placebo-controlled studies have shown that local treatment of herpes labialis has little benefit. In recurrences, the attack can sometimes be partially suppressed if the patient begins local treatment with an antiviral cream (e.g. aciclovir) during the prodromal phase. Because the recurrence frequency is not affected by local therapy, and the duration of the symptoms only slightly, this treatment is generally not indicated.

If the crust stage has begun, treatment with aciclovir will no longer help, and a moisturizer is sufficient. If impetiginization occurs, treatment with a local antibiotic (e.g. fusidic acid cream 2%) is indicated (see Chapter 13).

PREVENTION AND ADDITIONAL INFORMATION

If the episodes recur frequently, the GP should explore possible predisposing factors, so that these can be avoided. If desired, the patient can start using aciclovir cream in the prodromal phase of any recurrence.

The lesions are contagious until they have dried out. Patients must avoid having other body parts come into contact with the contents of the blisters (as far as possible), and practice proper hygiene to avoid spreading the virus to the fingers or eyes. For this reason, cleaning contact lenses with saliva is strongly discouraged.

Key points

- Between 20% and 40% of people have suffered cold sores at some time.
- HSV-1 and HSV-2 cannot be accurately distinguished purely on the clinical picture.
- The primary infection with HSV-1 can manifest as acute gingivostomatitis in young children and as ulcerating glossitis in adolescents.
- Various placebo-controlled studies have shown that local treatment of herpes labialis has little benefit.

Literature

Baker D, Eisen D. Valacyclovir for prevention of recurrent herpes labialis: 2 double-blind, placebo-controlled studies. *Cutis* 2003;**71**(3):239–42.

Emmert DH. Treatment of common cutaneous herpes simplex virus infections. *Am Fam Physician* 2000;**61**(6):1697–706.

Lin L, Chen XS, Cui PG, Wang JB, Guo ZP, Lu NZ, Bi ZG, Jia H, Yang XY. Topical Penciclovir Clinical Study Group. Topical application of penciclovir cream for the treatment of herpes simplex facialis/labialis: a randomized, double-blind, multicentre, aciclovir-controlled trial. *J Dermatol Treat* 2002;**13**(2):67–72.

Raborn GW, Grace MG. Recurrent herpes simplex labialis: selected therapeutic options. *J Can Dent Assoc* 2003;**69**(8):498–503.

Rothbarth Ph.B. Antivirale therapie: 1 [Antiviral therapy: 1]. *Geneesmiddelenbulletin* 1993;**27**(4):26–8.

Spruance SL, Kriesel JD. Treatment of herpes simplex labialis. *Herpes* 2002; **9**(3):64–9.

Spruance SL, Nett R, Marbury T, Wolff R, Johnson J, Spaulding T. Acyclovir cream for treatment of herpes simplex labialis: results of two randomized, double-blind, vehicle-controlled, multicenter clinical trials. *Antimicrob Agent Chemother* 2002;**46**(7):2238–43.

57

DRY MOUTH/XEROSTOMIA

DEFINITION

The symptom of dry mouth resulting from decreased secretion of saliva is called xerostomia. This develops if saliva production falls below 100 ml/day.

AETIOLOGY/PATHOGENESIS

A healthy adult produces on average 1–2 l/day of saliva. Dry mouth occurs most commonly in older patients, apparently because of changes in the physiology of the salivary glands. This idiopathic xerostomia should be distinguished from the other types – it should not always be assumed that old age is the primary cause, because a large number of the causes of xerostomia occur in older people.

Iatrogenic causes include medications and the use of radiotherapy in the head/neck area. The major groups of medications responsible are antihistamines (e.g. promethazine), anticholinergics (e.g. anti-Parkinson's remedies such as benzatropine), spasmolytics (e.g. propantheline), antihypertensives (clonidine, beta blockers, and, to a lesser extent, ACE inhibitors), antidepressants (tricyclics) and antipsychotics (e.g. chlorpromazine).

There are also disorders that indirectly affect the salivary glands or drainage ducts, such as systemic illnesses influencing fluid balance (e.g. diabetes mellitus), Sjögren's syndrome (rarely), impaired general health, cachexia, dehydration, nervous system disorders, cerebral malignancies, trauma, nasopharyngeal obstruction (e.g. due to tumours), hypertrophy of the adenoids, allergy and infections.

In rare cases, decreased saliva secretion is due to disorders that directly affect the salivary glands or their drainage ducts, such as infections, trauma to a salivary gland or drainage duct, salivary gland tumours, obstruction of the drainage canal (salivary stone or tumour) and congenital hypoplasia. Disorders of the oral mucous membrane, such as gingivitis, stomatitis and fungal infections, can also result in xerostomia.

In addition, patients may subjectively experience 'dry mouth' without an objective decrease in salivary secretion and for which no cause can be determined. Psychological factors, such as tension, stress, fear and depression, can, sometimes acutely, cause the tongue to stick to the roof of the mouth.

Xerostomia is usually one symptom among many, rather than being the primary reason for consultation.

PRESENTATION

Patients complain of a dry feeling in the mouth or difficulties with swallowing, especially dry food, such as biscuits. Other subjective symptoms include a feeling of thirst, loss of taste, difficulties when chewing and talking, a burning or painful tongue and mucous membranes, and difficulty with wearing dentures.

EPIDEMIOLOGY

Xerostomia occurs often, particularly in older people, and more frequently in women than in men. The prevalence figures vary significantly.

HISTORY

The GP asks:

- about medication use and any underlying disorders
- about local radiotherapy of the head/neck area
- about symptoms indicating diabetes or other systemic disorders.

EXAMINATION

The mouth is inspected for atrophy of the mucous membranes, fissures and ulcers, *Candida* infection, gingivitis, dental plaque, infection of the salivary glands and salivary stones.

Laboratory tests can confirm or rule out underlying illnesses, such as diabetes mellitus. Diagnosis of Sjögren's syndrome (an autoimmune illness characterized by the triad xerostomia, xerophthalmia and rheumatoid arthritis) or other autoimmune disorders can be supported by the appropriate laboratory tests. (For additional examination/tests relevant to the mouth, see Chapter 59.)

TREATMENT

First, any underlying cause or illness should be eliminated or treated. The symptoms can be alleviated by replacing any medication causing xerostomia with an alternative, although this will often be difficult. Symptomatic treatment focuses on relieving the symptoms by drinking lots of water, avoiding dry, heavy food, avoiding alcohol, not smoking, and stimulating saliva production by chewing (e.g. chewing gum) or by using/consuming sour substances (e.g. citrus products).

Artificial saliva usually contains carboxymethylcellulose or mucin as a lubricating agent. The preparations containing mucin seem to be the most effective. However, no type of artificial saliva will relieve symptoms for more than 2 hours.

Pilocarpine and carbachol are used for xerostomia after radiotherapy. However, these substances can have unpleasant side-effects (sweating, diarrhoea, nausea, bradycardia) and are only effective if functional salivary gland tissue is still present. The advantages and disadvantages of the treatment must therefore be carefully considered.

PREVENTION AND ADDITIONAL INFORMATION

It is difficult to prevent the common age-related xerostomia; some of the aforementioned measures can be considered preventive. When prescribing, the GP should remember that xerostomia can occur as a side-effect.

Patients should be informed that xerostomia increases the risk of caries and gingivitis, so they should pay extra attention to their teeth and gums (this includes visiting the dentist).

Key points

- Dry mouth occurs most commonly in older patients, as idiopathic xerostomia.
- Iatrogenic causes include medications and the use of radiotherapy in the head/neck area.
- Other subjective symptoms in patients with dry mouth include a feeling of thirst, loss of taste, difficulties when chewing and talking, a burning or painful tongue and mucous membranes, and difficulty with wearing dentures.
- No type of artificial saliva will relieve symptoms for more than 2 hours at a time.

Literature

Brennan MT, Shariff G, Lockhart PB, et al. Treatment of xerostomie: a systemic review of therapeutic trials. *Dent Clin N Am* 2002;**46**:847–56.

Daniels TE. Evaluation, differential diagnosis, and treatment of xerostomia. *J Rheumatol* 2000;**61**(Suppl):6–10.

Diaz-Arnold AM, Marek CA. The impact of saliva on patient care: a literature review. *J Prosthet Dent* 2002;**88**(3):337–43.

Frydrych AM, Davies GR, Slack-Smit LM, Heywood J. An investigation into the use of pilocarpine as a sialagogue in patients with radiation induced xerostomia. *Austr Dent J* 2002;**47**(3):249–53.

Guggenheimer J, Moore PA. Xerostomia: etiology, recognition and treatment. *J Am Dent Assoc* 2003;**134**(1):61–9.

Scully C. Drug effects on salivary glands: dry mouth. *Oral Dis* 2003;**9**(4):165–76.

Ship JA, Pillemer SR, Baum BJ. Xerostomia in the geriatric patient. *J Am Geriatr Soc* 2002:**50**:535–43.

58

PERIORAL DERMATITIS

DEFINITION

Perioral dermatitis is a skin problem that occurs around the mouth, resulting in burning, redness, papules and pustules.

AETIOLOGY/PATHOGENESIS

The aetiology of the disorder is unknown, but there seems to be a relationship with the use of creams containing corticosteroids. The clinical picture is sometimes considered a variant of rosacea.

PRESENTATION

The patient presents with a red skin rash around the mouth, and often complains of a burning or painful itching. The skin is very sensitive to external stimuli.

EPIDEMIOLOGY

This skin disorder primarily occurs in young women – less than 10% of patients are men. It is occasionally diagnosed in children. There are no known specific figures from general practice research.

HISTORY

The GP asks:

- about how long the current rash has been present and the duration of previous skin disorders of the face
- about the use of ointments and creams, especially corticosteroid cream.

EXAMINATION

The diagnosis is usually easy to make because of the typical distribution. There is usually erythema around the mouth, except for a small border just around the edges of the lips. Small, red, sometimes flaky papules are visible. During an exacerbation, pustules may also be present. Further investigations such as allergy tests are not helpful.

TREATMENT

The cause is explained and the use of creams containing corticosteroids must be stopped. It is better to use lukewarm water, without soap, to clean the face. The GP should explain that the disorder may get worse before it gets better. A neutral non-greasy cream can be prescribed. If this is not effective and the symptoms significantly worsen, an oral course of tetracycline can be prescribed (e.g. tetracycline 250 mg four times daily for 3 weeks). If the patient cannot take tetracycline or it is contraindicated, preparations containing metronidazole (as used for rosacea) may be used, although these are less effective than tetracycline (see Chapter 70).

PREVENTION AND ADDITIONAL INFORMATION

This disorder can be considered in part an iatrogenic dermatosis: these patients should be told that, in principle, steroids should not be used (long-term) on the face, and that the disorder may sometimes recur.

Key points

- Perioral dermatitis results in burning, redness, papules and pustules around the mouth.
- Corticosteroid creams play a part in the aetiology, but stopping them may cause a temporary exacerbation.
- Less than 10% of patients are men.
- The diagnosis is usually easy to make because of the typical distribution.

Literature

Boeck K, Abeck D, Werfel S, Ring J. Perioral dermatitis in children – clinical presentation, pathogenesis-related factors and response to topical metronidazole. *Dermatology* 1997;**195**(3):235–8.

Goa KL. Clinical pharmacology and pharmacokinetic properties of topically applied corticosteroids. A review. *Drugs* 1988;**S5**:51–61.

Laude TA, Salvemini JN. Perioral dermatitis in children. *Semin Cutan Med Surg* 1999;**18**(3):206–9.

Malik R, Quirk CJ. Topical applications and perioral dermatitis. *Austr J Dermatol* 2000;**41**:34–8.

Veien NK, Munkvad JM, Nielsen AO, Niordson AM, Stahl D, Thormann J. Topical metronidazole in the treatment of perioral dermatitis. *J Am Acad Dermatol* 1991;**24**:258–60.

Wilkinson DS, Kirton V, Wilkinson JD. Perioral dermatitis: a 12 year review. *Br J Dermatol* 1979;**101**:245–57.

59

BURNING TONGUE/ GLOSSODYNIA/ BURNING MOUTH

DEFINITION

Glossodynia (pain in the tongue) is characterized by sensations of pain and/or burning in the tongue. The symptoms may not be limited to the tongue – they can extend to the mouth, hence the alternative name, 'burning mouth'. The term 'burning tongue' is used in this chapter. In addition, sensations such as a strange taste (e.g. metal) or a loss of taste may also be present.

A distinction should be made between burning tongue with a clear cause, and essential, idiopathic, or 'true' burning tongue. The complaint can only be considered true burning tongue if the symptoms have been present for longer than 6 months and no cause has been found.

AETIOLOGY/PATHOGENESIS

When the symptoms occur at a specific site in the mouth or when they are limited to one side, there is usually an underlying cause. Local disorders and, much less frequently, internal or neurological problems can result in this symptom. Local causes include primarily benign abnormalities of the mucous membrane, such as candidiasis, glossitis, lichen planus, stomatitis and papillitis, and various mucous membrane disorders of the tongue, such as geographical tongue, although these also often occur without the symptom of burning tongue. Other local causes include ill-fitting dentures or oversensitivity to metals used to repair the teeth. Only rarely is the cause a local malignant disorder or the preliminary stage thereof, such as leukoplakia.

Internal or neurological disorders such as iron-deficiency anaemia, pernicious anaemia, diabetes mellitus, neuralgia and a lesion of the lingual nerve can also cause tongue symptoms in rare cases.

A dry mouth, for example resulting from antidepressants or antihypertensives, or from Sjögren's syndrome, can exacerbate the burning-tongue sensation, although they do not represent the cause.

In the case of idiopathic burning tongue, the symptoms are usually located on both sides. Although the complaint occurs relatively frequently in women during and after the menopause, it has never been established that hormonal influences are to blame. Also, it is difficult to say whether psychosocial factors play a role. It is striking, though, that in a number of cases, the symptoms start soon after a major event in the patient's life.

PRESENTATION

The patient attends with symptoms of burning in the mouth, as if the tongue/mouth has been burnt by a hot liquid. Sometimes, the patient will describe a more dull, deep pain, a sharp, searing feeling or an itching sensation. In some cases, the symptoms are accompanied by a dry feeling in the mouth. The pain is often located on the edges or point of the tongue, and often also in the upper or lower lip. The symptoms are generally bearable in the morning, but increase as the day goes on, until they become unbearable in the evening. Nearly two-thirds of patients sleep badly as a result.

Some patients visit their dentist first, because they think there is a dental problem, or that the burning feeling started soon after dental work was done.

EPIDEMIOLOGY

Epidemiological data are scanty. It is known, however, that peri- and post-menopausal women suffer more often from this complaint than men.

HISTORY

Try to determine whether the problem is local, or a symptom of an internal or neurological disorder. By definition, the duration of symptoms is important in making the diagnosis. The GP asks:

- how long ago the symptoms started
- whether the patient has any ideas about the cause of the symptoms
- what the symptoms are precisely
- where they are located in the mouth
- whether the patient has noticed any abnormalities in the mouth
- whether the patient wears dentures
- about symptoms of an internal or neurological disorder
- about the use of medications.

EXAMINATION

The physical examination consists primarily of careful inspection of the mouth. Dentures must be taken out completely. The examination begins with the inspection of the tongue (top and bottom); the patient must also stick the tongue out so that the sides can be properly examined. The mucous membranes and the teeth are also inspected and, depending on the site of the symptoms, the tongue, bottom of the mouth and mucosa of the cheek are palpated.

Attention should be paid to localized abnormalities, the colour of the mucous membrane, and the consistency and extent of any disorder noted. If it is suspected that a neurological or internal disorder is the cause, the examination should be expanded appropriately.

If candidiasis is suspected, a bit of the mucosal surface scraped from the mouth and mixed with a potassium hydroxide solution can be examined under a microscope to see if any fungal hyphae are visible. More extensive tests are necessary if it is suspected that the candidiasis is caused by another disorder, such as a human immunodeficiency virus (HIV) infection.

If the mucous membrane is completely normal, tests such as a trial exclusion diet, blood tests and allergy tests do not contribute to making the diagnosis. With possible neurological or systemic pathology, additional tests are carried out accordingly.

TREATMENT

If *Candida* or another local cause is present, the appropriate treatment should be used. For idiopathic burning tongue, there is no therapy that has been proven effective. Naturally, the GP must show that these sometimes very significant symptoms are being taken seriously. The subject of a possible relationship with a psychological cause should be carefully raised. A referral along these lines is only helpful if the patient acknowledges a clear relationship between the symptom and tension, anxiety, depression or other psychosocial factors.

PREVENTION AND ADDITIONAL INFORMATION

Clearly, if no cause can be determined and it cannot be predicted who will develop this disorder, general prevention is not possible. Anticipating the symptoms in people who have had this disorder in the past, such as when prescribing medications or considering oral surgery, can be helpful.

If idiopathic burning tongue is suspected, it is important to focus sufficient attention on the complaint (e.g. starting with a careful examination). If no abnormalities are present, the patient should be warned about the hopeless task of consulting one specialist after another.

Key points

- The symptoms may not be limited to the tongue.
- A distinction should be made between burning tongue with a clear underlying cause, and essential, idiopathic, or 'true' burning tongue.
- The complaint can only be considered true burning tongue if the symptoms have been present for longer than 6 months and no cause has been found.
- In the case of idiopathic burning tongue, the symptoms are usually present on both sides of the tongue.
- The symptoms are generally bearable in the morning, but increase as the day goes on, until they become unbearable in the evening.
- Overreferral of patients with idiopathic burning tongue should be avoided.

Literature

Kapur N, Kamel IR, Herlich A. Oral and craniofacial pain: diagnosis, pathophysiology, and treatment. *Int Anesthesiol Clin* 2003;**41**(3):115–50.

Marbach JJ. Medically unexplained chronic orofacial pain. Temporomandibular pain and dysfunction syndrome, orofacial phantom pain, burning mouth syndrome, and trigeminal neuralgia. *Med Clin North Am* 1999;**83**(3):691–710.

Van der Reijden JA, De Jongh TOH. Glossodynie en mondbranden [Glossodynia and burning mouth]. *Modern Med* 1993;**17**:777–9.

60
APHTHOUS ULCERS

DEFINITION

Aphthous ulcers are painful, solitary or multiple ulcers in the oral mucous membrane. They result in a recurring inflammation of the non-keratinized oral mucous membrane, in which a few to many aphthous lesions are present.

AETIOLOGY/PATHOGENESIS

Aphthous ulcers appear in three forms, which can occur simultaneously. In the most common, minor, form, ulcers are 2–5 mm in size. These lesions are covered with a greyish-white layer and are surrounded by a red border; they usually appear in the mucous membrane of the cheek, inside the lips and on the tongue frenulum. They disappear spontaneously within 2 weeks.

In the major form of aphthous ulcers, one to several, very painful ulcers (1–3 cm in size), are present. The ulcer consists of a deep crater with a raised edge. This type heals slowly (1–2 months) and leaves scars.

The third form is herpetiform stomatitis, in which many ulcers the size of a pinhead, covered with a yellow layer, are present. There may be more than 100 ulcers, and they can converge into larger ulcers with rough edges. As the name indicates, this form looks like herpes stomatitis. Distinguishing features are the site (herpes lesions usually occur on the keratinized mucosa, gingiva and hard palate) and the appearance (herpes lesions begin as a vesicle and the erosion is not covered by a layer or surrounded by a red border).

To date, none of the research on aphthous ulcers has revealed a cause. The following are considered possible culprits: autoimmune processes, such as in Behçet's disease; infections or poor oral hygiene; allergies to or intolerances of certain substances in food; and iron and vitamin deficiency (especially folic acid and vitamin B_{12}). However, none of these causes have been proven. Psychological, hereditary and hormonal factors may also play a role – in women, the lesions often occur premenstrually. Aphthous ulcers are sometimes considered part of the symptom complex in acquired immunodeficiency syndrome (AIDS).

If the patient has a fever and generally feels unwell, other ulcerating disorders of the oral mucous membrane must be considered, such as herpetic gingivostomatitis (a herpes-simplex infection) and herpangina (a coxsackievirus infection). In terms of differential diagnosis, ulcers in the mouth can be caused by disorders that are quite rare and which are therefore diagnosed at a relatively late stage. These include: lichen planus (chronic ulcerations primarily found on the cheek mucous membrane and bordered by reticular, white stripes, the so-called Wickham's striae), pemphigus vulgaris (weak bullae that break open and converge into superficial ulcerations with a clear red base, often also bullae on the skin), benign mucosal pemphigoid (thick-walled, red bullae of the gingiva; the abnormalities are chronic and accompanied by erosion of the nasal mucosa and the conjunctiva), lupus erythematosus (ulcers causing relatively few symptoms in the centre of a large red plaque; recovery takes years), Behçet's disease (also ulcers on the genitalia and eye abnormalities) and squamous cell carcinoma.

PRESENTATION

Pain in the mouth, especially when eating dry foods, is the main reason the patient consults the GP; the patient may well be aware that there is no cure, but may, for example, wonder if new treatment is available.

EPIDEMIOLOGY

Point prevalence has been reported as 2%, and between 5% and 10% in children. Up to 66% of adults report a previous history of these ulcers.

HISTORY

The GP asks:

- about previous episodes of these symptoms, in view of the recurring character of the disorder
- about the presence of general symptoms of illness and fever, which might point to an alternative diagnosis.

EXAMINATION

When inspecting the mouth, superficial defects typically measuring 2–5 mm are typically visible on the oral mucosa. Lesions as previously described will be visible. They are painful to the touch. The regional lymph nodes are not swollen. If the lymph glands are swollen and fever is present, infection due to the herpes-simplex virus or coxsackievirus must be considered.

TREATMENT

Most aphthous ulcers heal spontaneously within 14 days. In view of the unknown aetiology, cure is impossible. Many different therapies are described in the literature, but none of them have been proven effective. Typical treatments tried include salicylic acid gels and steroid-based lozenges or pastes; the latter may reduce the duration of the attack and hasten pain relief. Rinsing the mouth with chlorhexidine 0.2% mouthwash may relieve the pain and shorten the episode, but will not affect the risk of recurrence. A tetracycline mouthwash may be helpful, particularly in the immunosuppressed.

PREVENTION AND ADDITIONAL INFORMATION

There is no treatment to prevent recurrences. Providing information about the harmless yet recurring character is advisable. To detect a possible hypersensitivity, it may be helpful for the patient to keep a diary of foods eaten and match this with episodes of aphthous ulcers.

Key points

- Aphthous ulcers appear in three forms: minor, major and herpetiform.

- To date, none of the research on aphthous ulcers has revealed a cause.

- If the patient has a fever, enlarged nodes and generally feels unwell, other ulcerating disorders of the oral mucous membrane must be considered, such as herpetic gingivostomatitis and herpangina.

Literature

Huizing EH, Snow GB (eds). *Leerboek keel-, neus- en oorheelkunde* [*Textbook for throat, nose and ear medicine*]. Houten: Bohn Stafleu Van Loghum, 1993.

McBride DR. Management of aphthous ulcers. *Am Fam Physician* 2000;**62**(1):149–54.

Porter S, Scully C. Aphthous ulcers (recurrent). *Clin Evid* 2003;**9**:1499–505.

Rogers RS 3rd. Common lesions of the oral mucosa. A guide to diseases of the lips, cheeks, tongue, and gingivae. *Postgrad Med* 1992;**91**(6):141–8.

Wielink G. Adviezen bij aften [Advice for aphthous ulcers]. *Huisarts Wet* 1997;**40**:389–95.

61

ORAL THRUSH IN INFANTS AND ADULTS

DEFINITION

Oral thrush is an acute pseudomembraneous candidal infection of the oral mucous membrane.

AETIOLOGY/PATHOGENESIS

Thrush is caused by *Candida*, a yeast, which is found in many people (up to 40%) as a commensal on the skin and mucous membranes (mouth, vagina) and in the stomach/intestinal tract. It is possible to isolate *Candida* from the mouth of the newborn only a few days after birth. *Candida albicans* is the most common form; however, other strains do exist.

In many cases, colonization of the skin and mucous membranes does not lead to the clinical picture of thrush infection. This can occur, however, under circumstances favourable to *Candida*, such as through the use of broad-spectrum antibiotics; *Candida* is therefore a true opportunist.

Newborns, whose immune system is not fully developed, will apparently develop thrush more readily; oral thrush is also associated with immunosuppression in older patients. Inhaled steroids may be a significant aetiological factor.

In addition to the acute pseudomembranous form, there is a chronic atrophic and a chronic hyperplastic form of candidiasis. Chronic atrophic candidiasis may affect the tongue and the area under the upper dentures; it also causes angular cheilitis. This chronic form affects approximately 40% of denture wearers.

In terms of differential diagnosis, the GP must consider leukoplakia. In this case, the top layer of the lesion cannot be scraped off, and it is usually clearly defined. It is usually painless, although it may be sensitive to touch or spicy food. Lichen planus is another possibility: this disorder does not usually cause any symptoms when it affects the mouth, but a white reticular pattern may be visible.

PRESENTATION

In newborns, the parents may have noticed one or more white patches in the mouth. Otherwise the child will appear completely healthy – pain generally seems to be mild or absent, although occasionally there may be feeding problems. An adult patient may have noticed a white patch on the oral mucosa, but may have no further symptoms. The patches can sometimes be painful. In general, however, pain is not a prominent symptom (in contrast to aphthous stomatitis, see Chapter 60). The patient's sense of taste may have decreased, and difficulty swallowing may sometimes be present. Chronic forms sometimes develop without symptoms, but are usually accompanied by dryness, burning and a bad taste in the mouth.

EPIDEMIOLOGY

In neonates and young children, prevalences of 0.5–20% have been reported; approximately 4% of all newborns (especially sick infants and premature babies) apparently experience thrush. It is less common in older children and adults, although it is rather more likely in the elderly and those in hospital (especially the immunosuppressed).

HISTORY

For infants and small children, the GP asks:

- about the type of feeding (breast or bottle) and about nipple problems, such as irritation and redness, as an infected nipple or teat may be the source of the problem
- about pain or problems with feeding
- about recent illnesses
- about use of medications (antibiotics, corticosteroids)
- about abnormalities in the nappy area.

For older children and adults, the GP asks:

- about smoking habits
- about oral hygiene
- whether the patient wears dentures, and about denture maintenance/hygiene
- about the use of inhaled steroids.
- about any pointers to immunosuppression.

EXAMINATION

The examination consists of careful inspection of the mouth. If acute thrush is present, a number of (greyish) white, somewhat raised, clearly defined patches are seen on the oral mucous membrane (especially the cheek, tongue and upper palate, but also on the gums). These patches consist of a layer adhering to the mucosa, and have a tendency to converge. In chronic atrophic candidiasis, white patches are often missing; pinkish-red maculae may be visible instead. When inspecting the mouth, pay attention to the condition of the teeth, and the fit of dentures, if present. It is important to remove the dentures and inspect the upper palate: in chronic candidiasis, the roof of the mouth is reddened. Also, patients with dentures frequently suffer from angular cheilitis (see Chapter 55). The GP can use a spatula to establish whether the visible layer can be scraped off.

TREATMENT

First, steps should be taken to eliminate any predisposing factors and to treat any underlying disorder. If no such factors are present, bear in mind that oral candidiasis is often self-limiting. However, treatment with antimycotics can accelerate resolution. Local treatment is nearly always sufficient; systemic therapy is only indicated in immunodeficient patients or for frequent recurrences. There is evidence that gels are more effective than suspensions in infants.

In infants, the treatment options are miconazole gel 20 mg/g, 2.5 ml four times daily, or nystatin suspension 100,000 units/ml, 1–2 ml after feeding four times daily.

In children and adults, there is a choice between local treatment with miconazole gel 20 mg/g, 2.5–5 ml four times daily, nystatin suspension 100,000 units/ml, 4–6 ml four times daily, amphotericin suspension 100 mg/ml, 1 ml four times daily, or amphotericin lozenges 10 mg four times daily. Gels and suspensions should be held in the mouth as long as possible before swallowing. Local treatment must be continued for at least 2 days after the lesions have disappeared. In practice, treatment lasting 7–10 days is usually sufficient. Side-effects are rare.

If there is doubt about the condition of the teeth and gums, it is desirable to obtain the opinion of a dentist or dental hygienist. Dentures should temporarily be left out as much as possible. They should also be disinfected, and corrected if necessary.

If local treatment is not effective, or in the case of frequent recurrences or immunodeficiency (such as due to acquired immunodeficiency syndrome (AIDS)), a systemic therapy is chosen (e.g. fluconazole 50–100 mg once daily for 7–14 days, or itraconazole 100 mg once daily for 14 days). If this treatment is not successful, additional tests for an underlying disorder must always be considered (e.g. a human immunodeficiency virus (HIV) test).

PREVENTION AND ADDITIONAL INFORMATION

Thrush can be prevented to a certain extent through the proper (but not over-rigorous) hygiene of nipples and teats, proper dental and denture hygiene, and so on. Information provided to the patient consists primarily of an explanation of the cause, nature and prognosis of the disorder, and how to prevent reinfection. Steroid inhalers, as used for asthma, can cause candidal infections of the mouth. Each time the steroid is inhaled the patient should rinse the mouth; spacer devices may help, too.

Key points

- There are three forms of oral thrush: acute pseudomembranous, chronic atrophic and chronic hyperplastic.
- It tends to occur in the newborn, those with impaired immunity and patients using inhaled steroids.
- In terms of differential diagnosis, the GP must consider leukoplakia. In this case, the top layer of the lesion cannot be scraped off, and it is usually clearly defined.
- Local treatment is nearly always sufficient; systemic therapy is only indicated in immunodeficient patients or for frequent recurrences.

Literature

Appleton SS. Candidiasis: pathogenesis, clinical characteristics, and treatment. *J Calif Dent Assoc* 2000;**28**(12):942–8.

Epstein JB, Polsky B. Oropharyngeal candidiasis: a review of its clinical spectrum and current therapies. *Clin Ther* 1998;**20**:40–57.

Fotos PG, Lilly JP. Clinical management of oral and perioral candidosis. *Dermatol Clin* 1996;**14**:273–80.

Van der Schroeff JG. Lokale antimycotica [Local antimycotics]. *Geneesmiddelenbulletin* 1995;**29**(7):69–71.

62

GINGIVITIS

DEFINITION

Gingivitis is an inflammation of the gums. It is nearly always chronic. Other types, such as acute gingivitis, chronic desquamative gingivitis and plasma cell gingivitis are rare.

AETIOLOGY/PATHOGENESIS

Gingivitis is almost always related to an increase in dental plaque, in which both the number of bacteria and the plaque composition change. At a microscopic level, dental plaque consists of bacteria, food particles, epithelial cells and leukocytes. Poor oral hygiene, breathing through the mouth, improperly fitting fillings and smoking are all factors that promote plaque. It is assumed that the bacteria in dental plaque result in the inflammation of the gums. An increase in anaerobic Gram-negative bacteria seems particularly important. Pregnancy, endocrine disorders, blood disorders, cirrhosis of the liver, anticonvulsant medication and general poor health can exacerbate the problem.

Another, infamous form of gingivitis is necrotizing/ulcerative gingivitis. This involves swollen, painful gums that have a strong tendency to bleed. Herpes-simplex virus can also cause gingivo-stomatitis, mainly as a primary infection in young children (see Chapter 56).

Periodontitis – infection of the bone and ligaments supporting the teeth – is always preceded by gingivitis. Although not every case of gingivitis progresses to this serious disorder, the GP should be aware of this possible complication.

PRESENTATION

Bleeding of the gums or pain when brushing the teeth are usually the reasons for the patient consulting the GP or dentist. Alternatively, the disorder may be detected while the mouth is being examined for some other reason.

EPIDEMIOLOGY

Epidemiological data are scanty, but it can be estimated that chronic gingivitis presents two or three times per year in general practice (many will not present, or will attend the dentist). One study revealed that 85% of the population had suffered gingivitis.

HISTORY

The GP asks:

- about problems with the teeth
- about the most recent visit to the dentist
- about the gums having an increased tendency to bleed when the teeth are brushed
- if the onset was acute
- about smoking habits
- about other factors, such as stress, chronic illnesses, pregnancy and medication.

In the acute form, and especially in acute necrotizing/ulcerative gingivitis, the patient may feel very unwell and usually has a fever. Increased salivation may also be present.

EXAMINATION

The examination begins by inspecting the teeth, then the gums. In chronic gingivitis, the gums change colour at an early stage (from light to dark red) as a result of hyperaemia. In addition, the gums are often swollen; swelling of the interdental papillae may give the gums a bullous appearance.

In the acute form of gingivitis, watch out for: oral fetor; reddening, swelling and tenderness of the gums; necrosis of the interdental papillae; painful cervical lymphadenopathy. The infection sometimes spreads to the oral mucosa and the clinical picture of gingivostomatitis develops. In this situation, the differential includes a spreading streptococcal throat infection.

Additional investigations are not necessary for chronic gingivitis. For acute necrotizing gingivitis and recurrences, it is sensible to carry out blood tests to rule out endocrine and blood disorders.

TREATMENT

The proper treatment of chronic gingivitis involves having a dentist remove the source of infection – dental plaque. This almost always results in healthy gums. In addition, advice about caring for the gums is necessary. The benefit of mouth rinses has not been demonstrated.

For acute gingivitis, the first course of action is to relieve the pain, prior to plaque removal. Rinsing (1–2 minutes twice daily) with 10 ml chlorhexidine 0.2% mouth rinse is advised. If there is general malaise due to a bacterial infection, a short course of a broad-spectrum antibiotic can be considered (e.g. amoxicillin 500 mg three times daily for 5 days, or metronidazole 400 mg three times daily for 5 days).

PREVENTION AND ADDITIONAL INFORMATION

Regular dental check-ups and proper care of the gums are the most important preventive measures, especially in view of the 'complication' of periodontitis. Brushing between the teeth, flossing and consistent use of toothpicks help prevent plaque.

Key points

- Gingivitis is almost always related to an increase in dental plaque.
- Poor oral hygiene, breathing through the mouth, improperly fitting fillings and smoking are all factors that promote plaque.
- In chronic gingivitis, the gums change colour at an early stage (from light to dark red) as a result of hyperaemia, and the gums are often swollen.

Literature

Abbas F, Van der Velden U, Rodenburg JP. Gingivitis en parodontitis: diagnostiek van plaque gerelateerde aandoeningen [Gingivitis and parodontitis: diagnosis of plaque-related disorders]. *Ned Tijdschr Geneeskd* 1990;**97**:152–6.

Bauroth K, Charles CH, Mankodi SM, Simmons K, Zhao Q, Kumar LD. The efficacy of an essential oil antiseptic mouthrinse vs. dental floss in controlling interproximal gingivitis: a comparative study. *J Am Dent Assoc* 2003;**134**(3):359–65.

De Jong A, Streefkerk JG. Theorie en praktijk bij gingivitis en parodontitis [Theory and practice in gingivitis and parodontitis]. *Modern Med* 1994;**18**:101–7.

Grundemann LJ, Timmerman MF, Van der Velden U, Van der Weijden GA. Reduction of stain, plaque and gingivitis by mouth rinsing with chlorhexidine and peroxyborate. *Ned Tijdschr Tandheelkd* 2002;**109**:255–9.

Hubbard TM. Periodontal disease and the family physician. *Am Fam Physician* 1991;**44**(2):487–91.

Novak MJ. Necrotizing ulcerative periodontitis. *Ann Periodontol* 1999;**4**(1): 74–8.

Research, Science and Therapy Committee of the American Academy of Periodontology. Treatment of plaque-induced gingivitis, chronic periodontitis, and other clinical conditions. *J Periodontol* 2001;**72**(12): 1790–800.

Sharma NC, Charles CH, Qaqish JG, Galustians HJ, Zhao Q, Kumar LD. Comparative effectiveness of an essential oil mouthrinse and dental floss in controlling interproximal gingivitis and plaque. *Am J Dent* 2002;**15**(6):351–5.

Quirynen M, Avontroodt P, Peeters W, Pauwels M, Coucke W, Van Steenberghe D. Effect of different chlorhexidine formulations in mouthrinses on *de novo* plaque formation. *J Clin Periodontol* 2001;**28**: 1127–36.

Van Winkelhoff AJ, et al. Tandvleesontstekingen; microbiologie en samenhang met elders in het lichaam voorkomende infecties [Infection of the gums; microbiology and relationship with infections elsewhere in the body]. *Ned Tijdschr Geneeskd* 1992;**136**:679–81.

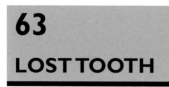

63

LOST TOOTH

DEFINITION

A tooth is usually lost because of contact trauma or a fall. The tooth can come loose from the jaw either broken or as a whole.

AETIOLOGY/PATHOGENESIS

Injuries to the teeth usually occur in children while they are playing contact sports, such as boxing, hockey, ice hockey, basketball and football. The injury involves falling, being hit with a hard object, being punched or, in rare cases, biting or chewing on a hard object.

PRESENTATION

The child, its caregivers or someone who witnessed the event explains that one or more teeth have broken off, are loose or have come out, after the child fell or was hit in the mouth with a hard object. Heavy bleeding of the mouth or lips may also be a prominent symptom.

EPIDEMIOLOGY

GPs are confronted with this problem only rarely – about once every 4 years. Clearly, the majority will attend the dentist or the local casualty department. Boys are three times more likely than girls to experience trauma to the teeth, with peaks around age 4, 8–11 and 14 years old. Injuries to baby teeth tend to cause displacement, while in permanent teeth a break of the crown or root is more common.

HISTORY

The GP asks:

- whether the tooth is a baby or permanent tooth

- how long ago the accident happened
- what happened
- whether the child can close the mouth with the upper and lower teeth in the correct position on top of each other, as before the injury
- whether the child can open the mouth wide without pain
- whether the child can move the lower jaw up and down without pain.

EXAMINATION

Inspect the entire mouth: cheeks, tongue, gums and lips. Also examine for any exposed bone, foreign bodies and loose pieces of tooth. Check whether the entire tooth has come out, or if part of it is still in the mouth. If a tooth is broken, palpate the lips to ensure there are no pieces of tooth in the lip: this can cause unpleasant scarring. Examine the face and the upper and lower jaw for possible fractures. The best way to carry out palpation of the cranium and facial bones is to sit behind the patient and use both hands. Palpate all the teeth for mobility and for possible crepitation. Always bear in mind the possibility of child abuse. If the trauma affects only the teeth, additional investigations are generally unnecessary.

TREATMENT

The assumption here is that a situation has arisen where the only help available is the GP. The patient ought to be seen by a dentist, particularly if dental assistance is available rapidly.

Telephone advice is as follows: if the lost tooth is a baby tooth and has come completely out of the jaw, do not replace it because this could damage the bud of the permanent tooth. Advise the patient to attend for an examination to assess further. In the case of a subluxed baby tooth or a broken baby tooth, refer the patient to the dentist.

In the case of avulsion of a permanent tooth, advise the patient to immediately put the tooth back in the socket and to avoid any further manipulation. If the repositioning is not successful, have the parent/patient put the tooth in a cup of milk (preferred option) or between the patient's cheek and molars (or the parent/caregiver could oblige), and to attend.

At the GP's surgery, it should be remembered that the longer the tooth is out of the mouth, the smaller the chance of permanent recovery. If the trauma took place less than half an hour previously, the chance of recovery is 90%. If the trauma occurred more than 2 hours before, this figure is only 10%.

In the case of avulsion, the GP cleans the mouth well with physiological salt or, if need be, with tap water, and removes any blood clots. The tooth is gently rinsed with physiological salt or it can be sucked clean in the mouth: it should not be washed under fast running water or brushed. Watch out for damage to the root membrane. Then put the tooth back in its socket – not much force is needed. Next, firmly compress the tooth socket between the thumb and index finger. If necessary, for pain, inject a solution of lignocaine and adrenaline right next to the bone. Then secure the tooth. The easiest and best way to do this is to use histoacryl tissue adhesive to affix the tooth to the teeth next to it. An alternative is to secure the tooth between the patient's thumb and index finger and have him go to the dentist like this.

In the case of subluxation, put the tooth back into place with the thumb and finger, and then compress the tooth socket with the thumb and index finger. Check the position of the teeth by having the patient carefully close their mouth. The subluxed tooth should never be the only tooth that makes contact. The patient should visit the dentist as soon as possible.

In the case of a broken tooth/teeth, having checked for other injury, refer the patient to the dentist – make sure the patient takes along all parts of the tooth.

Always send the patient to a dentist for assessment and follow-up, even if the repositioning and fixation of the tooth seems to be successful. Dentists are far better equipped than GPs and have the proper knowledge to assess and treat the teeth and related body parts.

If a fracture is present or suspected, the patient should be referred to an oral surgeon as quickly as possible.

PREVENTION AND ADDITIONAL INFORMATION

For risky sports, a mouth or teeth guard is essential.

Key points

- Injuries to baby teeth tend to cause displacement, while in permanent teeth a break of the crown or root is more common.

- If a tooth is broken, palpate the lips to ensure there are no pieces of tooth in the lip: this can cause unpleasant scarring.

- With this type of injury, it is important to examine the face and the upper and lower jaw for possible fractures.

- Always bear in mind the possibility of child abuse.

- If the lost tooth is a baby tooth and has come completely out of the jaw, do not replace it because this could damage the bud of the permanent tooth.

- In the case of avulsion of a permanent tooth, advise the patient to immediately put the tooth back in the socket and to avoid any further manipulation. It should be remembered that the longer the tooth is out of the mouth, the smaller the chance of permanent recovery.

- In the case of a broken tooth/teeth, having checked for other injury, refer the patient to the dentist – make sure the patient takes along all parts of the tooth.

Literature

Lohr JA. *Pediatric outpatient procedures*. Philadelphia: Lippincott 1991.

Roberts G, Scully C, Shotts R. ABC of oral health. Dental emergencies. *BMJ* 2000;**321**(7260):559–62.

Tung TC, Chen YR, Chen CT, Lin CJ. Full intrusion of a tooth after facial trauma. *J Trauma* 1997;**43**(2):357–9.

Wesselink PR. *Traumata van gebitselementen; paot-cursus Endodontologie: II* [*Traumas of the teeth: paot course Endodontology II*]. Amsterdam: Academisch Centrum Tandheelkunde Amsterdam, 1988.

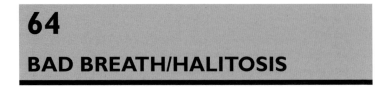

64

BAD BREATH/HALITOSIS

DEFINITION

Halitosis is an unpleasant smell in exhaled air. The individual affected does not usually notice this odour.

AETIOLOGY/PATHOGENESIS

Bacterial, metabolic and chemical factors can all play a role in this problem. Stasis in the oral cavity during the night causes a shift from predominantly Gram-positive to more Gram-negative flora in the mouth, which can result in the familiar bad breath on waking. Gram-negative anaerobic bacteria are found in the gum crevices. These bacteria produce sulphur-containing substances with a strong odour, especially in the presence of gingivitis and periodontitis. The vast majority of cases of halitosis are, in fact, linked with poor dental hygiene.

Infection in the throat cavity and paranasal sinuses, which the patient may not be aware of, is another cause. Similarly, foreign bodies in the nose can provide an explanation for the problem.

Malignancies in the oropharynx, airway and digestive tract can be accompanied by putrefaction, and an anaerobic infection in the lung can also cause a putrid odour. Certain bacteria in the large intestines can sometimes form methane compounds, which are reabsorbed and exhaled through the lungs. In addition, an insufficient cardiac sphincter of the stomach can allow unpleasant fumes to escape from the stomach.

Enzymatic digestion of the body's own protein and fat (when hungry or dieting) is accompanied by the release of substances that pass through the bloodstream to the lungs and end up being exhaled, giving an unpleasant smell to the breath. Similarly, some metabolic disorders can be linked with a certain breath odour. Examples include acetone in diabetes mellitus and metabolic acidosis (diarrhoea and vomiting) and fetor hepaticus with hepatic coma. The rare body malodour syndromes, such as fish-odour syndrome owing to decreased oxidation of trimethylamine, are also metabolic disorders.

Certain medications can cause halitosis, such as penicillin, isosorbide dinitrate and disulfiram.

Clearly, there are also substances which, after being consumed or inhaled, can cause halitosis, such as alcohol, smoking and garlic.

PRESENTATION

The nasal mucosa contain an adaptation mechanism in which, after a time, odours are no longer noticed by the person involved. So the patient is often sent to the GP by other people. Alternatively, the patient may attend for some other reason and the GP notices the problem coincidentally. Talking about the symptom may be difficult. It is important to pay attention to how and why the patient has attended. The patient may be ashamed about it, feel isolated or avoid contacts. Sometimes the complaint is only subjectively present. If the patient thinks he smells his own bad breath, but this cannot 'objectively' be confirmed by others around him, there is usually a psychological basis to the symptom.

EPIDEMIOLOGY

There are no figures available concerning the epidemiology of GP attendance for this symptom. Many patients will see their dentist about the problem. Past studies report prevalences of 8% in people under the age of 20 years to 24% of people aged 70 years and older. It is unknown how many of these had a specific underlying cause.

HISTORY

The GP asks about non-pathological clues:

- age
- morning and hunger bad breath
- diet

- medications, tobacco and alcohol.

The GP also asks about symptoms that might indicate pathological explanations:

- mouth – teeth, gingivitis/periodontitis, stomatitis, glossitis, salivary gland disorders, tumours, dehydration
- nose and paranasal sinuses – foreign bodies, symptoms of infection and tumours
- pharynx – tonsillitis, pharyngitis, foreign bodies, tumours, pouches
- digestive tract – reflux, digestive problems
- respiratory tract – symptoms of chest pathology, such as infection or neoplasm
- systemic disorders – diabetes, ketoacidosis in general, liver and kidney insufficiency, body malodour syndromes
- psychological/psychiatric – anxiety, psychotic features, hallucinations (frontal lobe abnormalities).

When taking the history, it is important to remember the patient's underlying concern and presentation. Halitosis, as a complaint for which the patient wants a solution, requires a different approach than the situation in which the symptom reflects an underlying disorder. This last group goes beyond the scope of this book; besides, in nearly all such cases, the patient already knows about the illness causing the symptom, and bad breath is not the predominant complaint.

EXAMINATION

It is important to verify the fetor objectively – and therefore to smell it. The GP should also inspect the teeth and gums, examine the rest of the mouth and check the nose and sinuses. If indicated, further physical examination (digestive tract, respiratory tract) should be carried out and additional tests (gastroscopy and chest X-ray) should be conducted, although these will seldom be necessary.

TREATMENT

Partly because the social consequences are often serious (isolation, avoidance behaviour), the, real or supposed, problem should be taken seriously.

The following measures can be recommended. For morning bad breath, patients are advised to increase their fluid intake; any nasal obstruction that might cause the patient to mouth breathe at night should be managed as appropriate. In the case of poor oral hygiene, gingivitis or periodontitis, the following are necessary: measures to remove dental plaque; rinsing with 0.2% chlorhexidine mouth rinse and combating any bacterial or mycotic infection. These recommendations should be reinforced and expanded via a consultation with a dentist or oral hygienist.

Drinking plenty of fluid is helpful for halitosis related to the diet. Limiting the amount of protein (in milk, cheese and eggs) and fat, as well as certain foods (garlic, herbs) can contribute to solving the problem. Sensible dietary advice about avoiding 'crash diets' can help.

Halitosis resulting from medications, alcohol or nicotine can be dealt with by avoiding or replacing the relevant substances.

Any underlying cause should be identified and treated as appropriate. In the case of 'non-objectifiable' halitosis, a psychological cause is likely and treatment is oriented accordingly.

If the fetor is untreatable and bothersome, the patient can try remedies from the chemist to mask the odour.

PREVENTION AND ADDITIONAL INFORMATION

As this symptom is usually caused by abnormalities on and around the teeth, it is important to emphasize the importance of oral and dental hygiene (brushing, flossing), and regular dental check-ups.

Recommendations about fluid intake (e.g. drinking enough water), as well as simple dietary advice, should be discussed when appropriate. The untreatable character of halitosis in some illnesses makes resolving the complaint next to impossible. In such a case, providing information to the family and caregivers is useful, to prevent the patient from becoming isolated. Masking the bad breath with lozenges or mouth rinses can make life easier for the patient and those around him. A good-quality air freshener can also be used.

Key points

- The vast majority of cases of halitosis are linked with poor dental hygiene.
- It is important to objectively verify the fetor – and therefore to smell it.
- Additional investigations will seldom be necessary.
- As this symptom is usually caused by abnormalities on and around the teeth, it is important to emphasize the importance of oral and dental hygiene (brushing, flossing), and regular dental check-ups.

Literature

Ratcliff PA, Johnson PW. The relationship between oral malodor, gingivitis, and periodontitis. *J Periodontol* 1999;**70**:485–9.

Replogle WH, Beebe DK. Halitosis. *Am Fam Physician* 1996;**53**(4):1215–18.

Scully C, Porter S, Greenham J. What to do about halitosis. *BMJ* 1994;**308**:217–18.

65

VIRAL CROUP

DEFINITION

Viral croup is a disorder of young children that involves shortness of breath, inspiratory stridor and a barking cough resulting from an infection of the mucosa of the larynx and trachea.

AETIOLOGY/PATHOGENESIS

The disorder is viral – usually the parainfluenza virus, but other causes include influenza A virus, influenza B virus, adenovirus and respiratory syncytial virus. The interior wall of the larynx swells up, particularly in the mucosal folds just under the vocal cords. Because of the cartilage rings, the swelling can only expand in the lumen of the larynx, and not to the periphery. This narrowing high up in the airway causes the shortness of breath, cough and the often very audible inhalation. Mucus accumulation may also be present, in addition to the inflammation of the mucous membrane. The child's agitation only serves to make the shortness of breath worse. Viral croup is usually a harmless disorder. However, rarely, the lumen can become entirely occluded in a relatively short time.

PRESENTATION

There is a typical pattern to the presentation. The GP is often called in the evening. The parent reports that the child played normally during the day, but had a bit of a cold. The child then went to bed at the normal time, but after sleeping an hour or more, woke up with shortness of breath and a cough like a seal's bark. Anyone who has ever heard this will recognize it easily, even over the phone. Parents who have never heard it before are often very worried.

EPIDEMIOLOGY

Viral croup is a disorder that usually occurs in young children aged 3 months to 3 years. It occurs very occasionally in children of school age. The incidence is 0.7–3.5 per 1000 children under 6 years old per year. It is more common in boys than girls. As for the typical seasonal peaks of virus infections, viral croup occurs more often when there is an 'R' in the month – especially in the autumn.

HISTORY

The GP asks:

- when the child began experiencing shortness of breath
- if there were symptoms earlier (during the day)
- whether the child makes noises when breathing
- whether fever is present (there may or may not be fever with viral croup, but it would be unlikely to produce a temperature above 40°C)
- whether the child has (previously) had asthmatic symptoms
- if there is any possibility of a foreign body.

EXAMINATION

Auscultation usually reveals nothing apart from the conduction of the inspiratory stridor. Rhonchi can be heard if tracheobronchitis is present, in which case the child's temperature is usually higher. An important differential is epiglottitis. In such a case, the onset is sudden, and the child is older, sicker, paler and calmer than a child with pseudo-croup. Usually, the child is unable to lie down and (characteristically) drools because he cannot swallow. If epiglottitis is suspected, the throat should not be examined.

TREATMENT

In the first (telephone) contact, the GP recommends that the parents sit with the child in a steamy bathroom or shower. It is important that the child sees the parents are calm – agitation will aggravate the problem. The parents usually accept that this will help settle the situation. It is unclear what part of this treatment is the most effective: the steam or the 'calm'. If the parents are satisfied with this reassuring advice, the GP asks them to call back to inform him about the child's progress.

However, if the parents remain anxious, or there is any diagnostic doubt, the GP should arrange to see the child to assess further. In rare cases, viral croup can cause significant airways obstruction, for which hospitalization and even intubation may sometimes be necessary.

Treatment with steam has not been scientifically evaluated, although it is not harmful – and in daily practice, steaming has often already been started by the parents before they call the GP. It is not known if it is in spite of, or thanks to, steaming that less than 5% of children with croup have to be referred to hospital. The effect of treatment with (inhaled) steroids has only been evaluated in selected populations. The guideline *Acute Coughing* from the Dutch College of General Practitioners advises, for more severe croup with stridor and tachypnoea, a once-only dose of steroid (e.g. 5 to 10 puffs with fluticasone via a spacer).

PREVENTION AND ADDITIONAL INFORMATION

When giving information to the parents, emphasize the good prognosis of viral croup and the value of the most frequently recommended remedies – steam and rest.

Key points

- Viral croup is a disorder of young children that involves shortness of breath, inspiratory stridor and a barking cough resulting from an infection of the mucosa of the larynx and trachea.
- The barking cough is instantly recognizable, even over the phone, but it may worry parents if they have never heard it before.
- An important differential diagnosis is epiglottitis.
- In rare cases, viral croup can cause significant airways obstruction.

Literature

Folland DS. Treatment of croup. Sending home an improved child and relieved parents. *Postgrad Med* 1997;**101**(3):271–3.

Kerstens JM, et al. Pseudo-kroep opnieuw bezien [Another look at pseudo croup]. *Ned Tijdschr Geneeskd* 1994;**138**(11):545–7.

Roorda RJ, Walhof ChM, Brand PL. Behandeling van laryngitis subglottica (pseudo-kroep): steroïden in plaats van stomen [Treatment of subglottic laryngitis (pseudo croup): steroids instead of steaming]. *Ned Tijdschr geneeskd* 1998;**142**:1658–62.

Rosekrans JA. Viral croup: current diagnosis and treatment. *Mayo Clin Proc* 1998;**73**(11):1102–6.

Verheij ThJM, Salome PhL, Bindels PJ, Chavannes AW, Ponsioen BP, Sacks APE, Thiadens HA, Romeijnders ACM, Van Balen JAM. NHG standaard: acuut hoesten [NHG standard: acute cough]. *Huisarts Wet* 2003;**46**(9):496–506.

66

HOARSENESS/DYSPHONIA

DEFINITION

Hoarseness is an impairment of the voice, in which the basic sound produced by the glottis has more the character of a rustle or murmur than a tone. Dysphonia includes other voice problems, such as a raspy, quiet or 'broken' voice.

AETIOLOGY/PATHOGENESIS

Hoarseness can have a number of causes. The most common are discussed below.

Acute laryngitis usually occurs as the result of an upper respiratory infection, or by heavy overtaxing of the voice during a short period.

Chronic laryngitis is mainly caused by smoking. Voice overuse can also give rise to irritation and oedema of the larynx.

Polyps, cysts and nodules are benign tumours of the vocal cords. The first two occur in people of all ages, and the last is seen particularly in children, and is probably caused by improper use of the voice.

Laryngeal carcinoma is a rare, but very important, cause of hoarseness. This symptom is an early pointer, and early treatment has a relatively good prognosis.

Paralysis of the vocal cords is caused by damage of the laryngeal nerves. This tends to happen on one side and, in general, the position of the paralysed vocal cord (medial, intermediate or lateral) determines the remaining function. The most common cause of this type of injury is iatrogenic (e.g. thyroidectomy). Other causes include trauma, tumours, neurological disease or muscular disorders.

Functional causes are quite common. Psychological stress creates increased muscle tone in the larynx. This can give rise to symptoms, such as hoarseness, a sensation of a lump in the throat, the need to clear the throat and a nervous tickly cough.

Various medications, such as diuretics, anticholinergics and antihistamines, can affect the function of the vocal cords. The use of inhaled corticosteroids can cause irritation.

Hormonal disorders, such as thyroid and growth hormone problems, or the use of anabolic steroids, can affect the larynx and thereby the voice.

Intubation (during anaesthesia) can cause damage to the larynx, which can result in short-term dysphonia.

Ageing can cause the voice to weaken, but account should be taken of the fact that the risk of tumours increases with age.

Anatomical variations can affect laryngeal structure, resulting in a weak or hoarse voice.

PRESENTATION

The patient attends with the complaint of hoarseness, raspiness or loss of the voice. The GP will sometimes also detect this disorder in a patient presenting with an entirely different complaint.

EPIDEMIOLOGY

The incidence of hoarseness in general practice is seven per 1000 patients per year; women attend with this complaint twice as often as men. There are about 3670 cases of laryngeal cancer each year in the UK. This means the average GP will see one new case every 8 years. It almost always affects those aged 50–70 years.

HISTORY

The GP asks:

- how long the symptom has been present and whether it developed acutely or gradually
- about any connection with an upper respiratory infection
- about smoking habits

- whether the patient uses inhaled medications
- about emotional stress and other psychological factors
- about any straining/overtaxing of the voice
- about symptoms of hormonal problems
- whether the patient has recently undergone anaesthesia with intubation
- whether the patient has had problems with hoarseness his entire life.

EXAMINATION

For acute hoarseness, examination of the vocal cords is not usually necessary, at least initially, as the diagnosis can be made based on the history and by listening to the voice. The GP can check for signs of an upper respiratory infection.

Additional investigations must be carried out if the hoarseness persists for longer than 3 weeks in patients aged 50 years or more, because of the risk of laryngeal carcinoma. Thorough visualization of the larynx will usually require referral to an ear, nose and throat (ENT) specialist.

TREATMENT

Acute laryngitis is generally viral and can be treated by resting the voice, using steam inhalations and not smoking. Antibiotics (e.g. amoxicillin) may be prescribed if there is secondary bacterial infection. In young people with gradually developing hoarseness, the cause is almost always chronic laryngitis. The patient should stop smoking and not overuse or force the voice.

Long-term hoarseness in children can be successfully treated by a speech therapist. The vocal nodules that sometimes accompany this are reversible, so referral to an ENT specialist is not essential. Nowadays, primary school children with voice or speech problems are often directly referred for speech therapy.

Hoarseness that is clearly functional in adults can be treated by the GP providing advice about relaxation and stress reduction.

In other cases, the treatment will depend on the underlying cause.

PREVENTION AND ADDITIONAL INFORMATION

As can be seen from the above, much of the treatment is also preventive: providing information about proper speech technique, use of medications, smoking and stress management.

Key points

- Laryngeal carcinoma is a rare but very important cause of hoarseness. Additional investigations must be carried out if the hoarseness persists for longer than 3 weeks in patients aged 50 years or more.

- Acute laryngitis is generally viral and can be treated by resting the voice, using steam inhalations and not smoking.

- Long-term hoarseness in children can be successfully treated by a speech therapist – it does not require the attention of an ENT specialist.

Literature

DaCosta SP, Damsté RH, Gerritsma EJ, et al. Stem- en spraakstoornissen [Voice and speech disorders]. *Bijblijven* 1992;**4**.

Rosen CA, Anderson D, Murry T. Evaluating hoarseness: keeping your patient's voice healthy. *Am Fam Physician* 1998;**57**(11):2775–82.

Sinard RJ. The aging voice: how to differentiate disease from normal changes. *Geriatrics* 1998;**53**(7):76–9.

67

SNORING

DEFINITION

Snoring is the production of upper airway noise via breathing during sleep.

AETIOLOGY/PATHOGENESIS

Snoring originates in those parts of the upper airway where there is no rigid support to counteract compression from outside or collapse from inside. This narrowing leads to local acceleration and turbulence of the air breathed. This, in turn, causes vibration of the floppy pharyngeal wall. The structures implicated are the soft palate, uvula, tonsils, base of the tongue, pharyngeal muscles and pharyngeal mucosa.

Many factors contribute to snoring. The palate, tongue and pharyngeal muscles play a part in keeping the airway open during the inspiratory phase of the breathing cycle. If, during the deep sleep phase, and especially during REM sleep, the muscle tone is insufficient, the tongue can fall backward due to gravity, and vibrate against the soft palate, the uvula and the pharynx. This occurs particularly in the supine position. Anatomical abnormalities can limit the passage of air in the oropharynx and the hypopharynx – such abnormalities include enlarged tonsils and adenoids, fatty tissue in the pharynx (due to obesity), and a relatively large tongue (in the case of retrognathia, micrognathia and acromegaly). A particularly long palate and uvula also narrow the nasopharyngeal opening during inspiration. An overly narrow nasal passage causes an increase in negative pressure during inspiration, which increases the effect on the floppy pharyngeal tissue. This explains why people who normally do not snore may do so when they have a cold or allergic rhinitis. Septal abnormalities, nasal polyps and tumours can also contribute to constriction.

Alcohol and hypnotics can intensify the overall effect, as can hypothyroidism and neurological disorders.

PRESENTATION

Snoring patients usually attend because their bed partner complains about the problem. They may also experience unexplained tiredness or sleepiness during the day. The snoring noise can sometimes be as loud as 50–70 dB, which is similar to the noise of a low-flying jet plane. The result may be disrupted social activities and relationship problems (and even divorce).

Sometimes, the person snoring also will stop breathing temporarily (sleep apnoea), which can be very alarming for the partner – this may be the reason for seeking help.

EPIDEMIOLOGY

Snoring is common. Research has shown that 23% of men over 35 years old snore (almost) daily. The percentage is lower for women. Of a group of women aged 50 and above, 13% snored (almost) daily. Different researchers have found evidence that hypertension, angina pectoris, myocardial infarction and cerebrovascular accidents (CVAs) may occur more often in people who snore than in those who do not – it seems that people who snore are more than three times as likely to have a CVA than people who do not.

HISTORY

The GP asks (the patient or a witness to the snoring):

- how long the snoring has been going on
- whether the snoring has recently become worse
- whether the patient's breathing stops temporarily, and is then accompanied by loud sounds when the breathing starts again
- about symptoms during the day, such as tiredness and sleepiness, or unexplained car accidents
- about the patient's occupation (especially if a public service vehicle driver)

- whether the snoring depends on the sleeping position
- about a dry throat or other symptoms on waking
- about allergies
- about weight gain
- about cardiovascular problems
- about alcohol and/or hypnotic use
- about smoking habits.

EXAMINATION

Attention is paid to the ear, nose and throat (ENT) area, particularly the tonsils, palate, uvula and tongue. Check also for nasal polyps, swollen turbinates, septal deviation, hyperreactive nasal mucosa, and abnormal anatomy of the lower jaw (relatively too small or recessed). Further examination might include weighing the patient and measuring the blood pressure. If hypothyroidism is suspected, the thyroid stimulating hormone level should be checked.

TREATMENT

If, based on the history or examination, no abnormalities that require treatment or further investigation are found, general measures can be suggested. These include: losing weight if necessary; avoiding lying on the back if the snoring is position-dependent (e.g. by attaching a tennis ball to the back of the pyjama top); and, as appropriate, discouraging smoking, alcohol consumption and the use of hypnotics. If significant ENT abnormalities are present, referral to an ENT specialist is indicated.

Any underlying causes or contributory factors, such as hypothyroidism or allergies, should be dealt with.

Mechanical devices placed in the nose and mouth only reduce snoring to a limited extent. If, in the case of habitual snoring, the patient's partner indicates that the patient temporarily stops breathing and/or the patient reports that he is sleepy and tired during the day, sleep apnoea syndrome must be considered. Referral is necessary for further assessment and treatment, particularly if simple measures result in no improvement.

PREVENTION AND ADDITIONAL INFORMATION

Attention to weight, smoking, alcohol and hypnotics, and avoiding sleeping on the back are effective preventive measures. Reassurance is sometimes appropriate, particularly if there are groundless fears about sleep apnoea.

Key points

- Snoring may disrupt social activities and cause relationship problems, so its impact should not be underestimated.
- The possibility of sleep apnoea should be considered.
- If significant ENT problems are discovered, referral is indicated.
- General measures to improve the situation include: losing weight, if necessary; avoiding lying on the back if the snoring is position-dependent; stopping smoking; reducing alcohol consumption; and stopping hypnotics.

Literature

Knuistingh Neven A, De Backer W. Snurken en het slaapapneusyndroom [Snoring and sleep apnoea syndrome]. In: Van Ree J, Lammers JWJ (eds). *Praktische Huisartsgeneeskunde: longziekten* [*Practical general practice: lung illnesses*]. Houten: Bohn Stafleu Van Loghum, 1999.

Littlefield PD, Mair EA. Snoring surgery: which one is the best for you? *Ear Nose Throat J* 1999;**78**:861–5, 868–70.

Rappai M, Collop N, Kemp S, de Shazo R. The nose and sleep-disordered breathing: what we know and what we do not know. *Chest* 2003;**124**(6):2309–23.

Trotter MI, D'Souza AR, Morgan DW. Simple snoring: current practice. *J Laryngol Otol* 2003;**117**(3):164–8.

68
SALMON PATCH/STORK MARK

DEFINITION

Salmon patches, also known as stork marks, are flat capillary haemangiomas seen on the newborn, primarily on the bridge of the nose and the eyelids, and on the neck (occasionally also on the sacrum).

AETIOLOGY/PATHOGENESIS

The aetiology is unknown. The lesion must be distinguished from the much darker naevus flammeus (port-wine stain): this is a capillary haemangioma, which can be found anywhere on the body (although especially on the head and neck) and which does not disappear spontaneously. A salmon patch does not enlarge and tends to regress spontaneously during the first year of life. The patches on the face usually disappear more quickly than those on the neck or sacrum. The naevus does not disappear completely in approximately 50% of cases. There are no known predisposing factors.

PRESENTATION

The parents of the newborn are usually worried about the nature and prognosis of the naevus. The baby is not bothered by it at all.

EPIDEMIOLOGY

Little epidemiological information is available. However, it is estimated that 30–40% of all newborns have one or more salmon patches.

HISTORY

The GP asks:

- whether the haemangioma was present at birth and, if so, whether it has increased in size.

EXAMINATION

On examination, the GP will find a flat pink patch, caused by dilated capillaries, on the eyelids and sometimes in a V-form on the forehead. A similar lesion may be found on the neck or sacrum. In contrast, a naevus flammeus is a deeper, more purplish red. The latter usually covers a larger area, is permanent and may be cosmetically disfiguring. A one-sided naevus flammeus may, especially if located on the forehead, accompany an intercranial haemangioma on the homolateral side (Sturge–Weber syndrome, which is very rare). This combination has never been reported for salmon patches.

TREATMENT

The lesions often disappear spontaneously. Even if they do not, they are almost never considered cosmetically disfiguring. A wait and see policy accompanied by reassurance for the parents is appropriate.

PREVENTION AND ADDITIONAL INFORMATION

The most important point is to inform the parents that in most cases the patch will disappear spontaneously.

Key points

- Salmon patches are flat capillary haemangiomas on the bridge of the nose and the eyelids, and on the neck (occasionally also on the sacrum) of the newborn.
- It is estimated that 30–40% of all newborns have one or more salmon patches.
- The naevus does not disappear completely in about 50% of cases.
- A salmon patch should be distinguished from a naevus flammeus – the latter is a deeper, more purplish red, covers a larger area, is permanent and may be cosmetically disfiguring.

Literature

Brown RL, Azizkhan RG. Pediatric head and neck lesions. *Pediatr Clin North Am* 1998;**45**(4):889–905.

Fishman SJ, Mulliken JB. Hemangiomas and vascular malformations of infancy and childhood. *Pediatr Clin North Am* 1993;**40**(6):1177–200.

Jolly H, Levene X. *Diseases of children*. Oxford: Blackwell, 1990.

Van Vloten WA, Degreef HJ, Stolz E, Vermeer BJ, Willemze R (eds). *Dermatologie en venereologie* [*Dermatology and venereology*]. Utrecht: Bunge, 1996.

69
CHLOASMA/MELASMA

DEFINITION

Chloasma is a type of hyperpigmentation of the face. Synonyms are melasma, melanoderma and 'mask of pregnancy' (as the hyperpigmentation may be present during pregnancy). Chloasma is derived from the Greek word *cloazein*, which means 'to be green'. The Greek *melas* means 'black', so melasma is the more correct name for this problem.

AETIOLOGY/PATHOGENESIS

The main aetiological factors are pregnancy, oestrogens and progestogens (e.g. in oral contraceptives), sunlight, cosmetics and medications. There is also a genetic predisposition. In addition, food ingredients, systemic illness, parasitic infection and nutritional deficiencies have been cited as causes. These last two factors are particularly important in countries outside Europe, but are becoming more relevant due to continuous migration.

The mechanism that causes melasma is not completely understood. It is clear, however, that sunlight plays an important role, together with hormonal factors and a familial predisposition. The end result is an increased activity of melanocytes, leading to a higher melanin production. Melasma occurs on the face because this area of skin has a high density of melanocytes and is also exposed the most to sunlight.

PRESENTATION

Patients attend with the symptom of persisting dark skin discoloration on the face, which may have been present for several years. The lesions are usually first noticed during the summer, or after a period of increased exposure to sunshine. They may have been commented on by a friend or relative, leading to a consultation.

EPIDEMIOLOGY

The exact incidence and prevalence of melasma is not known, but the condition is certainly common. It is present in varying degrees in approximately 50–75% of all pregnant women, and so can be considered part of the normal physiological changes that occur during pregnancy. Melasma is primarily seen in people with a darker skin type, especially in (dark-haired) women. The disorder occurs almost exclusively during the fertile period, and rarely in the postmenopause. Research has shown that men with melasma have the same clinical–histological characteristics as women.

HISTORY

The GP asks:

- about the duration, development and location of the lesions
- about sun exposure
- about pregnancy or gynaecological abnormalities
- about medications (oral hormone preparations, other systemic or local medications)
- about cosmetic use (face lotions, perfumes, sprays and sunscreens)
- whether family members have similar symptoms
- about any special diet
- about any symptoms of systemic illnesses.

EXAMINATION

The characteristic site and symmetry, colour and pattern of the disorder will generally lead to the diagnosis. The patchy macular hyperpigmented areas are clearly defined, initially light brown (sometimes greyish-brown) and gradually become darker. They may have a predominantly linear or a more confetti-like pattern. Additional symptoms are sometimes present, such as a burning sensation, itching or discomfort.

If the history does not suggest any systemic or gynaecological disorder, additional tests are not necessary.

TREATMENT

Because a cure is rarely possible in practice, the GP should focus on an explanation and preventive measures. The patient should be informed about the benign nature of the disorder, the treatment options and limitations, and the prognosis. If provoked by pregnancy, it is likely to resolve after delivery. If provoked by the pill, then the prognosis is more guarded.

To obtain a result that is cosmetically acceptable to the patient, a topical combination containing hydroquinone 2%, tretinoin 0.05% and hydrocortisone 1% (the latter to counteract the burning, erythema and flaking which the tretinoin can cause) can be tried. This should be applied initially every 2–3 days to limit the side-effects; the frequency can be increased later if necessary. After 4–5 weeks, the patient can expect an initially patchy, and later a more diffuse, and finally an even depigmentation. This treatment is contraindicated during pregnancy and lactation.

Particular care should be taken in darker skinned patients because of the risk of patchy depigmentation. It is recommended that the cream or lotion is first applied to a less visible area of the skin to assess the effect.

In general, treatment will have to be continued for months; the result can be pleasing and permanent if the patient uses optimum sun protection. The patient should be warned, however, of overly optimistic expectations. On pigmented skin in particular, these bleaching creams have varying results. To prevent patchy depigmentation, it may even be better not to treat the disorder. An entirely different, 'palliative', treatment is camouflage. The effect can be flawless if the cosmetics are applied carefully.

PREVENTION AND ADDITIONAL INFORMATION

When prescribing oral contraceptives, the GP can ask if there is a familial predisposition to melasma, especially in patients with dark hair. Providing information to such patients about sun habits and the use of sunscreens is advisable. Even if melasma is already present, it is a good idea to avoid direct sunlight as far as possible. The use of sunscreens with a high sun protection factor is recommended.

Pregnant women with a predisposition to melasma can be given similar recommendations. Even if a woman did not suffer from melasma during pregnancy, there is no guarantee that she will not develop it when using oral contraceptives. Women who have had melasma during pregnancy have an increased risk of this disorder if they use oral contraceptives.

Key points

- The mechanism that causes melasma is not completely understood. It is clear, however, that sunlight plays an important role, together with hormonal factors and a familial predisposition.

- The characteristic site and symmetry, colour and pattern of the disorder will generally lead to the diagnosis.

- Because a cure is rarely possible in practice, the GP should focus on an explanation and preventive measures.

- Patients with, or with a history of, this problem are well advised to avoid direct sunlight as far as possible.

Literature

Fleischer AB, Schwartzel EH, Colby SI, Altman DJ. The combination of 2% 4-hydroxyanisole (Mequinol) and 0.01% tretinoin is effective in improving the appearance of solar lentigenes and related hyperpigmented lesions in two double-blind multicenter clinical studies. *J Am Acad Dermatol* 2000;**42**:459–67.

Griffiths CE, Finkle LJ, Ditre CM, Hamilton TA, Ellis CN, Voorhees JJ. Topical tretinoin (retinoid acid) improves melasma. A vehicle-controlled, clinical trial. *Br J Dermatol* 1993;**129**:415–21.

Haddad AL, Matos LF, Brunstein F, Ferreira LM, Silva A, Costa D Jr. A clinical, prospective, randomized, double-blind trial comparing skin whitening complex with hydroquinone vs. placebo in the treatment of melasma. *Int J Dermatol* 2003;**42**(2):153–6.

Van Stralen-Bohlmann AG, Streefkerk JG. Kleine kwalen in de huisartsgeneeskunde: chloasma of zwangerschapsmasker [Minor ailments in general practice: chloasma or mask of pregnancy]. *Ned Tijdschr Geneeskd* 1995;**139**:1971–5.

70
ROSACEA

DEFINITION

Rosacea is a chronic inflammatory dermatosis that occurs on the face. It is characterized by the symmetrical presence of erythema, oedema, telangiectasia, papules and pustules on the cheeks, chin, nose and ears. The eyes can also be affected, usually with conjunctivitis and blepharitis. In men, a follicular thickening of the nose can also occur (rhinophyma).

AETIOLOGY/PATHOGENESIS

The cause of rosacea is unknown. Climatological, immunological and pharmacological factors may play a role. It can be aggravated by factors that cause vasodilatation, such as alcohol, highly spiced food or hot foods and drinks. Psychological factors (increase in flushing), vasodilatory medication, cosmetics and local corticosteroids (stronger than class 1) also aggravate the problem. Rosacea can get worse in the winter or the summer, especially during the transition from cold to warm weather, and vice versa. Bacteria probably do not play a role in the aetiology, despite the fact that antibiotics are an appropriate and effective treatment.

PRESENTATION

Only a small percentage of people with rosacea consult their GP, usually for help with the cosmetic problems caused by telangiectasia and papulopustules.

Patients with rhinophyma may receive unwelcome comments about their nose. These nasal abnormalities have traditionally been associated with alcohol use, but no such relationship exists.

EPIDEMIOLOGY

Rosacea occurs primarily in people aged 30–60 years and is more frequent in women than men; one study showed a prevalence of 14% in women and 5% in men. It occurs primarily in people with white skin. There are no good epidemiological data available from general practice.

HISTORY

An important part of the history is oriented towards establishing how much the patient is affected by the skin disorder. The GP asks:

- how long the patient has had the problem
- about any particular triggers
- whether the patient uses any topical treatment
- if the patient has sought medical help in the past, and what treatment was used at that time
- whether the patient has tried special diets for the disorder
- how other people react to it
- what medications are being used
- whether the patient has ever had significant eye symptoms.

EXAMINATION

The GP will note the symmetry of the erythema, papules, pustules and telangiectasia on the cheeks, chin, nose and ears. Differential diagnoses include acne vulgaris (comedones are present) and seborrhoeic eczema (flakiness on the scalp, in the eyebrows and in the nasolabial folds). In view of the distribution of the rash, lupus erythematosus should be considered.

TREATMENT

Rosacea is a chronic skin disorder that can be alleviated but not cured by treatment; this should be explained to the patient. It should also be pointed out that the problem may flare up again after stopping medication. Before choosing a treatment, it is important to find out which skin lesions predominate: erythema, telangiectasia and rhinophyma do not respond to local or systemic antibiotic treatment.

In a mild case with papules and pustules, the preferred remedy is metronidazole cream or gel, applied thinly twice daily for 4–6 weeks.

In more severe cases, or if local treatment is not sufficient, oral therapy with tetracycline is indicated. The initial dose is 250 mg three to four times daily for 2 weeks; this dose can gradually be reduced after 6–8 weeks, depending on the response. An alternative to oral tetracycline is oral metronidazole.

Isotretinoin is sometimes prescribed if the rosacea is very resistant to therapy – this should be initiated by a dermatologist. Rhinophyma also responds to isotretinoin, which means that plastic surgery can sometimes be avoided. Isotretinoin has potentially serious side-effects (hepatotoxicity and teratogenesis), and therefore proper information and follow-up are essential. Further detail about this treatment is beyond the scope of this book.

The patient can be referred to a dermatologist or plastic surgeon for treatment of permanent disfiguring skin abnormalities complicating rosacea. Telangiectasia can be treated with laser therapy; rhinophyma can be corrected by a plastic surgeon. The possibility of cosmetic camouflage should also be pointed out to the patient.

PREVENTION AND ADDITIONAL INFORMATION

For most patients, the frequency and intensity of the exacerbations decrease over the years. Advice should be provided about avoiding triggers that could lead to vasodilatation, and which could therefore aggravate the problem. A strict dietary regimen does not contribute significantly to the prognosis. The use of corticosteroids stronger than class 1 can make the symptoms deteriorate and should be avoided.

Key points

- Bacteria probably do not play a role in the aetiology, despite the fact that antibiotics are an appropriate and effective treatment.
- The nasal abnormalities associated with rosacea have traditionally been linked to alcohol use, but no such relationship exists.
- Differential diagnoses include acne vulgaris and seborrhoeic eczema.
- Rosacea is a chronic skin disorder that can be alleviated but not cured by treatment; this should be explained to the patient.
- Erythema, telangiectasia and rhinophyma do not respond to local or systemic antibiotic treatment.
- The use of corticosteroids stronger than class 1 can make the symptoms deteriorate and so should be avoided.

Literature

Berg M, Liden S. An epidemiological study of rosacea. *Acta Dermatol Venereol* 1989;**69**:419–23.

Blount BW, Pelletier AL. Rosacea: a common, yet commonly overlooked, condition. *Am Fam Physician* 2002;**66**(3):435–40.

Carroll S. Rosacea. *Update* 1993:542–9.

De Groot AC. De behandeling van rosacea [The treatment of rosacea]. *Geneesmiddelenbulletin* 1998;**32**(9):101–5.

Millikan L. Recognizing rosacea. Could you be misdiagnosing this common skin disorder? *Postgrad Med* 1999;**105**:149–58.

71

HEAD TREMOR IN THE ELDERLY/ TITUBATION

DEFINITION

A tremor is a rhythmic contraction of voluntary muscles, usually resulting in movement. The classic head tremor in the elderly (titubation) occurs when the patient sits erect or stands. Other names are 'senile', 'benign' and 'familial' tremor.

AETIOLOGY/PATHOGENESIS

Head tremor represents an amplified physiological tremor (frequency 1–5 Hz). The cause is unclear, but it may be due to a reduction in the availability of certain neurotransmitters. Emotion, stress and fatigue aggravate the problem. It is an autosomal-dominant disorder with variable penetration, and is classified as an essential (primary) tremor: a postural or movement tremor that occurs often (at least several times a week) or is present at all times, and is not caused by any systemic or neurological disorder, or by a drug side-effect. Being a postural tremor, it is not present when the head is supported or lying down, but does occur when the person sits erect, stands or walks.

The head tremor consists primarily of a 'yes–yes' movement, but may also occur as a 'no–no', or a combination of the two; over time, the tremor can also switch between the two.

PRESENTATION

Usually, patients consult the GP to ask if the tremor is due to Parkinson's disease, particularly as the head tremor may well be accompanied by a similar tremor of the hands/arms. The head tremor rarely leads to any functional problem.

EPIDEMIOLOGY

There is little epidemiological information available. A GP with an average list could expect to have a couple of patients with this disorder. In these cases, there may well be a family history.

HISTORY

The GP asks:

- when the tremor started and how it has developed
- whether the tremor runs in the family
- whether symptoms improve with alcohol use (alcohol characteristically relieves this type of tremor)
- when the tremor occurs – mainly when sitting or standing, or when the patient is at rest (a tremor when the patient is at rest does not support the diagnosis; consider Parkinson's disease).

EXAMINATION

Observation is usually sufficient as a diagnostic tool, particularly given the clues already gleaned by the history. Supplementary tests are rarely necessary.

To rule out other neurological disorders, watch out for signs of bradykinesia and muscle rigidity; also look for abnormal posture, and cerebellar signs, such as disturbed coordination and an abnormal gait. Have the patient stand without support. Is the head position normal? A head tremor (if the position is abnormal) can occasionally be the first symptom of spasmodic torticollis.

TREATMENT

Explanation is the cornerstone of treatment. Patients will need reassurance that this is not Parkinson's disease. They should also be informed that the clinical picture usually remains fairly stable, although it can worsen to a degree in some.

Medication is only advised if the tremor limits the ability to carry out certain activities. The first choice is propranolol. This can be used continuously or intermittently. The successful use of continuous electric thalamus stimulation has been described, although this is obviously a highly specialized treatment.

Referral to a neurologist is required only if the patient requires further reassurance, there is uncertainty about the diagnosis or there is a suspicion of an underlying dystonia.

PREVENTION AND ADDITIONAL INFORMATION

It is important to provide information and reassurance, as appropriate.

Key points

- Head tremor represents an amplified physiological tremor.
- It is not present when the head is supported or lying down, but does occur when the person sits erect, stands or walks.
- The head tremor consists primarily of a 'yes–yes' movement.
- Patients will need reassurance that this is not Parkinson's disease.

Literature

Anouti A, Koller WC. Tremor disorders. Diagnosis and management. *West J Med* 1995;**162**(6):510–13.

Dauer WT, Burke RE, Greene P, Fahn S. Current concepts on the clinical features, aetiology and management of idiopathic cervical dystonia. *Brain* 1998;**121**:547–60.

Smith DL, DeMario MC. Spasmodic torticollis: a case report and review of therapies. *J Am Board Family Pract* 1996;**9**(6):435–41.

72

BELCHING/ERUCTATION

DEFINITION

Belching, or eructation, is a physiological phenomenon in which excess air or gas from the stomach is expelled via the oesophagus through the mouth. It is clearly a normal everyday experience, but it may be viewed as a problem if it happens, or appears to happen, to excess.

AETIOLOGY/PATHOGENESIS

Chapter 91 explains the normal physiology of gas metabolism in the digestive tract. The digestive tract normally contains 100–200 ml of air/gas. Every time a person swallows, some air is swallowed as well. Without physiological belching of this swallowed gas, stomach dilatation and excess flatulence would result. Because swallowed air, as well as excess intestinal gas (which consists almost exclusively of varying proportions of nitrogen, oxygen, carbon dioxide, hydrogen and methane) has no odour, belched air is usually odourless.

The causes of abnormal belching can be divided into two main groups: gastrointestinal and psychological. Both can be subdivided into serious and harmless.

If the patient has serious gastrointestinal disorders, such as a gastric or duodenal ulcer or a malignancy, belching is seldom the only symptom. Further discussion of these pathologies is beyond the scope of this book. The significance of belching with vomiting will depend on the underlying problem – again, belching is unlikely to be the presenting complaint.

Non-sinister gastrointestinal causes include excess gas in the bowel. The digestion of carbohydrates, other complex polysaccharides (cellulose, pectin), and disaccharides (lactose, fructose) varies between individuals. The result can sometimes be significant amounts of gas in the large or small intestine. These can push on the stomach and so indirectly cause eructation. Excess gas can also be iatrogenic: lactulose, bulk-forming laxatives, and medications that affect intestinal mobility often disrupt the 'gas balance'.

Psychological, non-serious, subjective belching is often caused by eating and drinking habits: rushing, agitation, anxiety and gluttony result in air being swallowed in amounts larger than the stomach can deal with. True aerophagy – swallowing only air, without food or drink – can be a harmless cause of eructation. However, the situation is different in the rare situation where the swallowing of air is compulsive; this may be associated with a globus sensation, a food fixation, or a fear of starving in obsessive/compulsive or phobic states.

PRESENTATION

In most cases, it is the symptom itself that bothers patients (or those around them). Occasionally, the patient may fear significant underlying pathology and so require explanation and reassurance. In some cases, belching may be just one of several other somatic symptoms.

EPIDEMIOLOGY

There are no reliable data about the frequency of this symptom – epidemiological studies usually combine it with other gastrointestinal symptoms.

HISTORY

The history is focused on establishing the aetiology. The GP asks:

- about serious gastrointestinal symptoms
- about the relationship with eating and drinking
- whether the abdomen feels bloated
- about eating habits that could be the reason for excess gas
- whether the patient drinks a lot of fizzy drinks (carbon dioxide, fructose, sorbitol)
- about the use of medications, such as laxatives (lactulose).

EXAMINATION

If the GP suspects a serious somatic disorder, a focused physical examination and additional investigations should be arranged as appropriate. In such a case, eructation will usually be accompanied by other symptoms. The same is true for a psychological cause.

In most other cases, no abnormalities are found. Because the patient's main agenda may be reassurance, a careful abdominal examination is a good idea.

TREATMENT

Provide an explanation and reassurance: give instructions if the patient has incorrect eating and drinking habits; dietary advice can help control the complaint if the patient's 'food history' indicates that dietary habits may be to blame (see also Chapter 91).

In the case of minor psychological causes, an explanation giving the patient insight into the problem can be helpful.

If serious somatic or psychological causes (for which belching is very rarely a significant or sole complaint) are suspected, referral to a specialist is advised.

PREVENTION AND ADDITIONAL INFORMATION

The treatment described above, which consists primarily of the provision of information, will have a preventive effect.

Key points

- The causes of abnormal belching can be divided into two main groups: gastrointestinal and psychological.
- If the patient has significant pathology, belching will seldom be the sole symptom.
- Many patients with belching will require little more than explanation and reassurance.

Literature

Cassani VL 3rd. Anesthesia for the pediatric patient with asthma. *CRNA* 1996;**7**(4):200–6.

Rao SS. Belching, bloating, and flatulence. How to help patients who have troublesome abdominal gas. *Postgrad Med* 1997;**101**(4):263–9.

Suarez FL, Levitt MD. An understanding of excessive intestinal gas. *Curr Gastroenterol Rep* 2000;**2**(5):413–19.

Talley NJ, Stanghellini V, Heading RC, Koch KL, Malagelada JR, Tytgat GN. Functional gastroduodenal disorders. *Gut* 1999;**45**(Suppl 2):II37–42.

73

SWALLOWED COIN

DEFINITION

The concept of a 'swallowed coin' speaks for itself. The vast majority of cases involve young children.

AETIOLOGY/PATHOGENESIS

As is commonly known, small children go through a developmental stage where they tend to put everything within reach directly in their mouths. These objects are sometimes swallowed. Once a coin has passed the cardia, it will always be expelled from the body without further problems. There is a small risk that the coin could get stuck in the oesophagus: complications include fistula development, stricture and even perforation of the oesophagus. However, these serious complications occur very rarely. Problems usually only occur if the coin swallowed is larger than 20 mm in diameter.

PRESENTATION

Most swallowed coins do not cause any symptoms. The parents will be worried about whether the coin will pass through or cause any damage. If the coin has become stuck in the oesophagus, the child may complain of pain, vomiting, excessive salivation and pain when swallowing.

EPIDEMIOLOGY

It is unknown how often GPs are confronted with patients who have swallowed coins. Various studies have shown that coins are the most frequently swallowed foreign objects. This usually occurs in children younger than 7 years old. The proportion of coins that become stuck in the oesophagus varies in the literature from less than 1% to 20%.

HISTORY

The GP asks:

- when the coin was swallowed (it is important to ensure that the coin was indeed swallowed rather than inhaled)
- about the size of the coin
- whether the patient is experiencing pain, excessive salivation, shortness of breath or vomiting (bearing in mind possible oesophageal complications).

EXAMINATION

If there are no symptoms, additional tests are not indicated, except if it is certain that the coin swallowed is larger than 20 mm in diameter, in which case an X-ray should be taken of the oesophagus (two views) to see if the coin has stuck.

TREATMENT

If, in the case of a coin less than 20 mm in diameter, no symptoms are present, a wait and see approach is advised. Most coins will pass without complications. Checking the faeces is unpleasant and inaccurate, and therefore not useful. The parents must look out for any relevant symptoms, which can sometimes develop a few days after the event. If, within 3 days, there are complaints of pain, vomiting, excessive salivation, unexplained poor appetite or shortness of breath, an X-ray of the oesophagus is indicated. There are then three possibilities. If a coin is visible in the upper part of the oesophagus, it must be removed. If it is in the distal oesophagus, it is reasonable to observe for a further 24 hours, as the coin may still progress. Finally, if no coin is visible, it is possible to continue to observe if the symptoms settle rapidly; if the symptoms persist or are severe, the child must be referred to the surgical team.

PREVENTION AND ADDITIONAL INFORMATION

It is better to prevent than cure this situation: make sure no coins are lying around if small children are in the area. If a coin is swallowed, the GP can explain to the parents and the child that the coin will almost always pass through the entire digestive tract and be expelled from the body without problems.

Key points

- Problems usually only occur if the coin swallowed is larger than 20 mm in diameter.
- Once a coin has passed the cardia, it will always be expelled from the body without further problems.
- Most swallowed coins do not cause any symptoms.
- It is important to ensure that the coin was indeed swallowed rather than inhaled.
- Relevant symptoms can sometimes take days to develop.

Literature

Conners GP, Chamberlain JM, Ochsenschlager DW. Symptoms and spontaneous passage of esophageal coins. *Arch Pediatr Adolesc Med* 1995;**149**(1):36–9.

Lehmann CU, Elitsur Y. Keep the change, doc! Coins in the upper GI tract of children. *W V Med J* 1995;**91**(1):13–15.

Stringer MD, Capps SNJ. Rationalising the management of swallowed coins in children. *BMJ* 1991;**302**:1321–2.

74

TIETZE'S SYNDROME

DEFINITION

Tietze's syndrome, also called costochondritis, is characterized by pain at the costochondral junction, usually affecting the upper ribs. It is caused by a non-purulent inflammation of the rib cartilage.

AETIOLOGY/PATHOGENESIS

The exact cause of Tietze's syndrome is unknown. It may be triggered by heavy physical labour or trauma to the rib cage. Other possible aetiological factors are respiratory tract infections, minor injuries and the presence of polyarthritis.

The rib cartilage may remain swollen for several months to 3 years, even if the pain has long since disappeared.

PRESENTATION

The patient complains of pain in the chest. Swelling may appear later. If the pain is acute and on the left side of the chest, the patient may fear a myocardial infarction.

EPIDEMIOLOGY

Tietze's syndrome is a relatively rare disorder, which can occur at any age. Accurate epidemiological data are sparse.

HISTORY

Tietze's syndrome, which is harmless, must be distinguished from other disorders – some serious – which can cause pain in the chest.

The GP asks:

- when the pain began
- how it has developed
- what brings the pain on or aggravates it
- if the pain is present all the time
- where the pain is located and about any radiation
- whether the patient has ever experienced this pain in the past
- whether the patient has noticed palpitations, shortness of breath, sweating or nausea
- whether the patient is coughing up sputum
- whether the patient has a fever.

EXAMINATION

In general, there are no objective findings. Occasionally, there may be a warm swelling or local redness of one or more costosternal joints. The upper ribs are usually affected. Often, the only physical sign is tenderness on firm palpation. Further physical examination (blood pressure, pulse, heart and lungs) may be necessary to check for other disorders that can cause similar symptoms.

TREATMENT

Tietze's syndrome is a harmless disorder. The treatment consists first of reassuring the patient. Painkillers (e.g. paracetamol or non-steroidal anti-inflammatory drugs) may also be advised or prescribed.

PREVENTION AND ADDITIONAL INFORMATION

Prevention is not possible, as Tietze's syndrome usually develops unexpectedly and acutely. The patient should be reassured about the harmless character of the disorder and that the rib cartilage may remain swollen for a long time, even after the pain has disappeared.

Key points

- Tietze's syndrome is an inflammation of the costochondral joint, usually affecting the upper ribs.
- The swelling of the rib cartilage may persist for months or even years.
- The syndrome is harmless but must be distinguished from other – potentially more serious – causes of pain in the chest.

Literature

Aeschlimann A, Kahn MF. Tietze's syndrome: a critical review. *Clin Exp Rheumatol* 1990;**8**:407–12.

Jurik AG, Graudal H. Sternocostal joint swelling – clinical Tietze's syndrome. Report of sixteen cases and review of the literature. *Scand J Rheumatol* 1988;**17**(1):33–42.

75
CRACKED NIPPLES

DEFINITION
Cracked nipples are cracks in the skin of the areola and nipple.

AETIOLOGY/PATHOGENESIS
Cracked nipples only occur in women during lactation. Various factors play a role. The most important is incorrect positioning of the nipple in the baby's mouth – this relates to how the baby is held to the breast. The baby often lies too low and with the head turned to its mother's breast, which means the nipple is 'pulled on' in two directions. Other factors include the constant moisture of the nipple and areola due to lactation, suckling on tender skin (a nipple that is not yet 'hard'), and overly dry, chapped skin. The presence of infection (e.g. fungal) is rare.

PRESENTATION
The complaint of painful nipples usually arises soon after the baby's birth. True cracked nipples can develop in the days that follow. The woman will say that the pain is most severe during breast-feeding.

EPIDEMIOLOGY
There are no reliable data about the incidence of cracked nipples. They occur in most nursing mothers, especially after the first child. The problem develops very rapidly and usually lasts several days.

HISTORY
The GP asks:

• about how the baby is held to the breast

- about symptoms of dry, chapped skin
- about whether the patient's bra is too tight
- whether the nipples are dry between feeds
- if absorbent pads are changed when damp between feeds
- whether disinfectant sprays, ointments or creams are used (which may cause hypersensitivity reactions).

EXAMINATION

First, the nipple and the areola are inspected. The GP checks for visible lesions, moisture, maceration or dryness, and signs of allergic skin reactions or skin infections. In addition, the GP checks for signs of mastitis. The baby's mouth is examined for oral infections such as thrush.

Further investigation is usually unnecessary.

TREATMENT

The presence of cracked nipples, however painful they may be, is seldom a reason to stop breast-feeding completely. The most important action is to explain the correct way to hold the baby to the breast. Typical advice is as follows: use a pillow to lay the baby on, or hold the baby under the arm, with its head right in front of the nipple and the legs under the mother's arm. It is better to breast-feed more often, and to begin with the least painful breast, than to postpone feeding in an attempt to give the breast a sufficient recovery period – if this is done, the baby will suck even harder and negate any improvement that may have occurred. The usefulness of nipple ointments, nipple protectors, etc. has not been demonstrated.

Local skin infections with *Candida albicans* – and thrush in the baby's mouth – should be treated (e.g. with miconazole).

PREVENTION AND ADDITIONAL INFORMATION

Preventive measures reflect the action advised above in 'Treatment'. Information and instruction about properly holding the baby to the breast is the key – the midwife or health visitor will be invaluable here. This type of information can be provided during the pregnancy, too – again via the midwife or health visitor, or through the numerous other support agencies. Using chlorhexidine to prevent cracked nipples has not been shown to be more effective than normal washing with water.

Key points

- The most important aetiological factor is incorrect positioning of the nipple in the baby's mouth, and this relates to how the baby is held to the breast.
- Fungal infection, as a cause, is rare.
- It is better to breast-feed more often, and to begin with the least painful breast, than to postpone feeding.

Literature

Oldenziel JH, Flikweert S, Giessen PHJ, et al. NHG-standaard: zwangerschap en kraambed [NHG standard: pregnancy and the period after birth]. In: Thomas S, Geijer RMMM, Van der Laan JR, Wiersma TJ (eds). *NHG-standaarden voor de huisarts* [*NHG standards for the general practitioner*]. Utrecht: NHG, 1996.

Olsen C, Gordon R. Breast disorders in nursing mothers. *Am Fam Physician* 1990;**47**:1509–16.

Prachniak GK. Common breastfeeding problems. *Obstet Gynecol Clin North Am* 2002;**29**(1):77–88.

Tait P. Nipple pain in breastfeeding women: causes, treatment, and prevention strategies. *J Midwifery Womens Health* 2000;**45**(3):212–15.

76

MASTOPATHY/ PAINFUL BREASTS

DEFINITION

'Mastopathy' is a collective description of various problems of one or both breasts, which can occur both in women and men. For the purposes of this chapter, mastopathy describes breast tissue that feels firm, nodular and irregular, which is tender when palpated and sometimes spontaneously painful, especially premenstrually in women. This definition includes both patient symptoms and examination findings. Terms such as 'mastalgia', 'mastodynia' and 'fibrocystic breast disease' are sometimes used, but these only represent a part of the problem. Some are strongly in favour of calling the complaint simply 'pain in the breasts'.

AETIOLOGY/PATHOGENESIS

Mastopathy can be divided into: cyclical symptoms, non-cyclical symptoms and pain in the chest wall. Both hormonal and psychological mechanisms are often regarded as causes, although clear evidence is lacking.

Cyclical symptoms. Cycle-related symptoms in both breasts are often reported, primarily during the premenstrual phase. Such patients can sometimes suffer from the symptoms for several weeks. It is assumed that the changing levels of oestrogens, progestogens and prolactin influence the sensitivity of the breast glandular tissue. The increased premenstrual circulation and fluid retention are simply physiological processes.

Non-cyclical symptoms. In a minority of women, the complaints are actually reported independent of the menstrual cycle. The symptoms are then often present in one breast and are usually easy to locate. Previous trauma or infection, or the presence of a (fibro)adenoma or cyst may provide the explanation.

Pain in the chest wall. The cause of the pain is not the breast itself, but the surrounding tissue, such as ribs (Tietze's syndrome, see Chapter 74) and muscles.

Mastopathy in itself is not associated with a higher risk of developing breast cancer. However, women with a family history of breast cancer (especially under the age of 50 years) have a higher risk, and therefore should be assessed particularly carefully.

PRESENTATION

The patient complains of pain in one or both of the breasts, which may vary in intensity during the menstrual cycle. Usually, the concern is the symptom itself, but in some cases fear of breast cancer may be significant. Women sometimes have such severe symptoms that problems develop with work, sport and relationships.

EPIDEMIOLOGY

Research in the USA indicates that breast symptoms occur very frequently in selected populations, but GPs see a relatively small number of women with symptoms in one or both breasts. The prevalence of mastopathy is age-dependent: the highest prevalence is found in the 45- to 54-year-old age group, with 41 cases per 1000 persons. In those over the age of 45 years, about 70% suffer breast pain sufficient to cause distress or interfere with their daily routine. Two-thirds have cyclical pain, the remainder non-cyclical.

HISTORY

The GP asks:

- about the relationship with the menstrual cycle
- about the character of the pain – diffuse in one or both breasts, or pain that can easily be localized – and about pain severity
- about whether the symptoms are dependent on position or movement, which can indicate an extra-mammary problem
- whether the patient has noticed a lump or nipple discharge
- about the use of hormonal treatments
- whether breast cancer runs in the family.

EXAMINATION

It is obviously important to differentiate between mastopathy and a breast carcinoma. The GP assesses whether there is a difference in appearance between the breasts, such as colour differences or skin retraction. Examination should focus on excluding a discrete lump.

In the case of mastopathy, during palpation the breasts are usually tender, nodular and irregular. It is important to determine whether there is one localized painful or tender spot. During this examination, the GP should also assess whether the axillary glands are palpable.

TREATMENT

The presence of a discrete lump necessitates referral.

Patients who have clear cycle-dependent symptoms, in whom the examination findings (tender, nodular, irregular) reinforce the diagnosis of mastopathy, should be reassured with a clear explanation and advice about analgesia. A variety of treatments (e.g. tamoxifen, danazol, bromocriptine, progestogens, evening primrose oil, diuretics and vitamin E or B_6) have been tried for mastopathy, but no beneficial effect has been scientifically proven.

Mild non-cyclical pain also requires only reassurance. Severe, diffuse non-cyclical pain may require treatment such as non-steroidal anti-inflammatory drugs or danazol. Severe localized non-cyclical pain warrants referral, although pain is only very rarely a presenting symptom of breast cancer.

Hormonal contraceptives can often reduce the symptoms of mastopathy. Conversely, a link can sometimes be made between the symptoms and hormonal treatments, in which case the treatment may need to be changed or stopped.

PREVENTION AND ADDITIONAL INFORMATION

An explanation and reassurance are important if the symptoms are clearly cycle related and bilateral, and if no palpable abnormalities are found in the examination. Pain in the breast is only rarely a pointer towards malignancy.

Key points

- Mastopathy can be divided into cyclical symptoms, non-cyclical symptoms and pain in the chest wall.
- In some cases, fear of breast cancer may be significant and should be addressed.
- The prevalence of mastopathy is age-dependent: the highest prevalence is found in the age group 45–54 years.
- The presence of a discrete lump necessitates referral.
- Severe localized non-cyclical pain warrants referral, although pain is only very rarely an initial symptom of breast cancer.

Literature

Austoker, Mansel. Guidelines for referral of patients with breast problems. Department of Health Advisory Committee on Breast Cancer Screening. London: Department of Health.

Den Heeten GJ, Van Rooij WJJ, Roukema JA. Echografie is van belang als aanvullend onderzoek bij mammografie [Echography is important as an additional test for mammography]. Ned Tijdschr Geneeskd 1993;**137**: 2378–83.

El-Wakeel H, Umpleby HC. Systematic review of fibroadenoma as a risk factor for breast cancer. Breast 2003;**12**(5):302–7.

Knuistingh Neven A, De Bock GH. Mastopathie [Mastopathy]. Modern Med 1999;**23**(5):447–50.

Mehta TS. Current uses of ultrasound in the evaluation of the breast. Radiol Clin North Am 2003;**41**(4):841–56.

Miers M. Understanding benign breast disorders and disease. Nurs Stand 2001;**15**(50):45–52.

Roukema JA, Van der Heul C. Pijn in de borsten [Pain in the breasts]. Ned Tijdschr Geneeskd 1998;**142**:628–33.

77

ENLARGED BREASTS IN MEN/ GYNAECOMASTIA

DEFINITION

The term 'gynaecomastia' is generally used if there is clear hypertrophy of the mammary gland in a male. The most useful practical definition is: the presence of a palpable disc of breast tissue in men, measuring a minimum of 2 cm in diameter. If the breast is enlarged due to fat accumulation, this is referred to as 'pseudo-gynaecomastia'.

AETIOLOGY/PATHOGENESIS

It is generally assumed that gynaecomastia occurs due to a disruption in the hormonal balance between oestrogens and androgens. A preponderance of oestrogen results in stimulation of the growth of mammary gland tissue. The cause varies according to the age group. In neonates, the breast glands in both girls and boys often become enlarged due to the effect of maternal oestrogens. It is frequently possible to squeeze some fluid out of the nipple. This type of swelling disappears spontaneously over several weeks. Gynaecomastia in (pre)puberty can usually be explained by a temporary change in the aforementioned hormonal balance. It is also possible that, in some boys, breast gland tissue is hypersensitive to the influence of oestrogens. In older men, the phenomenon occurs due to a gradual decrease in androgen production, with a concomitant increase in oestrogen. So, in the great majority of cases, gynaecomastia is physiological in nature – even in severe cases, no demonstrable cause is present in 50–75% of patients.

The GP should be aware of organic causes, such as primary hypo-gonadism (e.g. Klinefelter's syndrome), secondary hypogonadism (e.g. testicular atrophy, orchitis, hypophyseal tumour), elevated oestrogen or gonadotrophin production (e.g. testicular tumour, adrenal cortex tumour, obesity), medications (e.g. sex hormones, finasteride, spironolactone, cimetidine, verapamil) and the use of marijuana and amphetamines. Other rare causes include hyperthyroidism, liver disorders and breast carcinoma.

PRESENTATION

Other than the apparent swelling, gynaecomastia is asymptomatic and, in most cases, bilateral. In newborns, the parents often attend concerned about the discharge from the child's breasts (the 'witches' milk'). In puberty, the reason is usually worry about the cosmetic appearance. If the symptom occurs on one side, then fear of breast cancer may be the reason for consultation.

EPIDEMIOLOGY

No reliable figures are available. The prevalence in puberty varies from 5% to 64%, depending on the diagnostic criteria. Gynaeco-mastia occurs most often at age 14 years, after which the incidence declines rapidly. After age 20 years, the frequency increases again, and enlarged breast glands are often found in men over 60 years old (72%). Only a small percentage of affected men visit their GP with the symptom of gynaecomastia. A study of men aged 20–30 years revealed an incidence of 2 to 3 per 1000 patients per year.

HISTORY

The GP asks:

- about the reason for the visit, such as cancer fear or cosmetic problems
- about pain and/or nipple discharge
- about the use of medications or illicit drugs
- about symptoms of liver disorders (remember alcohol) and thyroid disorders
- whether the patient has gained or lost a lot of weight.

EXAMINATION

The GP assesses whether unilateral or bilateral enlargement is present, whether the swelling is irregular or firm, and whether enlarged lymph glands are present. Be aware of obesity and/or weight loss, signs of hyperthyroidism, abnormal masses in the abdomen (hepatic enlargement, adrenal gland tumour); the testicles should be palpated for asymmetry, swelling or atrophy.

Only if the history or physical examination has suggested a pathological process, or if the swelling is unilateral, should additional tests or a referral be organized. Primary breast cancer is rare if no other palpable or visible abnormalities are present.

TREATMENT

If the history and examination suggest no underlying cause, the GP can reassure the patient and possibly conduct a follow-up check in 3–6 months. Gynaecomastia during puberty spontaneously disappears within 2 years in 92% of cases. If the abnormality has been present for a longer period, further tests may be carried out or the patient can be referred. In gynaecomastia in older men, spontaneous regression does not occur.

For idiopathic gynaecomastia causing significant cosmetic problems, surgery can offer a solution. Medical treatment has not yet been properly evaluated, although encouraging results have been reported for treatment with the anti-oestrogens clomiphene and tamoxifen and the anti-gonadotrophin danazol.

PREVENTION AND ADDITIONAL INFORMATION

After a careful evaluation, the management of gynaecomastia will in most cases consist of emphasizing the physiological and harmless character of the abnormality. Gynaecomastia does not result in an increased risk of breast cancer at a later stage.

Key points

- The most useful definition of gynaecomastia is: the presence of a palpable disc of breast tissue in men, measuring a minimum of 2 cm in diameter.

- In the great majority of cases, gynaecomastia is physiological.

- Only if the history or physical examination has suggested a pathological process, or if the swelling is unilateral, should additional tests or a referral be organized.

- For idiopathic gynaecomastia causing significant cosmetic problems, surgery may be indicated.

- Gynaecomastia during puberty spontaneously disappears within 2 years in 92% of cases.

Literature

Daniels IR, Layer GT. Gynaecomastia. *Eur J Surg* 2001;**167**(12):885–92.

Lazala C, Saenger P. Pubertal gynecomastia. *J Pediatr Endocrinol Metab* 2002;**15**(5):553–60.

Mathur R, Braunstein GD. Gynecomastia: pathomechanisms and treatment strategies. *Horm Res* 1997;**48**(3):95–102.

Meijman FJ. Gynaecomastie bij jong volwassenen [Gynaecomastia in young adults]. *Huisarts Wet* 1987;**30**:138–40.

Meyboom RHB, et al. Galactorroe en gynaecomastie als bijwerking van geneesmiddelen [Galactorrhoea and gynaecomastia as a side effect of medications]. *Ned Tijdschr Geneeskd* 1993;**137**:2498–503.

Warmerdam PE, Mulder Dzn JD. Kleine kwalen in de huisartsgeneeskunde; gynaecomastie [Minor ailments in general practice; gynaecomastia]. *Modern Med* 1989;**13**:1047–51.

78

UMBILICAL PROBLEMS IN INFANTS

DEFINITION

Umbilical problems in infants involve the presence of fluid or abnormal tissue in the navel area after the umbilical cord has fallen off. Such problems include an umbilical hernia, an infection of the navel area, a polyp and an umbilical granuloma.

AETIOLOGY/PATHOGENESIS

The umbilical cord starts to dry up several hours after birth. It will come loose from the underlying skin after about 5 days, and the navel stump normally falls off by the ninth day. If this does not happen, an umbilical hernia may develop, in which the peritoneum bulges out through the defect.

Despite careful drying and cleaning, the navel can remain moist after the tenth day. There may be discharge in the form of pus or mucus – and, rarely, urine and/or faeces.

Granulation tissue indicates chronic inflammation. Very rarely, a bright red polyp will produce mucus or a faecal discharge – this is likely to be a remaining part of the vitelline duct. In similarly obscure cases, the polyp is a remaining part of the urachus: mucosa from the urinary tract, covered in urothelium, which can result in the excretion of urine via the umbilicus.

PRESENTATION

Neither an umbilical hernia nor a navel granuloma are a problem for the infant, but they may concern the parents or caregivers. After 10 days, the navel should be dry and closed. If this is not the case, the parents will want to know what should be done. If a hernia is present, the parents are usually worried because of the abnormal appearance of the navel when the child cries or strains. In the case of a navel granuloma, the GP is usually consulted by the midwife, health visitor or practice nurse.

EPIDEMIOLOGY

There are no good epidemiological data on navel problems in infants in primary care. Figures from specialist practice report some degree of umbilical herniation in 20% of newborn babies. This prevalence is higher in premature babies and in situations involving increased abdominal pressure.

HISTORY

The questions are focused on distinguishing between the disorders mentioned. The GP asks:

- whether the skin around the navel bulges, is blue and/or feels harder if the child cries and strains (points toward an umbilical hernia)
- about general symptoms of illness, fever, malaise and possible weight loss
- whether the skin is noticeably pinkish-red and moist after the navel stump has fallen off (in the case of granuloma)
- whether there is bright red, abnormal tissue at the site of the navel stump (indicates a polyp).

EXAMINATION

For an umbilical hernia, the size of the defect is inspected and noted so the natural progression can be followed. If a navel infection is present, the infant may be unwell. An examination of the navel will reveal local inflammation; the surrounding skin is often infected as well. In the case of a navel granuloma, the infant is not ill. The spot where the navel stump has fallen off is moist and pinkish-red granulation tissue is present. Polyps are covered with mucosa and are bright red in colour.

TREATMENT

Most umbilical hernias close spontaneously, usually within the first year. Because improvement can also occur over the following 2 years, surgical intervention is not advised before the third year, unless the neck of the hernia is larger than 2 cm at the time of the child's first birthday, in which case spontaneous closure is very unlikely.

If the spot where the navel stump has fallen off is moist, the treatment involves cleaning the area, possibly with a disinfectant liquid (alcohol 70%, povidone iodine 10% solution, chlorhexidine 2.5% solution). Navel infections must be treated with an antiseptic dressing; parenteral administration of antibiotics is usually necessary. If the child is unwell, this treatment should preferably take place in consultation with a paediatrician.

Small granulations can be dabbed with silver nitrate two to three times daily; the surrounding skin should be protected with Vaseline. These small granulations usually also disappear without specific treatment, as long as the site is kept properly clean. If a navel granuloma does not improve despite treatment with silver nitrate, electrocauterization can be considered.

Surgical treatment is indicated for polyps.

PREVENTION AND ADDITIONAL INFORMATION

Careful cleaning and drying of the navel stump is the most important preventive measure. In the case of an umbilical hernia, a number of practical points must be discussed with the parents, such as the fact that most hernias spontaneously disappear and that it is safe to watch and wait. The thin skin will not tear, and strangulation virtually never occurs. It should be emphasized that the fact that the hernia feels harder when the child is crying is not a sign of pain.

Key points

- Neither an umbilical hernia nor a navel granuloma are a problem for the infant, but they may concern the parents or caregivers.

- If a navel infection is present, the infant may be unwell – liaison with a paediatrician, or referral, may be necessary.

- Surgery is not advised for umbilical hernias before the third year, unless the neck of the hernia is larger than 2 cm at the time of the child's first birthday, in which case spontaneous closure is very unlikely.

- It should be explained to worried parents that crying causes the umbilical hernia to protrude more, as they may interpret this the other way round.

Literature

Illingworth RS. *The normal child. Some problems of the early years and their treatment.* Edinburgh: Churchill Livingstone, 1991.

Jones PG, Woodward AA (eds). *Clinical paediatric surgery. Diagnosis and management.* Victoria: Blackwell Scientific Publications, 1989.

Wooltorton E. Noninvasive treatments for umbilical granulomas. *Am Fam Physician* 2003;**67**(4):698.

79
NAPPY RASH

DEFINITION

Nappy rash is a skin disorder in children that develops due to the use of nappies. The most common symptoms are redness, flakiness and itching.

AETIOLOGY/PATHOGENESIS

The skin under the nappy is usually wet: it is the function of the nappy to ensure that the infant's urine and faeces do not get all over the child's bed or clothes. The nappy shifts in relation to the skin as the child moves, and this friction damages the wet skin. The presence of urine raises the pH (i.e. lowers the acidity) of the environment on the skin under the nappy. Enzymes present in the faeces (proteinases and lipases) are activated by the increased pH and cause further harm to the damaged skin. There does not seem to be any specific link between ammonia and the occurrence of nappy rash. However, it has been found that *Staphylococcus aureus* and *Candida albicans* are much more likely to be present on the skin of infants who suffer from nappy rash than infants who do not. If the rash has been present for 3 days or more, the presence of *C. albicans* is almost inevitable. Acidic bile salts may also be a factor in this disorder, but the mechanism involved is not clear.

Research has been conducted on the effect of cotton and paper nappies, both combined with plastic pants. The study showed that paper nappies caused nappy rash less often.

PRESENTATION

The parents consult the GP because their child is crying and whimpering and has a red bottom. They may well be most bothered by the unpleasant appearance of the rash. The child may also be referred by the health visitor.

EPIDEMIOLOGY

Almost all babies have nappy rash at some time. Approximately one-third of parents consult their GP for this problem. However, because of the easy availability of anti-fungal and anti-yeast creams at the chemist, many cases are not presented. The incidence is highest in children aged 7–15 months.

HISTORY

The GP asks:

- if the symptoms (if any) appear to be the result of the rash (there may be some other reason why the child is crying or unsettled)
- what kind of nappies are used
- how often the child is changed
- about any other skin abnormalities.

EXAMINATION

Inspecting the skin is nearly always sufficient to make the diagnosis: there is diffuse erythema with vesicles, erosions, papules and nodules. Be sure to inspect all the baby's skin to check for other abnormalities, such as constitutional eczema. Secondary infection with *Candida* is characterized by a clearly defined edge with small patches outside of the area, the so-called 'satellite lesions'.

Additional tests are almost never necessary.

TREATMENT

The severity of the rash determines the therapy. In early nappy rash, zinc oxide cream may be sufficient. If there is a secondary infection with *Candida*, an antimycotic (e.g. miconazole cream) can be applied – or it can be added to zinc oxide cream. If the nappy rash is very severe or persistent, hydrocortisone cream may also be used.

PREVENTION AND ADDITIONAL INFORMATION

Preventive measures are aimed at minimizing irritation due to moisture, faeces, etc. as much as possible. Therefore, the time for which the baby wears a wet nappy should be kept as short as possible, so the baby should be changed frequently. The parents should also be advised to wash the infant's bottom with lukewarm water (not with soap) and rub in baby oil to reduce the friction between the nappy and the skin. If possible, cotton nappies should be replaced by paper nappies.

Key points

- Do not assume that nappy rash is the reason for a fretful of crying child.
- If nappy rash has been present for 3 days or more, the presence of *C. albicans* is almost inevitable.
- In prevention and treatment, the time the baby wears a wet nappy should be minimized.

Literature

Prasad HR, Srivastava P, Verma KK. Diaper dermatitis – an overview. *Ind J Pediatr* 2003;**70**(8):635–7.

Scowen P. Nappy rash: let's give mothers more help. *Prof Care Mother Child* 2000;**10**(1):26–8.

80
VAGINAL BLOOD LOSS IN INFANTS

DEFINITION

Vaginal blood loss in infants involves a macroscopically visible blood loss from the vagina in infant girls up to 1 year of age.

AETIOLOGY/PATHOGENESIS

Vaginal blood loss in infants is usually a physiological phenomenon in newborn girls. Shortly before birth, a female foetus has a well-developed endometrium due to the influence of the oestrogen and progestogen hormones formed in the placenta. Some of these maternal hormones cross over to the foetal blood system and, especially in the final weeks of pregnancy when the levels are highest, differentiation of the foetal uterine mucosa takes place. After birth, this atrophies because the hormonal stimulation is no longer present. Shedding of the mucosa, and secretion products formed before birth, cause a vaginal mucus discharge in the newborn. Occasionally, this mucus can be mixed with a little blood.

Much rarer causes of vaginal blood loss in infants include trauma, vulvovaginitis, genital tumours and hormonal disorders. Remember sexual abuse as a cause of traumatic lesions in infants under 1 year of age. Foreign bodies in the vagina can produce a bloody discharge, but are rare in infants.

Blood loss from the vagina must be differentiated from rectal blood loss and haematuria. Urate in an infant's urine can be similar in appearance to blood, causing a brick-red discoloration in the nappy. On occasion, dermatological disorders of the anogenital region can also be the cause of blood in the nappy.

PRESENTATION

The child's parent or caregiver consults the GP because blood was found in the infant's nappy. The nappy is often brought along as evidence of the blood loss.

EPIDEMIOLOGY

Physiological vaginal blood loss occurs in an estimated 3–10% of newborn girls. This blood loss begins between the second and tenth day after birth, and continues for a maximum of a week. The amount of blood lost is usually small; heavier bleeding can occur sporadically. There are no data available about the incidence in general practice. Often, the midwife or health visitor will be the person the parents first consult about the symptom. Pathological causes of vaginal blood loss in infants must be considered if the bleeding begins more than 2 weeks after birth.

HISTORY

The GP asks:

- when (postpartum) the bleeding started
- about the amount and duration of the blood loss
- how certain the parents are of the source of the blood loss
- about a possible cause (e.g. lesions caused by safety pins)
- about the presence of vaginal discharge and its colour and consistency.

EXAMINATION

If, based on the history and inspection of the nappy, it seems likely the vaginal blood loss is physiological, no further assessment is necessary. If there are deviations from the physiological pattern (first manifestation more than 2 weeks after birth, a large amount or long duration, doubt about the source of the bleeding) further examination is necessary. The GP inspects the genital and anal region to check for injuries, signs of infection, skin abnormalities, urethral prolapse, haemangiomas, warts, abnormal bumps/swelling or discharge. If traumatic injuries are present, the possibility of sexual abuse must always be considered. The GP should check for secondary sex characteristics in order to detect any hormonal disorders. In the case of discharge, swabs are taken to rule out the sexually transmitted diseases gonorrhoea and chlamydia. If haematuria is suspected, a urine test is performed; possible faecal loss requires faecal blood testing.

TREATMENT

In the case of physiological blood loss in newborns, the GP should simply offer explanation and reassurance. Although perhaps not strictly accurate (it is actually withdrawal bleeding), explaining the blood loss as 'a kind of menstruation' may provide an explanation most mothers will understand and accept. A wait and see approach is justified. If the bleeding does not stop after a few days, or it recurs, further evaluation is necessary. In the case of pathological blood loss in the first year, there may well be doubt about the origin or cause of the bleeding. In this case, referral to a paediatrician or another specialist with knowledge of paediatric gynaecology is indicated. The blood loss could imply a serious problem. If sexual abuse is suspected, urgent consultation with a paediatrician is mandatory.

PREVENTION AND ADDITIONAL INFORMATION

Providing information about the possible occurrence of vaginal blood loss in newborn girls and an explanation about the cause (e.g. during antenatal classes) can prevent a great deal of unnecessary worry.

Key points

- Blood loss is usually the result of hormonal stimulation and subsequent hormonal withdrawal.
- Physiological vaginal blood loss occurs in an estimated 3–10% of newborn girls.
- Pathological causes of vaginal blood loss in infants must be considered if the bleeding begins more than 2 weeks after birth.
- Remember sexual abuse as a cause of traumatic lesions in infants under 1 year of age.

Literature

Baldwin DD, Landa HM. Common problems in pediatric gynaecology. *Urol Clin North Am* 1995;**22**:161–76.

Eijkelenboom PR, Mulder Dzn JD. Kleine kwalen in de huisartsgeneeskunde; vaginaal bloedverlies bij pasgeborenen [Minor ailments in general practice; vaginal blood loss in newborns]. *Ned Tijdschr Geneeskd* 1987;**131**:1166–7.

81

TIGHTENING OF THE FORESKIN/PHIMOSIS

DEFINITION

Phimosis is a tightening of the opening of the foreskin.

AETIOLOGY/PATHOGENESIS

In the embryonic phase, the head of the penis and the foreskin form one structure. The 'splitting' process generally starts after birth, and can continue until the age of 17 years. In the child's first few years, the foreskin being stuck to the head of the penis is physiological, and rolling it back completely is often impossible. The term 'adhesion' incorrectly suggests that this is an abnormality. Even after these so-called adhesions have disappeared, it is not always possible to actively retract the foreskin. It is the retraction of the foreskin that results in a small opening developing in the foreskin. Phimosis is pathological when the opening is too small to let urine pass freely. On attempted micturition, the space between the foreskin and the head of the penis fills up like a second bladder, and the foreskin balloons out until sufficient pressure builds up to allow the urine to pass.

PRESENTATION

For pathological phimosis, the parents explain to the GP that the child has problems urinating; they will have noticed that a swelling develops at the end of the penis when the child tries. Physiological phimosis can be presented in a variety of ways. The parents sometimes think that the head of the penis should be able to be exposed completely, and they want to know why their son's foreskin cannot be retracted completely. If balanitis is present, they may well assume that the foreskin is abnormally tight. The 'elephant trunk' type of foreskin also gives rise to these anxieties. Each of these types of presentation may be accompanied by a request for circumcision.

EPIDEMIOLOGY

In only 4% of newborns can the foreskin be completely retracted. Even in 6 to 9 year olds, full retraction is not possible in up to 60%. The figures available detailing how often this problem presents to GPs vary widely. The physiological type of phimosis represents the majority; the incidence of true (pathological) phimosis is unknown.

HISTORY

The main purpose of the history is to make a distinction between pathological and physiological phimosis. The GP asks:

- about difficulties with urination
- if the foreskin balloons out
- about symptoms of balanitis (see Chapter 82).

EXAMINATION

To inspect the opening in the foreskin, the foreskin is gently pulled away from the body and held slightly open. If the foreskin is pushed backwards, an opening the size of a pinhead will be seen; if the foreskin is instead pulled to the front, an opening is visible that is normally large enough to be viewed as normal for that age. Over time, the opening will enlarge until it has reached an adult size (by about the age of 17 years).

TREATMENT

The information provided above under 'Aetiology/pathogenesis' explains why it is not necessary to expose the head of the penis in young boys. Also, forced manipulation of the foreskin is strongly discouraged: this may ultimately result in fear of masturbation and coitus. For physiological phimosis, providing an explanation and hygiene guidelines are sufficient.

In the case of pathological phimosis, surgery is often indicated. Recurrent balanitis can also warrant surgery. Dorsal slits or complete circumcision are the main options. The choice depends on the anatomical situation, the parents' beliefs and the surgeon's views. Circumcision can lead to sexual problems, and should therefore only be performed when strictly necessary.

An effective alternative to surgery for the treatment of phimosis is topical steroids (0.05% bethamethasone cream) twice daily for 1 month. After a week of topical application parents are told to retract the prepuce and are given hygiene routine instructions. This avoids or delays circumcision.

PREVENTION AND ADDITIONAL INFORMATION

True prevention is not possible. Explanation is the key. The 'splitting' process can continue until the boy reaches puberty; forcibly pushing back the foreskin is not recommended. In addition, hygiene advice is important. Material can accumulate between the foreskin and the head of the penis, so regular cleaning is important. This should be carried out as follows: twice weekly, retract the foreskin back as far as possible without using force, and clean the exposed parts with plenty of water. This is easiest in a lukewarm bath or the shower.

Key points

- Phimosis is pathological when the opening is too small to let urine pass freely.
- Even in 6 to 9 year olds, full retraction is only possible in 40%.
- Forced manipulation of the foreskin is strongly discouraged.
- Physiological phimosis requires only explanation and hygiene guidelines.
- Surgery is indicated only for pathological phimosis and in some cases of recurrent balanitis.

Literature
Ashfield JE, Nickel KR, Siemens DR, MacNeily AE, Nickel JC. Treatment of phimosis with topical steroids in 194 children. J Urol 2003;**169**(3):1106–8.

Gordon A, Collin J. Save the normal foreskin. *BMJ* 1993;**306**:1–2.

Huntley JS, Bourne MC, Munro FD, Wilson-Storey D. Troubles with the foreskin: one hundred consecutive referrals to paediatric surgeons. *J R Soc Med* 2003;**96**(9):449–51.

Kirby RS. The joy of uncircumcising! [book review]. *BMJ* 1994;**309**:679.

82

INFLAMMATION OF THE GLANS PENIS/BALANITIS

DEFINITION

Balanitis is an inflammation of the epithelium of the glans penis, which usually also affects the foreskin.

AETIOLOGY/PATHOGENESIS

In young boys, inflammation can result from debris accumulating beneath the foreskin. A foreskin that is narrow and shaped like an elephant's trunk is most likely to accumulate such debris.

Phimosis (see Chapter 81) is an important factor in patients who are older. Also, the foreskin or the glans can suffer mechanical damage from sexual activity – inflammation can then result through secondary infection of these (often small) lesions. In the majority of such cases, *Candida albicans* is the pathogenic micro-organism. The GP should bear in mind the possibility of diabetes mellitus, especially in older men. Sexually transmitted diseases can also be accompanied by balanitis.

PRESENTATION

Because the patient is often a small child, the parents usually present the problem. This usually involves: a painful glans penis and foreskin (and also often the rest of the penis as well); a pus-like discharge from the opening of the foreskin; crusts around and/or in this opening; and swelling, often with redness, around the entire glans. If the glans is small in relation to the shaft, this swelling can appear to affect half of the penis.

Adult patients usually present with one or more of the following symptoms: pain in the glans or the entire penis, especially when

retracting the foreskin; itching; a burning feeling and redness
of the glans and/or foreskin; heavy, sometimes moderate,
discharge from under the foreskin; crusts around the opening
of the foreskin; and flakiness and redness of the glans and
sometimes the foreskin.

EPIDEMIOLOGY

Detailed epidemiological data are scanty. The incidence of balanitis in
boys up to 4 years of age can be estimated at 1 to 2 per 1000 patients
per year; and in adults aged 25–64 years around 1 per 1000 patients
per year.

HISTORY

The GP asks:

- about hygiene habits and about whether or not the foreskin can be
  retracted
- in adults, about sexual activities.

EXAMINATION

In young boys, the glans can be inspected by carefully pulling
(lengthwise) the foreskin open, away from the penis. Attempts to
retract the foreskin over the glans should be strongly discouraged. In
adults, too, retracting an infected foreskin should take place carefully
and never with force. After the glans has been exposed, it is inspected
for small wounds and sores.

Additional tests, such as a culture, are not usually necessary in the
first instance – although, if the history and the patient's sexual
habits suggest a possible sexually transmitted disease the relevant
investigations should be performed (preferably at the local genito-
urinary medicine clinic). If diabetes mellitus is suspected, the blood
sugar is measured.

TREATMENT

In many cases, explanation, reassurance and recommendations about
hygiene are sufficient. In troublesome situations, irrigation under the

foreskin three times daily with a syringe can be helpful: carefully insert the syringe containing 10 ml of lukewarm water in the opening of the foreskin and then empty the syringe. The water should be spurted along the glans. The first treatment should be carried out by the GP to demonstrate the technique to the parents. Debris can also be removed by gently inserting a moistened cotton bud beneath the foreskin. If inflammation is persistent or recurs, surgery may be necessary (see Chapter 81). *Candida* balanitis (characterized in particular by itching and redness) is treated with antifungal cream applied for at least a week. The treatment of sexually transmitted diseases is beyond the scope of this chapter.

PREVENTION AND ADDITIONAL INFORMATION

Depending on the situation, hygiene measures may need to be reinforced or increased. Explain that material can accumulate between the foreskin and the glans, and that regular cleaning is therefore important. This involves retracting the foreskin as far as possible without using force, and cleaning the exposed parts with lots of water. This should be done twice weekly in a lukewarm bath or the shower. Parents often ask if circumcision is necessary. The main medical indication is true phimosis (see Chapter 81), although circumcision is sometimes indicated in very troublesome and recurrent balanitis.

In adults, the foreskin is sometimes too narrow to retract easily over the glans, especially if the penis is erect. In this case, the GP should provide reassurance and an explanation, especially when attempts at coitus are unsuccessful (or are in danger of being so). The patient can gradually increase the degree of retraction area himself with practice: each day, the patient retracts the foreskin five times in a row, possibly using a lubricant, up to the point that can be reached without difficulty.

Key points

- In young boys, inflammation can result from debris accumulating beneath the foreskin.
- Phimosis is an important factor in patients who are older.
- Secondary infection usually involves *Candida*.
- In many cases, explanation, reassurance and recommendations about hygiene are sufficient – circumcision is not usually required, although the parents may ask about this.

Literature

Dekker JH, Boeke AJP, Damme D, et al. NHG-standaard: fluor vaginalis [NHG standard: vaginal discharge]. In: Thomas S, Geijer RMM, Van der Laan JR, Wiersma TJ (eds). *NHG-standaarden voor de huisarts II* [*NHG standards for the general practitioner II*]. Utrecht: Nederlands Huisartsen Genootschap, 1996.

Jamin R. Schoonspoelen van de voorhuidszak [Irrigating the foreskin sac]. *Huisarts Wet* 1989;**32**:106–7.

Mayser P. Mycotic infections of the penis. Andrologia. 1999;**31**(Suppl 1):13–16.

83

BLOOD IN SEMEN/
HAEMOSPERMIA

DEFINITION

The definition of haemospermia, hematospermia or bloody semen is self-explanatory: blood in the ejaculate.

AETIOLOGY/PATHOGENESIS

A large variety of urogenital abnormalities are listed as possible causes of haemospermia, but a direct causal relationship is not always clear. In most cases, the haemospermia is incidental – cause unknown. Infections such as prostatitis, posterior urethritis and infection of the seminal vesicles are well-recognized causes. Less likely possibilities include carcinoma of the prostate or seminal vesicles (and, occasionally, of the bladder or testicles). Trauma (injury or prostatectomy), blood vessel anomalies in the urethra, urethral stricture, tuberculosis and bilharzia are rare causes of bloody semen.

PRESENTATION

The patient attends with the complaint that he has bloody or red semen – this is the only symptom in 40% of patients. The rest have additional symptoms such as dysuria, pain during orgasm, urinary problems (frequency, small amounts, post-micturition dribbling) and blood in the urine. It is an alarming phenomenon that can cause worry and many questions, especially about the possibility of malignancy and sexually transmitted disease.

EPIDEMIOLOGY

There are no known figures on the incidence in general practice or elsewhere. According to urologists, the symptom is quite common. A rough estimate is that a GP would see an average of one patient a year with this problem. It occurs in sexually mature men of all ages. In 15% of patients it only occurs once, although most experience several episodes, and a few get recurrences for years.

HISTORY

The GP asks:

- about the presentation of the symptom (the presence of blood after coitus may represent postcoital bleeding, a gynaecological problem, rather than haemospermia)
- how and when the symptom began, and whether it has occurred once or several times
- about pain during orgasm
- about additional symptoms that could indicate an infection of the prostate, urethra or bladder
- about symptoms of prostatism
- about any recent trauma or any operation of the urogenital system
- about past infections, such as tuberculosis or gonorrhoea.

EXAMINATION

When inspecting the urethral orifice, check for any discharge from the urethra and any other local abnormalities. Palpation should involve checking the testicles and the local lymphatics. The digital rectal examination focuses on the prostate: the size, consistency, medial sulcus and any tenderness. The physical examination may be expanded according to any additional symptoms. Supplementary tests might include urinalysis, sperm analysis, a measurement of serum prostate-specific antigen (PSA) if prostate carcinoma is suspected, and a urine and/or sperm culture if a bacterial infection is possible.

TREATMENT

Management depends on the severity and duration of the complaint and the age of the patient. If the symptom has only occurred once and the assessment did not detect any abnormalities, no action needs to be taken unless it recurs or other symptoms develop. In this situation, the patient should be reassured about the harmless nature of the symptom. Any infection of the prostate and/or seminal vesicles should first be treated with antibiotics – this may resolve the problem. For persistent symptoms in young men, in which the physical examination and additional tests do not reveal any abnormalities, a trial treatment with an antibiotic (e.g. co-trimoxazole 960 mg twice daily for 7 days) is reasonable. If unexplained haemospermia persists after treatment, a urologist should carry out further tests. While the literature does report that haemospermia can be caused by a malignancy, the risk of this in men under 40 years old is virtually non-existent. However, if the patient is more than 40 years old, referral with a view to cystoscopy and prostate biopsy is appropriate.

PREVENTION AND ADDITIONAL INFORMATION

Any recommendations regarding prevention and explanation are determined by the (probable) cause. If no abnormalities are revealed, the patient should be reassured, and it must be explained that sexual activity is harmless for the patient and partner(s). Theoretically, prevention is only possible if the cause is a preventable infection. In that case, it is advisable to treat the patient's partner(s) also.

Key points

- In most cases of haemospermia, the cause is unknown.
- The risk of malignancy as a cause in a patient under 40 years old is virtually non-existent.
- Men over 40 years old should be referred to a urologist, particularly if the problem is recurrent.
- Empirical treatment with antibiotics is worthwhile in younger men with persistent symptoms.

Literature

Ganabathi K, Chadwick D, Fenely RC, Gingell JC. Haemospermia. *Br J Urol* 1992;**69**:225–30.

Jones DJ. Haemospermia: a prospective study. *Br J Urol* 1991;**67**:88–90.

Papp GK, Kopa Z, Szabo F, Erdei E. Aetiology of haemospermia. *Andrologia* 2003;**35**(5):317–20.

Thomas K, Emberton M. The patient with haemospermia. *Practitioner.* 2000;**244**(1614):778–80, 782–3.

84

CONSTIPATION IN CHILDREN

DEFINITION

Constipation is an abnormal pattern of defaecation in which the amount evacuated is too little, or the consistency too hard, or in which faeces are evacuated only with difficulty.

AETIOLOGY/PATHOGENESIS

The normal pattern of defaecation in children varies with age. A frequency of anything between three times daily to once every 3 days is considered normal. Cultural or family views tend to determine the limits of normality more strongly than medical or scientific insight.

Quantity and frequency of defaecation depend first of all on the quality and quantity of food and fluid consumed. Food with little plant-based fibre provides only minimal undigested matter in the colon, which means the capacity of the intestinal contents to absorb water is very small. This results in faeces consisting primarily of dead bacteria, so that, even if enough water is consumed, a small, dry mass is produced. Because this mass does not expand in the colon, there are minimal propulsive contractions, and transit is slow.

Normally, the faecal material is retained in the rectum and colon until sufficient stimuli are present to relax the upper anal sphincter. As the faeces enter the anal canal, there is an urge to defaecate. In addition, the external anal sphincter contracts to prevent undesired evacuation. Defaecation is only possible after this sphincter has been relaxed consciously. (For further description of the relevant anatomy and physiology see Chapter 87.)

This normal process can become disrupted due to anatomical, functional and psychological factors. In childhood, 90% of constipation is functional. Organic causes are usually discovered before the child's third year. The various aetiologies of constipation vary according to the child's age.

In infants up to 5 months old, constipation is usually related to the composition of the milk. Breast-feeding can result in relatively infrequent, hard faeces. Incorrectly prepared bottle formula (too much milk powder per unit of water) can also lead to constipation, and small anal fissures may aggravate the situation. Finally, there are several, very rare disorders that are accompanied by constipation in newborns and infants up to 2 months old, such as anal atresia, malrotation, Hirschsprung's disease (one in 5000 births) and meconium ileus.

Between 2 and 5 months of age a baby may simply have difficulty evacuating the faeces (its face turns red). The faeces are visible at the anal opening, but are not easily passed. Incomplete coordination of the various motor reflexes seems to be the cause. This 'problem' disappears spontaneously.

In children of pre-school age, constipation is usually caused by emotional or behavioural factors, although changes in diet and potty training may be relevant. Chronic constipation in children under 2 years of age, a constantly bloated abdomen and an empty rectum during a digital rectal examination, strongly suggest the diagnosis of Hirschsprung's disease. Early diabetes, lead intoxication, hypercalcaemia and various renal and metabolic disorders can also be the cause.

In school-age children, constipation usually presents as stomach ache. Only on inquiry is slow, infrequent defaecation reported. Peculiar dietary patterns, sometimes involving the entire family, are often found. Acute painful constipation may also be related to irritable bowel syndrome (IBS). Extreme cases of faecal soiling and encopresis, both usually the result of long-term overfilling of the colon and rectum, require a great deal of attention. The assistance of a paediatrician and/or a child psychologist may be valuable.

In puberty, most constipation results from an imbalanced diet. Anorexia nervosa can also play a role at this age: the resistance to food and the desire to lose weight can lead to minimal food intake, constipation and laxative use.

PRESENTATION

Very young children do not complain about constipation. Their parents, however, may be worried, and addressing their anxieties is just as important as examining the factors that are causing the constipation.

Some children may experience pain during defaecation, and the fear of this can cause them to suppress the urge to defaecate, thereby aggravating the problem.

In severe chronic constipation, symptoms may include a lack of appetite and general malaise.

Recurring stomach aches, urinary tract infections or 'paradoxical' diarrhoea can also be symptoms of constipation.

EPIDEMIOLOGY

In various primary care morbidity studies, an incidence of constipation in children up to 4 years old of 24 cases per 1000 patients per year has been reported. This drops to four cases in children aged 5–14 years. There is little difference between boys and girls. Most episodes are shorter than 4 weeks, and the GP is typically consulted once or twice during such an episode.

HISTORY

Depending on the child's age, the GP asks:

- about the duration of the symptoms
- about the frequency, type and consistency of the faeces
- about blood or pain during defaecation
- about any abdominal pain, vomiting or diarrhoea
- about the child's diet (high fibre, sufficient liquids, breast-feeding)
- about the child's appetite and general health
- about symptoms of urinary tract infection
- about the parent–child relationship
- about potty training
- about defaecation at school.

EXAMINATION

The abdomen is inspected to see if it is bloated, and the GP palpates for faeces in the colon and assesses whether these are hard. The anus may be inspected for anal fissures. If necessary, a digital rectal examination is carried out.

Additional tests (haemoglobin level, midstream urine, etc.) are carried out if indicated.

TREATMENT

The treatment depends on the cause, the child's age and the severity of the symptoms. It is important to distinguish between cases that can be dealt with by the parents and/or GP, and those that need to be referred.

First, establish that there really is a problem with constipation and address any parental fears. The history can be supported by having them keep a 'defaecation diary', in which they can also list all the foods eaten.

For infants, provide dietary advice: if bottle-feeding, add more water, possibly with a few teaspoons of orange juice or juice from soaked prunes – an alternative is a lactose-rich milk formula; in those on solids, vegetables, fruit (not too finely chopped) and brown bread should be encouraged. Children who consume a lot of milk and juice often have less appetite for solid foods with the necessary fibre.

Pay particular attention to potty training in preschool-age children. When trying to defaecate, they need to be able to sit with their feet on the floor to learn the normal 'pushing' process. The GP can advise the use of a footstool for this. Also, it is better to make a game of using the potty and to provide a clear reward for the child's achievement – long, unproductive periods on the potty should be avoided.

In the case of chronic constipation with faecal retention, the rectum first needs to be emptied. If a suppository or micro-enema is not successful, a volume enema with lukewarm water and physiological salt can be used – this may require attendance at the local hospital. Subsequently, the child may be treated with lactulose (although one disadvantage of this is that the child may develop stomach ache as a side-effect). In addition, for the first 1 or 2 months, a micro-enema (once daily or on alternate days) may be necessary. When mushy faeces are produced once daily, the dose and frequency can gradually be reduced. In many cases, chronic constipation needs to be treated for several months.

Newborns with atresia, malrotation and meconium ileus must be referred to the paediatrician. This also applies if Hirschsprung's disease or systemic abnormalities are suspected. For serious psychological problems (extreme faecal soiling, encopresis), referral to a child psychologist is indicated.

PREVENTION AND ADDITIONAL INFORMATION

Prevention involves dietary education, advice about normal potty training and attention to psychosocial factors. Parents, the health visitor and the GP can and should make a contribution to this.

Key points

- A frequency of defaecation of anything between three times daily to once every 3 days is considered normal.
- In childhood, 90% of constipation is functional. Organic causes are usually discovered before the child's third year.
- In infants up to 5 months old, constipation is usually related to the composition of the milk; in children of pre-school age, constipation is usually caused by emotional or behavioural factors.
- In the case of chronic constipation with faecal retention, the rectum first needs to be emptied.

Literature

Benninga MA. *Constipation and faecal incontinence in childhood* [dissertation]. Amsterdam: Universiteit van Amsterdam, 1994.

Clayden G, Keshtgar AS. Management of childhood constipation. *Postgrad Med J* 2003;**79**(937):616–21.

Ebelt VJ, Riddell D. Constipation in childhood. *Can Fam Physician* 1992;**38**:2167–74.

Fijn van Draat CJ, Keuzenkamp-Jansen CW, Douwes AC. Chronische functionele obstipatie bij kinderen [Chronic functional constipation in children]. *Ned Tijdschr Geneeskd* 1993;**137**:706–92.

85

CONSTIPATION IN THE ELDERLY

DEFINITION

Constipation is defined as an abnormal pattern of defaecation in which the faeces are too small, too hard and/or too difficult to pass.

AETIOLOGY/PATHOGENESIS

Food and liquid in the stomach and intestinal tract cause a gastrocolic reflex, which enables the contents of the intestines to be pushed in the direction of the anus via peristaltic contractions. Physical activity reinforces these propulsive contractions. Sufficient faeces in the sigmoid colon cause another reflex, by which the rectum is filled. Distension of the rectum in turn creates the urge to defaecate. The typical frequency of defaecation varies from three times daily to once every 3 days. However, significant variations on this norm exist, with personal habits playing a large role.

Liquids and fibre in food determine the consistency and volume of the faeces. Fibre stimulates the gut, shortening the transit time; also, fibre has the capacity to absorb water, making the faeces softer.

So, in summary, the following are needed for defaecation: intestinal contents, peristalsis, reflex mechanisms and intact motor skills. Also, the facility to 'defaecate at one's convenience' - in other words, a 'comfortable toilet experience' – is important. Problems can occur in all these areas, and constipation can be the result.

A practical classification of the types of constipation in the elderly, and their causes, follows.

Functional and/or habitual constipation. This type is the most common. Causes include: insufficient food intake (e.g. because of dental difficulties or decreased appetite); a low-fibre diet; insufficient fluid intake (e.g. because of being bedridden or the fear of having to urinate outside the home); inadequate physical exercise; ignoring the urge to defaecate; weakened abdominal muscles, which reduces 'pushing' strength; and poor or insufficient sanitary facilities (e.g. a toilet that is too high, an unheated toilet area or no privacy in the toilet).

Secondary, organic or symptomatic constipation. Here, a primary disorder is present to which the constipation is secondary; the cause can be intestinal or non-intestinal. Intestinal causes include obstruction due to carcinoma, stricture or volvulus. Non-intestinal causes include medication, spinal cord lesions, cerebrovascular accident, multiple sclerosis and Parkinson's disease.

Constipation due to motility disorders of the colon or rectum. The most well known of these is irritable bowel syndrome (IBS). Other causes include slow-transit constipation, which occurs primarily in young women (the transit time in the entire colon is increased, possibly due to a neurogenic cause), and outlet obstruction (rectal constipation, dyschezia), which is common in the elderly. If the urge to defaecate is repeatedly ignored, the defaecation stimulus is 'extinguished', and faeces accumulate in the rectum. The rectum then expands, resulting in faecal impaction in an atonic (mega)rectum.

PRESENTATION

The patient reports that his faeces are too hard, too difficult to produce or too infrequent. He usually needs information, reassurance and recommendations to improve matters. Other symptoms are sometimes present, such as abdominal pain, bloating, flatulence (see Chapter 91), a false urge to defaecate, anal pain, nausea, vomiting and a lack of appetite. Haemorrhoids (see Chapter 86), anal fissures (see Chapter 87) and rectal prolapse, which are the result of straining, can also prompt a consultation, as can paradoxical diarrhoea. In such cases, the patient may well request additional investigation and treatment. In elderly people who are confused, severe constipation may be the cause, although it is rarely volunteered.

EPIDEMIOLOGY

Only a very small percentage of people suffering from constipation consult their GP. In an average practice, 4.1 men and 7.6 women present with the complaint (in total 0.5%) per year. As people age, so does the likelihood of constipation. In hospitals and nursing homes, the complaint is very common. In western countries, 20% of the general population use laxatives sporadically and 3% do so regularly.

HISTORY

It must be clarified whether constipation is the sole complaint or is simply a symptom of another disorder – and whether any potentially serious abnormalities might be present. The GP should also establish what the patient considers as normal bowel movements, to decide whether constipation really is present. The GP asks:

- about the frequency (per day, per week), consistency and amount of faeces
- about the duration of the history
- how much the patient is bothered by the symptom
- about the presence of blood or mucus
- whether the patient strains when defaecating
- about symptoms of prolapse or haemorrhoids
- about false urges to defaecate and pain
- about whether the patient regularly postpones going to the toilet
- whether the diet is rich in fibre
- if the fluid intake is sufficient (at least 2 l/day)
- how regularly the patient eats
- about weight (loss), nausea and vomiting
- about anorexia and taste changes
- about other symptoms and the patient's previous history
- about the use of medications (see Aetiology/pathogenesis) and self-medication.

As a general rule of thumb (to be followed with caution), organic constipation often has a clear starting point, a progressive course, and may well be accompanied by pain and blood loss; whereas functional/non-organic constipation does not have a clear starting point, increases gradually or not at all, and is not accompanied by pain and/or blood loss.

EXAMINATION

Once again, this addresses the question of whether (serious) abnormalities might be present or whether the symptom is due to a non-organic cause. The following should be performed: inspection of the abdomen, inspection of the perianal area, percussion, palpation, auscultation and digital rectal examination. Additional investigations are indicated only if it seems likely that the constipation is non-functional. Further discussion of this falls beyond the scope of this book.

TREATMENT

Treatment depends on whether there is an organic cause. Any underlying cause of this sort should be managed as appropriate, and may well require referral. In the elderly, it is obviously important to have a low index of suspicion for significant pathology and to be cautious about making a functional diagnosis.

If, however, a functional cause has been established as the diagnosis, the following recommendations are appropriate.

Anxieties should be allayed – patients not only 'suffer' from constipation, they may also be very worried about it. Providing information about the physiology of the defaecation process and the ways in which their symptoms might have arisen helps reassure the patient. It also creates an understanding of why following a proper daily regimen (diet, toilet habits, etc.) is important.

The GP should explain that the patient should make physical exercise and routine a part of his normal lifestyle: for example, doing shopping himself, taking a daily walk, keeping a specific time for defaecation, not postponing defaecation, and taking the time to defaecate in a comfortable toilet area. It is also appropriate to focus attention on the defaecation position – a 'squatting' position is the best. If the patient must use an elevated toilet, the use of a footstool can be helpful.

Dietary advice is also important. Sufficient fluid should be taken, with a goal of 2 l/day. Patients should be advised to eat regular, sufficient, high-fibre meals. Elderly people often only consume 10 g/day of fibre, while the recommended daily dose is 10–30 g. The patient should first attempt to increase the natural fibres in his diet, by eating coarse wholemeal bread, rye bread, wholemeal pasta products, brown rice, raw vegetables and fruit. Foods that cause constipation should be avoided. This advice is usually sufficient, but it may be difficult to get elderly people to change their familiar low-fibre diet. A subsequent step involves adding bran to the diet (six tablespoons of bran is equivalent to 20 g of dietary fibre). Finally, bulk-forming laxatives, such as purified bran, psyllium seed or sterculia granules, can be advised. These remedies may only be used if sufficient fluid intake can be guaranteed (1.5–2 l/day). They will begin working after 2–3 days.

The patient's medication should be reviewed. Any constipation-inducing treatment should be reduced, eliminated or replaced, if possible.

If these general measures do not produce the desired result – and adequate time should be allowed for them to take effect – the use of a laxative should be considered. The first choice is an osmotic laxative, such as lactulose. These remedies have only mild side-effects and are safe. They work within 1–2 days and they are best taken in a single dose in the morning.

The second choice are stimulant laxatives, such as bisacodyl. If taken orally, these should work after 5–10 hours; it is best to take these in the evening. Bisacodyl has an effect in 15–60 minutes when administered rectally.

If faecal impaction is found during the digital rectal examination, an oral laxative is contraindicated. In such a case, a suppository (e.g. bisacodyl) or a (micro)enema should be administered first. A physiological salt enema is an alternative. If this is not successful, a phosphate enema (larger volume) should be tried. Sometimes, the faecal impaction is so extreme that the rectum must first be manually emptied. Subsequently, the patient should then try to re-establish the normal defaecation pattern (with the advice already mentioned above).

PREVENTION AND ADDITIONAL INFORMATION

Advice should be given about physical exercise and diet. This should include explanation about the benefit of fresh fruit and vegetables, sufficient fibre intake, adequate fluid (at least 2 l/day of fluid, equivalent to about 10–12 cups), and the importance of eating at regular times. If necessary, a dietician can provide expert advice and guidance.

The GP should also explain what a normal defaecation pattern is. Simple, but effective, recommendations are: acting on the urge to defaecate, taking time to defaecate and avoiding straining. An elevated toilet may seem ideal for elderly people, but this defaecation position promotes constipation. Warn the patient about long-term inexpert use of laxatives.

Risk groups among the elderly are: people who take too little exercise due to physical or psychological problems, and those who take medications.

Key points

- The typical frequency of defaecation varies from three times daily to once every 3 days.

- In general, organic constipation often has a clear starting point, a progressive course, and may well be accompanied by pain and blood loss.

- In the elderly, it is important to have a low index of suspicion for significant pathology and to be cautious about making a functional diagnosis.

- The patient's medication should be reviewed: any constipation-inducing treatment should be reduced, eliminated or replaced, if possible.

Literature

Abyad A, Mourad F. Constipation: common-sense care of the older patient. *Geriatrics* 1996;**51**(12):28–34, 36.

Laxantiagebruik door ouderen in de alledaagse praktijk [Laxative use by the elderly in daily practice]. *Geneesmiddelenbulletin* 1987;**10**:51–6.

Schaefer DC, Cheskin LJ. Constipation in the elderly. *Am Fam Physician* 1998;**58**(4):907–14.

Wilson JA. Constipation in the elderly. *Clin Geriatr Med* 1999;**15**(3):499–510.

86

PILES/HAEMORRHOIDS

DEFINITION

Haemorrhoids are distended veins in the anal area that are sometimes visible externally. A distinction is made between internal haemorrhoids (pathological, irreversible widening of the superior rectal plexus) and external haemorrhoids (affecting the inferior rectal plexus).

AETIOLOGY/PATHOGENESIS

Haemorrhoidal tissue consists of fibrovascular cushions that are suspended in the anal canal by a connective tissue framework derived from the internal anal sphincter and longitudinal muscle. The venous plexus of each cushion is fed by arteriovenous communications that allow for enlargement of the cushion to help control continence. With age and the passage of hard stools, the connective tissue supporting the cushions becomes weaker, so that these cushions may descend. Straining produces an increase in venous pressure and engorgement. The prolapsed cushion has an impaired venous return, which results in dilatation of the plexus and venous stasis. A decreased venous outflow can also result from, for example, spasm of the anal sphincter, straining and tumours in the pelvis. Alternatively, arterial inflow can increase via infection or alcohol. Inflammation occurs with erosion of the cushion's epithelium, resulting in bleeding. Haemorrhoids are the result of these pathological changes. This theory has superseded notions that piles were a form of varicose veins.

Internal haemorrhoids may be subdivided into the following grades based on severity: haemorrhoids that are only visible on proctoscopy (grade 1); those that prolapse when straining, but which reduce spontaneously (grade 2); those that spontaneously prolapse, but which can be reduced digitally (grade 3); and those that prolapse and cannot be reduced (grade 4).

External haemorrhoids result from straining; in women, other relevant factors may include the influence of hormones, pregnancy and the menstrual cycle.

PRESENTATION

The usual reason for consulting the GP is worry about the presence of blood during or after defaecation. If a haemorrhoid is damaged, rectal blood loss can sometimes occur independent of any bowel movement. Patients may also attend because they have felt a lump in the anal area. In approximately one-third of patients, itching is the reason for consulting (see Chapter 88).

EPIDEMIOLOGY

There are no reliable data about the actual incidence or prevalence of haemorrhoids. Many people have early, symptomless haemorrhoids. Also, many symptomatic patients do not consult a doctor. An average GP will probably see between 18 and 30 new cases a year. This problem occurs slightly more often in women than in men.

HISTORY

The history is aimed mainly at ruling out other causes of rectal blood loss or itching. The GP asks:

- how long the symptoms have been present
- about self-medication
- about toilet habits and constipation
- about any changes in bowel habit
- about the relationship between rectal blood loss and defaecation (the amount, whether it is bright or dark red, the presence of mucus, and whether the blood is only on the toilet paper, or also in, or on the surface of, the faeces)
- about any relationship with the menstrual cycle or pregnancy
- about medication (iron pills, laxatives, etc.)
- about pain (pain is not a symptom of uncomplicated haemorrhoids; if pain is present, this suggests an anal fissure (see Chapter 87) or a perianal haematoma)
- about risk factors for colonic carcinoma (positive family history for polyposis coli or colon carcinoma, long-term ulcerative colitis).

EXAMINATION

On inspection, the GP checks for perianal skin disorders (haemorrhoids often occur together with perianal dermatitis), abscesses, fistulae, scars, skin tags, external haemorrhoids and anal fissures (see also the chapters concerned). When the patient strains, the GP should look for prolapse of haemorrhoids or mucosa. The swelling of external haemorrhoids should be clearly visible. During palpation and the digital rectal examination, check for induration, sphincter tension (hypotonia, hypertonia), tumours, and abnormalities of the prostate, the uterus and the pouch of Douglas. Internal haemorrhoids are not usually palpable. They will, however, be visible on proctoscopy.

Additional tests are carried out based on the history and findings (e.g. full blood count, referral for bowel investigation). Further investigation is usually unnecessary for blood loss resulting from haemorrhoids in patients under 50 years old without risk factors for colonic carcinoma. However, it is indicated for rectal blood loss with existing haemorrhoids in patients above this age, to exclude co-pathology. Referral is also necessary if haemorrhoids are accompanied by anaemia.

TREATMENT

Haemorrhoids are extremely common and usually produce short-term symptoms that disappear spontaneously. They generally do not require treatment, as an explanation is usually sufficient. Advice should be given about a healthy diet (high fibre, adequate fluid intake; see also Chapters 85 and 90), toilet hygiene, acting on the defaecation reflex and not straining. Local therapy consists of treating the accompanying perianal dermatitis (see Chapter 88), cooling the area with ice (which reduces swelling, itching and pain), and warm baths, which relax the anal sphincter (thereby improving venous outflow) and protect the skin and mucous membrane.

Sclerotherapy or rubber-band ligation (for grades 1, 2 and 3) or surgical therapy (for grades 3 and 4) should only be carried out if there are persistent symptoms.

For the sake of completeness, the treatment of a perianal haematoma is also described here. Many cases will settle spontaneously. If active treatment is required, a radial incision is made, followed by expression of the clot. Local anaesthetics, mild astringents or steroids are often tried, but there is a lack of evidence to support their use. They only provide short-term relief from discomfort and do not affect the underlying pathological changes. Continuous application can cause eczema and sensitization of the skin around the anus; rectal absorption can lead to systemic side-effects.

Thrombosis of a prolapsed haemorrhoid is difficult for the GP to treat and will usually require referral.

PREVENTION AND ADDITIONAL INFORMATION

Common-sense recommendations are important for the prevention and treatment of haemorrhoids: avoiding straining and acting on the defaecation reflex are usually sufficient to prevent the problem.

Key points

- Further investigation is usually unnecessary for bleeding from haemorrhoids in patients under 50 years old without risk factors for colonic carcinoma.

- Patients over 50 years old with rectal bleeding should be referred for investigation, even if haemorrhoids are present.

- In patients with haemorrhoids, advice should be given about a healthy diet (high fibre, adequate fluid intake), toilet hygiene, acting on the defecation reflex and not straining.

Literature

Janssen LWM. Consensus hemorroïden [Consensus haemorrhoids]. *Ned Tijdschr Geneeskd* 1994;**138**:2106–9.

Neiger A. *Atlas of practical proctology*. Stuttgart: Hogrefe/Huber, 1990.

Nisar PJ, Scholefield JH. Managing haemorrhoids. *BMJ* 2003;**327**(7419): 847–51.

87
ANAL FISSURES

DEFINITION

Anal fissures are painful, linear, usually dorsally located lesions in the skin and/or the mucous membrane of the distal part of the anal canal. A distinction can be made between superficial/acute and deep/chronic fissures.

AETIOLOGY/PATHOGENESIS

The precise aetiology of anal fissures remains unclear. They seem to be initiated by trauma to the anal canal, usually due to overstretching when defecating too quickly or suddenly. This injury increases the tone of the internal sphincter, resulting in local ischaemia. This causes pain and also prevents the wound from healing. A vicious cycle results: hard faeces, fissure, pain, high sphincter tension, constipation, hard faeces, and so on.

The progression of an acute fissure to the chronic form takes place over 2–3 weeks and results from the ischaemia of the anorectal mucous membrane when the initial problem is inadequately managed. A chronic fissure is therefore, in fact, an ischaemic ulcer.

PRESENTATION

The patient's reason for attending is usually a sharp, stinging sensation in the anal area during the passage of faeces. In many cases, the symptoms occur not only during, but also after, defecation, possibly with a small amount of bright-red blood on the faeces or toilet paper (which raises the possibility of haemorrhoids, or other pathology).

EPIDEMIOLOGY

Anal fissures occur at every age, but usually in young children

(0–4 years) and in young and middle-aged adults. The gender division is approximately equal, with the exception of the youngest age category (0–4 years), in which the majority are girls. In an average practice, a GP will see new cases relatively frequently, about three to six times a year. The fissure is usually (80–90%) posterior, in the midline (it is anterior in 10% of fissures in women and only 1% in men). Due to better circulation elsewhere, fissures almost never occur outside the midline.

HISTORY

The GP asks:

- about the duration of the pain (longer than 3–4 weeks suggests a chronic fissure)
- about the duration and amount of blood loss (more than 'a little' on toilet paper or in the patient's underwear suggests a haemorrhoid; if this has been present for longer than 4 weeks, a lesion of the rectum or colon must be considered)
- about the defecation pattern (if this is changing, independent of anal pain, consider malignancy, especially in older age groups).

EXAMINATION

Careful examination of the anus is important. The fissure can easily remain hidden because the anal opening is pinched shut as a result of a sphincter spasm. This spasm can be overcome by careful, but firm, lateral spreading of the buttocks, possibly with the help of local anaesthetic, such as lidocaine gel. Based on the appearance and site, the GP can make a distinction between simple superficial and chronic fissures or other disorders in the area around the anus.

A superficial fissure is a straight lesion in the skin, which sometimes continues onto the mucous membrane of the rectum. In the case of a chronic fissure, the pale fibres of the internal sphincter are visible at the base. In some cases, a hypertrophied anal polyp may also be present, caused by oedema at the level of the dentate line (the transition from the anal mucous membrane to the skin of the anus); alternatively, a skin tag may be present ('sentinel pile').

Anal fissures must be differentiated from other disorders of the anal area, which can sometimes be very difficult. In pruritus ani, superficial lesions of the anal skin are often present, and these can be confused with a fissure – although this has few consequences for treatment. Other disorders that can produce lesions of the anal skin, and which look like anal fissures, include ulcerative colitis and Crohn's disease. In 7% of patients with ulcerative colitis, fissures are present that are multiple in number, wide, infected and located outside the median line. In Crohn's disease, the anal lesions are larger and the ulceration more extensive, and they are accompanied by oedema and large skin tags.

In the digital rectal examination, it should be established whether palpable abnormalities are present in the anus or rectum.

TREATMENT

Acute superficial fissures can spontaneously clear up within 2–3 weeks with the proper advice. It is extremely important to break out of the vicious circle described above.

An important recommendation is to act on the normal defecation reflex and to ensure the proper consistency of the faeces: a cellulose-rich diet (fruit, fresh or raw vegetables, brown bread and rye bread), possibly supplemented for a short time with volume-increasing laxatives (e.g. psyllium seed, sterculia gum). Warm baths after a bowel movement can help prevent and relieve the anal spasm.

The pain can be treated locally by short-term, sparing use of a local anaesthetic ointment, such as lidocaine. Long-term use can lead to allergic skin reactions and dermatitis. There is no use in continuing this remedy beyond 4 weeks, as the fissure is considered chronic at that point (and requires a different treatment).

However, conservative therapy with the application of topical glyceryl trinitrate ointment seems to lead to very good results. The patient is instructed to apply the ointment every 3 hours (not during the night) to the entire anal dermis. A follow-up check involving inspection is needed after 6 weeks, and can be repeated after another 6 weeks if necessary. If the fissure has not healed at that point, the patient must be referred for further tests, and possibly, in the most extreme cases, for surgery or for 'chemical denervation' of the internal sphincter (with botulinum toxin). An operation must also be considered for a fissure accompanied by an abscess or fistula.

For cases where there are specific underlying causes, the management is beyond the scope of this book.

PREVENTION AND ADDITIONAL INFORMATION

Information provided to the patient, especially with respect to diet, can help prevent the occurrence and recurrence of fissures.

Key points

- A chronic fissure is in fact an ischaemic ulcer.
- Do not overlook possible malignancy in the older patient with significant and persistent rectal bleeding.
- Acute superficial fissures can spontaneously clear up within 2–3 weeks with the proper advice.
- There is no point in continuing with a topical anaesthetic beyond 4 weeks, as the fissure is then considered chronic – glyceryl trinitrate ointment might help, or the patient may require surgery.

Literature

Jones M, Scholefield J. Annal fissure. *Clin Evid* 2004;**11**:533–43.

Linehan IP. The patient with anal problems. *Practitioner* 2000;**244**(1609):329–31, 333–4.

Schouten WR, Briel JW, Auwerda JJA, Boerma MO, Graatsma BH, Wilms EB. Intra-anale applicatie van isosorbidedinitraat bij chronische fissura ani [Intra-anal application of isosorbide dinitrate for chronic anal fissures]. *Ned Tijdschr Geneeskd* 1995;**139**:1447–9.

Utzig MJ, Kroesen AJ, Buhr HJ. Concepts in pathogenesis and treatment of chronic anal fissure – a review of the literature. *Am J Gastroenterol* 2003;**98**(5):968–74.

88

PRURITUS ANI

DEFINITION

Pruritus ani is itching around the anus, which can sometimes spread to the whole perianal area. Scratching can cause a traumatic dermatitis, which in turn also itches – a vicious cycle.

AETIOLOGY/PATHOGENESIS

The main cause of this symptom is faecal contamination of the perianal skin. The skin is irritated and inflamed by the alkaline faeces, causing itching and a risk of fungal and bacterial infection. If the skin is also too damp, maceration occurs, which aggravates the problem. A number of other factors can be involved in this process: rectal abnormalities, dermatological problems, systemic illnesses that may be accompanied by itching, and psychological issues.

Excessive perianal moistness can be caused by a number of factors, such as improper hygiene (cleaning the area too much or not enough), mechanical causes (deep anal folds), skin tags, poor mobility, excessive perspiration, insufficient ventilation (underwear, plastic chairs, obesity, nervousness), vaginal discharge and urinary incontinence.

Relevant anorectal problems that may cause or aggravate pruritus ani include perianal transudate (e.g. haemorrhoids, infections), discharge of mucus, pus and/or blood from the anus, anal fissures or fistulae, sphincter insufficiency (soiling), inflammatory bowel disease (in which the anus is involved), frequent defaecation or diarrhoea, and threadworm infection.

Dermatological abnormalities include itching skin disorders in general, contact dermatitis (allergic, toxic, irritative), fungal infections, and atrophy and maceration secondary to the use of corticosteroid ointments.

Any systemic illness that can cause itching (e.g. diabetes mellitus, hypothyroidism, uraemia, jaundice, haematological problems) may lead to pruritus ani. In most cases, however, the illness will already be known and anal itching will not be the first symptom.

Psychological factors also certainly play a role in causing or maintaining pruritus ani.

PRESENTATION

Patients with pruritus ani first complain about itching, and sometimes also about loss of mucus and/or blood. The itching can vary considerably in intensity: it may disrupt the patient's social functioning and sleep. It is located around the anus, but can spread to the entire perianal region.

EPIDEMIOLOGY

There are no reliable data available. It is estimated that a quarter of the adult population suffers from this symptom to varying degrees. It occurs four times more often in men than in women, and can be very persistent. Predisposing factors include: a sedentary profession, obesity, significant psychological stress/tension and a high consumption of alcohol and coffee.

HISTORY

The GP asks:

- about causes of perianal moistness (e.g. when the symptoms occur, toilet hygiene, defaecation habits, vaginal symptoms, discharge, urinary incontinence)
- about gastrointestinal problems and rectal disorders
- about allergies and/or skin disorders
- about other illnesses, medications and self-medication.

EXAMINATION

The aim is to detect any underlying problems. Aided by proper lighting, the GP inspects the perianal region and assesses the look of the skin (colour, eczema, excoriation, lichenification) and the presence of moisture, mucus, blood, pus and faeces. The GP also looks for fistulas, skin tags, prolapsed haemorrhoids, anal fissures, threadworms and the presence of a prolapse during straining. During the digital rectal examination, the GP checks the sphincter tension (hypotonia or hypertonia) and whether haemorrhoids and masses are present.

Proctoscopy may be indicated according to the symptoms. Also, based on the history or initial examination findings, supplementary physical examination may be performed (e.g. examination of the abdomen, vaginal speculum examination, digital vaginal examination). Any laboratory tests will be guided according to the findings. The following may be considered: a tape test for threadworm eggs, vaginal swab, and urinalysis (for infection and glucose). More extensive investigation, such as haematological tests and tests of liver, kidney and thyroid function, are sometimes necessary, depending on the differential diagnosis.

TREATMENT

If an underlying disorder is found, this should obviously be treated. Otherwise, the treatment should consist of preventing the inflammation of the skin by faecal matter and maceration. The following measures are helpful: proper hygiene, such as not using toilet paper, but instead dabbing the area with 'wet wipes', after which the skin is dried well; the patient should not wear tight trousers or pantyhose (loosely fitting cotton underwear is preferred); and the use of soap, bubble baths, etc. should be avoided. Fungal infection should be treated with an antifungal cream such as miconazole 2% or ketoconazole 2%, twice daily for 14 days. For a bacterial infection, fusidic acid cream, three times daily for 1 week is indicated. For severe (night time) itching, promethazine, such as 25 mg in the evening, is a symptomatic option.

PREVENTION AND ADDITIONAL INFORMATION

It is important to explain how the disorder develops and the rationale behind the treatment.

Key points

- Scratching can cause a traumatic dermatitis, which in turn also itches – a vicious cycle.
- A key point in the treatment of pruritus ani is the prevention of inflammation of the skin secondary to faecal contamination and maceration.
- Secondary fungal or bacterial infection also requires treatment.

Literature

Giordano M, Rebesco B, Torelli I, Blanco G, Cattarini G. Pruritus ani. *Minerva Chir* 1999;**54**(12):885–91.

Jones DJ. ABC of colorectal diseases. Pruritus ani. *BMJ* 1992;**305**:575–7.

Neiger A. *Atlas of practical proctology*. Stuttgart: Hogrefe/Huber, 1990.

Wigersma L. Adviezen bij aambeien en pruritus ani [Recommendations for haemorrhoids and pruritis ani]. *Huisarts Wet* 1997;**40**:204–9.

89
THREADWORMS

DEFINITION

Threadworms involve a parasitic infestation by *Enterobius vermicularis*. The worm is small: the male is 2–5 mm long with a diameter of 0.1–0.2 mm; the female is up to 15 mm long and is considerably 'thicker', up to 0.5 mm. The adult worm lives in the human caecum and appendix.

AETIOLOGY/PATHOGENESIS

The parasitic cycle is as follows. Swallowed eggs end up in the duodenum. The larvae migrate to the caecum, attach themselves to the intestinal wall, and develop into adult worms. After mating, the female can produce up to 10,000 eggs. The worm migrates to outside the anus (often at night) and lays a large number of sticky eggs on the perineum and around the anus. They are resistant to disinfecting agents.

Infection takes place via the faeco-oral route. Via the fingers, the eggs can end up on such objects as toilet seats, doorknobs, toys, floors, clothing and bed linen. As these objects are touched, the eggs are spread to the patient's or another person's fingers. The parasite cannot be transmitted by pets – threadworms can only live on humans.

In girls, vulvitis and vaginitis with discharge may occur. In very rare cases, threadworms can cause appendicitis.

PRESENTATION

In most cases, threadworms are asymptomatic. The patient, or his parents, usually consult because worms have been seen in the faeces. The main symptom is itching around the anus, especially at night and in the morning.

EPIDEMIOLOGY

Infestation with *E. vermicularis* is the most common helminthic infection in the UK. Research has shown that 10–30% of the population carries threadworms. The infection occurs slightly more often in children than adults. If one member of a family has threadworms, it can be assumed that the other children in the family (90%) and the parents (60%) will also be infected.

HISTORY

For symptoms of perianal itching or (in girls) itching of the labia and/or discharge, the GP should ask whether worms have been seen in the faeces. If a child sleeps restlessly and cries at night, the GP should consider threadworms as a possible cause.

EXAMINATION

Children and their parents may have seen small worms in the faeces, but a negative history of this sort does not rule out the diagnosis. The threadworms may be visible if the (peri)anal area is carefully inspected. The so-called 'scotch-tape test' is still the best method of demonstrating the presence of threadworms. In the morning, immediately upon waking, a piece of scotch tape is placed against the perineum or the perianal area, held there briefly, and then carefully removed before putting it on a slide. This is then examined at 100× magnification. If the diagnosis is correct, threadworm eggs, which are oval and flat on one side, should be visible.

TREATMENT

If there are no symptoms, all that is required is an explanation. It is not necessary to treat something that is harmless and does not cause any symptoms. Many parents and children consider the worms 'dirty' and will require appropriate reassurance. Nonetheless, proper instruction on simple hygiene measures is necessary to prevent reinfection or the spread of the problem. These measures consist of frequently washing the hands, cutting the fingernails short, changing clothes and bed linen often and washing them at a temperature of at least 60°C, and frequently cleaning the toilet, floors and toys. It is reasonable to inform the preschool or kindergarten teacher that threadworms have been detected; threadworm eggs may be spread (via stools or dirty hands) in the toilets, so the standard hygiene measures should be observed. It is important that the GP is honest in explaining that, even if the above measures are taken, there remains a high risk of reinfection from the surrounding environment.

If specific treatment is necessary, mebendazole is the preferred option in those over 2 years old: for children and adults, one 100-mg tablet repeated after 2 or 3 weeks if necessary. During pregnancy, this treatment should be prescribed only if absolutely necessary, because teratogenicity has not been ruled out. In children under 2 years old, piperazine may be used instead. Family members should be treated at the same time.

PREVENTION AND ADDITIONAL INFORMATION

The aforementioned hygiene measures have a preventive effect. The GP should also explain that threadworms are a harmless infection and that they do not cause other significant symptoms such as hunger or weight loss.

Key points

- In most cases, threadworms are asymptomatic.
- If one member of a family has threadworms, it can be assumed that the other children in the family and the parents will also be infected.
- A negative history of visible worms does not rule out the diagnosis.
- Proper instruction on simple hygiene measures is necessary to prevent reinfection or the spread of the problem.
- The GP should explain that threadworms do not cause other significant symptoms such as hunger or weight loss.

Literature
Elston DM. What's eating you? *Enterobius vermicularis* (pinworms, threadworms). *Cutis* 2003;**71**(4):268–70.

Russell LJ. The threadworm, *Enterobius vermicularis*. *Prim Care* 1991;**18**(1):13–24.

Tanowitz HB, Weiss LM, Wittner M. Diagnosis and treatment of common intestinal helminths. II: Common intestinal nematodes. *Gastroenterologist* 1994;**2**(1):39–49.

Vos F, Verheij TJM. *Enterobius vermicularis*, een ongenode gast [*Enterobius vermicularis*, an uninvited guest]. *Tijdschr Huisartsgeneesk* 1998;**15**:402–5.

90
PROCTALGIA FUGAX

DEFINITION

Proctalgia fugax is a severe cramp-like pain of the rectum, which can last from several seconds or minutes up to half an hour. It generally occurs at night, with intervals of weeks to many months. Proctalgia fugax is one of the most common causes of primary proctalgia – anorectal pain for which no cause is found.

AETIOLOGY/PATHOGENESIS

Little is known about the pathogenesis of proctalgia fugax. Recent research into the familial (autosomal-dominant) occurrence of this disorder points to a myopathy of the smooth muscle tissue (e.g. the internal anal sphincter). Electromyographic research has suggested a motor dysfunction of the internal sphincter. Another possibility is that the problem is caused by a neuropathy, in which case, it is regarded as a neuralgia of the pudendal nerve. An alternative theory is that proctalgia fugax occurs via congestion of the anal canal caused, for example, by internal haemorrhoids or proctitis. The literature also cites rectosigmoid intussusception and the accumulation of rectal gas as possible causes. Finally, the disorder is considered by some as an equivalent to vascular migraine.

PRESENTATION

Patients attend because of the pain. This is described as sharp and fleeting, or as a fierce cramp. The majority (84%) of the attacks apparently last less than 1 minute. There have been reports of the pain radiating to the gluteal area, the iliac fossa or the sacrum. The pain can be so intense that the patient collapses. Also, there are often accompanying symptoms, such as sweating, nausea and a false urge to defaecate. The attacks of anal cramps can occur at any time of the day, but they mainly take place at night. The patient is woken from sleep, is anxious and distraught, and displays significant motor agitation. He may try to relieve the pain by pushing on the anus with his fist, by crouching down with a fist in the lower abdomen or even by putting a finger in the anus. He sometimes succeeds in defaecating or passing wind, which may relieve the pain. The most frequently described triggers include orgasm and straining during defaecation.

EPIDEMIOLOGY

Epidemiological data are scanty. Based on a population study in the USA of people aged 15 years and older, it seems that 8% of people experience proctalgia fugax, although only a fraction of them consult a doctor. It occurs in all age groups from puberty, and to about the same extent in both women and men. The majority of patients (72%) have less than six attacks a year.

HISTORY

The clinical picture is so typical that distinguishing it from other rectal disorders should not be a problem. The GP asks:

- about the duration and frequency of the attacks of pain (see details above)
- how long the symptoms have been present
- about the site of the pain
- about other relevant symptoms.

EXAMINATION

The diagnosis of proctalgia fugax is made based on the typical history and the negative findings on physical examination, including inspection and a digital rectal examination. The GP checks for anal fissures or visible haemorrhoids. Other pathologies are excluded via the digital rectal examination.

TREATMENT

As proctalgia fugax usually spontaneously fades after several seconds or minutes, specific medical treatment has little to offer: in many cases, the episode will already have subsided before any medication could take effect. It is important to reassure the patient that this symptom does not indicate a serious disorder.

The literature describes several experienced-based techniques that may relieve the pain. The first is anal dilatation by means of manipulation via a finger in the anus. The second entails pushing upwards against the perineum using a closed fist. Another method involves a warm bath. However, convincing evidence for these methods is unavailable. Similarly, the apparently beneficial effects of clonidine, nitrates, nifedipine and diltiazem have been based on anecdotal reports rather than systematic studies. For this reason, these remedies are generally not recommended. One randomized, placebo-controlled cross-over study of patients with severe and long-term attacks, showed that inhaling salbutamol during an attack significantly shortens the duration of the episode. The mechanism of action is unclear; it does not seem advisable to prescribe such therapy for patients who only have a few attacks each year.

PREVENTION AND ADDITIONAL INFORMATION

Explanation about the nature of the disorder is very important in preventing unnecessary investigation and/or anxiety. In summary, the statement that 'proctalgia fugax is harmless, unpleasant and incurable' still seems to hold true.

Key points

- Proctalgia fugax is harmless, unpleasant and incurable; its cause is unknown.
- The clinical picture is so typical that distinguishing it from other rectal disorders should not be difficult.
- As proctalgia fugax usually spontaneously fades after several seconds or minutes, specific medical treatment has little to offer.
- Explanation and reassurance are important.

Literature

Babb RR. Proctalgia fugax. Would you recognize it? *Postgrad Med* 1996;**99**:263–4.

Matthijsen M, Knuistingh Neven A. Proctalgia fugax. *Modern Med* 1999;**23**(9):788–90.

Nidorf DM, Jamison ER. Proctalgia fugax. *Am Family Physician* 1995;**52**:2238–40.

Wald A. Functional anorectal and pelvic pain. *Gastroenterol Clin North Am* 2001;**30**(1):viii–ix, 243–51.

91
WIND/FLATULENCE

DEFINITION

In this chapter, 'wind' or 'flatulence' refer to the excessive passing of wind (as opposed to belching; see Chapter 72). Of course, this is only considered a problem if the wind bothers the person involved and/or others in the nearby environment, or if it is a symptom of an underlying illness. Normal flatus production is not insignificant – up to 2 l/day is normal. Belching (eructation), a 'full' feeling and flatulence can all have similar causes.

AETIOLOGY/PATHOGENESIS

Some details are given in Chapter 72. Gases in the gastrointestinal tract (normally 100–200 ml in total), consist almost entirely of nitrogen, oxygen, carbon dioxide, hydrogen and methane, in varying volume ratios. They end up there via swallowing, production in the bowel and diffusion from the blood.

Various actions can result in air being swallowed, such as chewing gum, drinking through a straw and smoking a pipe. People also swallow air when consuming food and drink: 20% of an apple consists of gas, and drinking a glass of water can result in an air/water ratio of 2:1 in the stomach. Fresh bread, beaten egg whites and carbonated drinks also contain air and gas. True aerophagy with anxiety is another cause of swallowed air.

Enzymatic and bacterial processes after a meal result in the production of approximately 15 l of gas. The vast majority in the small intestine is absorbed by the blood. Carbohydrates are mainly absorbed in the small intestines; the rest continues into the colon and undergoes fermentation by anaerobic flora. Malabsorption of carbohydrates will therefore result in excessive gas formation. Abnormalities such as lactase deficiency and the use of certain medications (e.g. lactulose, which is not broken down in the small intestine) can give rise to excessive gas formation via fermentation in the large bowel.

In the colon, anaerobic bacteria produce methane and hydrogen. Substances containing sulphur, and other compounds that cause the unpleasant odour, are mainly produced in the distal part of the colon.

With regard to diffusion, carbon dioxide, methane and hydrogen usually diffuse from the intestines to the blood; conversely, nitrogen and oxygen diffuse from the blood to the intestines. Oxygen is quickly used by the colonic bacteria, as a result of which the concentration in flatus is usually very low.

The elimination of intestinal gas takes place by belching and passing wind (an average of 10–20 times a day), by the use of gas by intestinal bacteria and by diffusion from the intestines to the blood.

If there is an imbalance between gas supply/production and elimination, excessive wind can occur, as can belching and a bloated feeling. An increased gas supply to the intestines can relate to aerophagy, diet or increased production in the intestines (food high in carbohydrates, malabsorption, bleeding in the gastrointestinal tract or achlorhydria). Other causes include a decreased diffusion of gas to the blood due to reduced intestinal motility – this can occur, for example, with an ileus or in hypotonia.

PRESENTATION

The complaint of flatulence is rarely expressed spontaneously. Because the audible or otherwise noticeable passing of wind is not considered polite in our society, it can be assumed that a patient's social background may play a role in consulting the doctor. On the other hand, a clear change in the flatus pattern may also be experienced and, therefore, presented as a problem. The GP needs to establish the reason for consultation: is it shame, with the fear of social isolation, or the fear of serious illness (such as cancer)?

EPIDEMIOLOGY

One study revealed that 21% of 315 'healthy' people had symptoms of flatulence. Because there is reluctance to consult a doctor with this symptom, or because the problem is not considered medically significant, it is undoubtedly underreported.

HISTORY

This is aimed at detecting both gastrointestinal abnormalities and psychosocial factors. The GP asks:

- about the patient's manner of eating (quickly/ravenously or relaxed)
- about the patient's diet (especially a large proportion of carbohydrates)
- about the bowel habit
- about previous operations on the gastrointestinal tract (which can sometimes result in accelerated intestinal passage, decreased absorption and increased fermentation in the colon)
- about certain relevant illnesses (Crohn's disease, lactase deficiency and chronic pancreatitis with disrupted carbohydrate digestion and absorption, resulting in abnormal gas formation)
- about psychosocial problems, which could be both the cause and the result of the flatulence.

EXAMINATION

This will depend on the patient's symptoms, concerns and the findings of the history. As a rule, it will comprise at least inspection while the patient is at rest, palpation and auscultation of the abdomen, and a digital rectal examination. It may also involve analysis of the faeces. Additional tests (e.g. X-rays, laboratory tests) should only be arranged if indicated.

TREATMENT

This will be oriented towards the reason for consultation and the findings after clinical assessment.

If an organic problem is suspected (previous operations, malabsorption, lactase deficiency, Crohn's disease, etc.), treatment is arranged as appropriate. Additional examination by a surgeon or gastroenterologist may be required.

If it seems that the cause is related to the patient's diet (unbalanced diet, food allergy, high-carbohydrate diet), the GP or a dietician can provide appropriate advice.

If it is evident that aerophagy is the main problem, explanation and advice may be sufficient.

Psychological components should be addressed; often, reassurance alone is sufficient.

PREVENTION AND ADDITIONAL INFORMATION

An explanation of the relationship between diet and flatulence can relieve the patient's anxiety, as well as the problem itself. Providing dietary information is part of the treatment for virtually all organic and non-organic disorders of the gastrointestinal tract.

Key points

- Flatulence is common, but rarely presented to the GP.
- The GP needs to establish the reason for consultation: this may be embarrassment, anxiety about a serious cause, or a simple request for treatment.
- Any underlying cause should be treated as appropriate; otherwise, management involves mainly dietary advice, explanation and reassurance.

Literature

De Ru VJ, Van Spronsen R. Onaangename lichaamsgeuren II: flatulentie [Unpleasant body odours II: flatulence]. Ned Tijdschr Geneeskd 1986;**130**:912–14.

Suarez FL, Levitt MD. An understanding of excessive intestinal gas. Curr Gastroenterol Rep 2000;**2**(5):413–19.

92
PULLED ELBOW

DEFINITION

Pulled elbow is a traumatic subluxation or dislocation of the head of the radius.

AETIOLOGY/PATHOGENESIS

Subluxation or complete dislocation of the head of the radius occurs if a child's arm is pulled while it is extended (e.g. when dressing the child, as its arm is pulled through the sleeve of a sweater, or pulling the child up by the arm when it falls over). In subluxation, part of the annular ligament slips over the head of the radius and shifts to the radiohumoral joint.

PRESENTATION

The child is usually crying and refuses to move the arm.

EPIDEMIOLOGY

Subluxation occurs commonly in children under 4 years old, usually between the ages of 1 and 3 years. It occurs slightly more often in boys and more often in the left elbow. Of all elbow injuries in young

children, 25% involve subluxation. No epidemiological data are
readily available.

HISTORY

It is a typical story: after the arm is pulled, the child begins to cry and
refuses to use it. The GP asks:

- how long ago it happened
- whether a 'click' was audible
- if the child appears to have pain in the wrist or shoulder.

EXAMINATION

During the inspection, the child usually holds the arm slightly flexed
in pronation against himself; the elbow is not swollen. The child
sometimes supports the painful arm with the other hand and refuses
to move the injured elbow.

Passive flexion and extension are not limited. Supination is limited
and very painful. There is local tenderness at the head of the radius
on the anterolateral side.

It is important to rule out a fracture – if there is doubt about this, the
child should be referred. Otherwise, for classic subluxation of the
head of the radius, X-rays are not indicated.

TREATMENT

If the subluxation has not spontaneously resolved by active or
passive supination of the forearm, the following action can be
taken. Explain to the parents that the procedure will be painful for
a moment, but that all pain will be gone immediately afterwards.
Move the arm to a 90° flexed position and securely hold the forearm
above the wrist. Place the thumb of your other hand at the level of
the head of the radius and exert light pressure. In this 90° flexed
position, quickly supinate the forearm. If this is successful, a 'click'
will be felt and heard. If this does not work, bend the forearm in
supination against the upper arm. Push on the head of the radius
until you hear a 'click'. The pain will disappear immediately, and
sometimes the child will start to use the arm again right away.
Neither a sling nor rest are indicated.

PREVENTION AND ADDITIONAL INFORMATION

Explain to the child's parents how the subluxation occurred, so that they can avoid provoking it again.

The prognosis is good. As stated above, the subluxation can spontaneously reposition itself. The chance of recurrence is approximately 5%. Of course, the risk of recurrence strongly depends on the actions of the child's parents.

Key points

- Subluxation or complete dislocation of the head of the radius occurs if a child's arm is pulled while it is extended (e.g. when dressing the child, as its arm is pulled through the sleeve of a sweater, or pulling the child up by the arm when it falls over).

- It is important to rule out a fracture – if there is doubt about this, the child should be referred. Otherwise, for classic subluxation of the head of the radius, X-rays are not indicated.

- Explain to the parents that the manoeuvre to cure a pulled elbow will be painful for a moment, but that all pain will be gone immediately afterwards.

- The chance of recurrence is approximately 5%.

Literature

Amir D, Frankl U, Pogrund H. Pulled elbow and hypermobility of joints. *Clin Orthopaed* 1990;**257**:94–9.

Dijk M, Streefkerk JG. Kleine kwalen in de huisartsgeneeskunde; zondagmiddagarmpje [Minor ailments in general practice; pulled elbow]. *Ned Tijdschr Geneeskd* 1993;**137**:1712.

Sankar NS. Pulled elbow. *J R Soc Med* 1999;**92**(9):462–4.

Visser JD. *Kinderorthopedie: pluis of niet pluis?* [*Paediatric orthopaedics: trustworthy or a scam?*] Groningen: Styx, 2003.

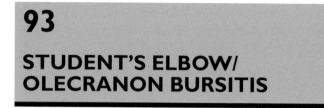

93

STUDENT'S ELBOW/ OLECRANON BURSITIS

DEFINITION

Olecranon bursitis is an inflammation of the olecranon bursa, which may be accompanied by infection in some cases. The non-septic bursitides (70%) include idiopathic olecranon bursitis (also known as student's elbow), traumatic bursitis and the bursitis present in systemic illnesses, such as rheumatoid arthritis and gout. Septic olecranon bursitis (30%) is the result of infection with bacteria, usually via the skin, and very rarely from the bloodstream.

AETIOLOGY/PATHOGENESIS

The olecranon bursa is located subcutaneously over the olecranon and is formed between the ages of 7 and 10 years. A bursa is filled with a small amount of synovial fluid, and its volume increases with age. It does not have a connection to the elbow joint. The olecranon bursa reduces the friction between the olecranon and the skin overlying it.

Idiopathic olecranon bursitis occurs due to chronic irritation (e.g. by repeatedly leaning on the elbow). Recurrent episodes of intrabursal bleeding may play a role in the pathogenesis of this form of bursitis. The presence of a bony spur on the olecranon may also play a role.

Traumatic bursitis can be the result of a blow to, or a fall on, the elbow, which causes bleeding in the bursa, and which can lead to an acute sterile inflammatory reaction.

Gout and rheumatoid arthritis are less frequent causes of non-infectious olecranon bursitis. In these situations, gouty tophi and rheumatoid nodules may be found intrabursally.

Septic olecranon bursitis is usually caused by the bursa becoming infected directly via skin trauma (e.g. scratching). In 90% of cases, the infection involves *Staphylococcus aureus* or *S. epidermidis*, and in 9% streptococci. Rarely, anaerobes, mycobacteria, fungi, *Haemophilus influenzae* or other Gram-negative micro-organisms are involved.

PRESENTATION

A person with olecranon bursitis notices a swelling on the point of the elbow, which can be painful when touched and sometimes feels warm. The questions the patient asks usually involve the cause and what can be done about the problem.

EPIDEMIOLOGY

Accurate epidemiological data are unavailable. A rough estimate would be one to two cases per average practice per year. The frequency of this problem generally increases with age; it also occurs more often in men than in women.

HISTORY

The history takes account of the likely aetiology of the bursitis. The GP asks:

- when the inflammation began
- if it was preceded by the patient continually leaning on the elbow (work, studies)
- how the symptoms arose (gradually and unnoticed, or acute and obvious)
- whether there was any trauma to the elbow
- whether the patient has a history of rheumatoid arthritis or gout
- whether the patient experienced any breach of the skin
- whether the patient has noticed warmth, redness or swelling.

EXAMINATION

Physical examination reveals a fluctuant swelling with a diameter of 2–6 cm. Maximal flexion of the elbow can be painful because of compression of the bursa. Further examination will be aimed at distinguishing between the different types of olecranon bursitis.

Local warmth and erythema can indicate gout. Redness, swelling, warmth and significant pain, peribursal cellulitis, swelling of the proximal forearm and regional lymphadenopathy, sometimes accompanied by general symptoms of illness such as fever, indicate septic bursitis.

Additional tests, at the earliest after a week, are mainly used for (and are only useful in) demonstrating sepsis. They consist of aspiration of the contents of the bursa. Purulent material indicates septic bursitis, and bacterial culture can confirm this.

TREATMENT

If the history and examination suggest a non-infectious cause, an explanation and a wait and see treatment are appropriate. If spontaneous recovery does not occur, one option is to aspirate and inject corticosteroids; a pressure bandage is then applied.

For septic bursitis, a course of flucloxacillin is sufficient. This may be preceded by aspiration of the contents of bursa.

If an abscess has formed, incision and drainage are indicated, followed by a pressure bandage.

The following circumstances should prompt referral to a surgeon: recurrence, chronicity or the presence of a loose body (after trauma). The treatment may be a partial or total bursectomy.

PREVENTION AND ADDITIONAL INFORMATION

For idiopathic forms, provide an explanation and instructions to avoid pressure and friction.

Key points

- Bursitis may be non-septic bursitides (70%) – including idiopathic olecranon bursitis, traumatic bursitis and the bursitis present in systemic illnesses, such as rheumatoid arthritis and gout – or septic (30%).

- Redness, swelling, warmth and significant pain, peribursal cellulitis, swelling of the proximal forearm and regional lymphadenopathy – sometimes accompanied by general symptoms of illness such as fever – indicate septic bursitis.

- The following circumstances should prompt referral to a surgeon: recurrence, chronicity or the presence of a loose body (after trauma).

Literature

Cardone DA, Tallia AF. Diagnostic and therapeutic injection of the elbow region. *Am Fam Physician* 2002;**66**(11):2097–100.

Keeman JN. *Kleine chirurgische ingrepen* [*Minor surgical procedures*]. Utrecht: Bunge, 1991.

Salzman KL, Lillegard WA, Butcher JD. Upper extremity bursitis. *Am Fam Phys* 1997;**56**(7):1797–806, 1811–12.

Vliet Vlieland TPM, Streefkerk JG. Kleine kwalen in de huisartsgeneeskunde; theorie en praktijk bij bursitis olecrani [Minor ailments in general practice; theory and practice for olecranon bursitis]. *Ned Tijdschr Geneeskd* 1991;**135**:837–9.

94

CARPAL TUNNEL SYNDROME

DEFINITION

Carpal tunnel syndrome (CTS) is a compression neuropathy of the median nerve. It can occur in one or both hands.

AETIOLOGY/PATHOGENESIS

The carpal tunnel is formed dorsally by a bony concave arch consisting of the carpal bones and, on the palmar side, by the transverse carpal ligament (retinaculum flexorum). The median nerve runs on the radial side of the superficial flexor tendons and under the tendon of the palmaris longus muscle. More distally, it passes under the transverse carpal ligament, so that the nerve rests on the bundle of the nine flexor tendons, which run through the carpal tunnel. The tunnel is narrowest where the ligament is thickest, approximately 2 cm distal from the opening of the carpal tunnel.

The disorder is due to an irritation or a constriction (often inter-mittent) of the median nerve in this rather rigid, osseofibrous carpal tunnel, resulting from an increase in the content or a decrease in the dimensions of the carpal tunnel. It is not usually clear how such constrictions develop in the carpal tunnel. Certain manual tasks probably play an important role. A relationship exists with intensive and repetitive wrist movements and activities in which the wrist is flexed or extended for a long time – which explains the frequency of CTS in craftsmen, typists and oral hygienists, and in those involved with certain pastimes, such as squash, golf or playing certain musical instruments.

Post-traumatic or postoperative fibrosis around the median nerve (after damage to the transverse carpal ligament) can also explain the development and/or recurrence of CTS. Obese, stocky people may have a higher risk of developing the problem. It is also associated with a variety of conditions, such as pregnancy, inflammatory arthritis, Colles' fracture, amyloidosis, hypothyroidism, diabetes mellitus, acromegaly, and the use of corticosteroids and oestrogens. Up to one-third of cases of CTS occur in association with such medical conditions.

There is also evidence suggesting a familial component. If no explanation can be found, the disorder is considered primary, essential or idiopathic CTS.

PRESENTATION

CTS is characterized by paraesthesiae, burning pain, numbness or the sensation that the fingers are thick and swollen (which may be accompanied by a ring becoming stuck), usually occurring in the area served by the median nerve and typically beginning in the dominant hand. Vasoactive phenomena may be present, causing clammy, cold or warm hands. The pain can be present in the palm, the lower and upper arm, and, rarely, even in the shoulder or neck region.

The symptoms occur mainly at night and in the early morning. The patient may experience difficulty in performing actions such as unbuttoning small buttons or wringing out a cloth. If the disorder progresses, it can eventually lead to permanent loss of sensitivity and strength in the thumb (abduction, opposition) due to paresis or paralysis of the thenar muscles. Most patients do not experience symptoms involving loss of motor function. The symptoms often occur in a cycle of remissions and exacerbations.

EPIDEMIOLOGY

Studies have revealed that the incidence of CTS is about 105 per 100,000 persons per year, so the average GP will see about two patients a year with CTS. The prevalence is about 3% in the general population. Sixty per cent of cases occur between the ages of 40 and 60 years. It is more common in women than men (especially in the older age groups). CTS also occurs more often premenstrually, and during the menopause and pregnancy (10%), in which case it usually arises after the sixth month and ultimately disappears.

HISTORY

The GP asks:

- about the type of symptoms and how they have progressed
- about symptoms at night
- about any loss of sensation or strength
- about disorders such as diabetes, hypothyroidism and rheumatoid arthritis
- about pregnancy
- about previous trauma and wrist operations.

EXAMINATION

The physical examination is focused on the potential loss of sensation or motor function. In the wrist extension test (maximal extension of the wrist joint) and Phalen's wrist flexion test (maximal volar flexion of the wrist joint), the median nerve is pressed against the transverse ligament for one minute. In Tinel's test the transverse carpal ligament is firmly tapped or pressed with a finger. The predictive value of these provocation tests, however, is limited, so they should be interpreted with caution. If the opponens pollicis muscle is weak, the patient may have difficulty placing the palmar side of the end of the thumb on the end of the little finger.

Blood tests are arranged if a rheumatic disorder, diabetes mellitus or a thyroid problem are suspected. In doubtful cases, a neurologist can carry out electrophysiological tests: the speed of conductivity can be delayed as a result of compression by the transverse carpal ligament.

TREATMENT

The natural progression of CTS justifies a wait and see policy. Only in the case of severe constriction is spontaneous improvement unlikely. If the symptoms are minor, conservative measures are advised. Actions that provoke the symptoms should be avoided. Treating the pain with paracetamol or similar analgesia may be helpful. A wrist splint, which holds the hand in a neutral or slightly extended position at night, is another option. The patient can put this brace on before bed, and hold it in place with a bandage or Velcro. The results are often limited and temporary.

The effect of steroid injection is often only transient; the risk of recurrence is high. The beneficial effect of physiotherapy, which may include massage, cryotherapy, thermotherapy and techniques such as massage and manipulation, has not been demonstrated. Non-steroidal anti-inflammatories, diuretics and pyridoxine have each been studied in small, randomized trials, with no evidence of efficacy.

If conservative therapy is not successful, and/or if thenar muscle wasting is present, surgical treatment is indicated. In most cases, decompression of the median nerve offers good results. The operation can be carried out by neurosurgeons, plastic surgeons, general surgeons or orthopaedic surgeons. The patient's symptoms usually resolve rapidly after the surgery. However, motor function may be restored less often than sensory loss.

PREVENTION AND ADDITIONAL INFORMATION

The risk of a recurrence can be reduced by avoiding factors that provoke the problem. So intensive and repetitive wrist movements and activities in which the wrist is flexed or extended for a long time should be avoided. This may mean stopping pastimes such as squash or golf, and giving up certain musical instruments.

Key points

- In up to one-third of cases, CTS is associated with an underlying condition, such as pregnancy, inflammatory arthritis, Colles' fracture, amyloidosis, hypothyroidism, diabetes mellitus or acromegaly, or the use of corticosteroids and oestrogens.

- The predictive value of Tinel's and Phalen's tests is limited, so they should be interpreted with caution.

- The natural progression of CTS justifies a wait and see policy. Only in the case of severe constriction is spontaneous improvement unlikely.

- If conservative therapy is not successful and/or if thenar muscle wasting is present, surgical treatment is indicated.

Literature

D'Arcy CA, McGee S. The rational clinical examination. Does this patient have carpal tunnel syndrome? *JAMA* 2000;**283**(23):3110–17.

Katz JN, Simmons BP. Clinical practice. Carpal tunnel syndrome. *N Engl J Med* 2002;**346**(23):1807–12.

Kuiper IA, Knuistingh Neven A. Het carpale tunnelsyndroom [Carpal tunnel syndrome]. *Modern Med* 1999;**23**(12):1006–11.

Lagro-Janssen ALM. Het carpale-tunnel syndroom [Carpal tunnel syndrome]. *Huisarts Wetenschap* 1989;**32**:370–5.

Padua L, Padua R, Lo Monaco M, Aprile I, Paciello N, Nazarro M, Tonali P. Natural history of carpal tunnel syndrome according to the neurophysiological classification. *Ital J Neurol Sci* 1998;**19**(6):357–61.

95

RING STUCK ON FINGER

DEFINITION

A pragmatic definition is a ring on a patient's finger that cannot be removed without the help of a medical professional.

AETIOLOGY/PATHOGENESIS

A ring that has been worn for a long time can become stuck because of swelling resulting from trauma, infection, allergic or toxic reactions, tumours or degenerative changes. Otherwise, this problem most commonly occurs when trying a ring on. The anatomy of the fingers makes it easy to push the ring onto the finger, but also renders it difficult to remove.

The manipulation involved in trying to remove a ring that is too tight can result in irritation and oedema, thereby aggravating the problem.

The main complication of a ring that has become stuck is possible or actual vascular occlusion. If the swelling expands in a proximal direction to the level of the ring, there is a risk of venous congestion. As a result, the swelling will further increase in size and ultimately lead to ischaemia of the finger.

PRESENTATION

The patient with a ring stuck on his finger will consult the GP mainly because of distress about the problem itself, or because of pain and/or swelling.

EPIDEMIOLOGY

It is not known how often people consult their GP for this problem. Many cases probably attend the casualty department.

HISTORY

The GP asks:

- how the ring became stuck
- what caused any swelling to develop
- if the patient or someone else has tried to remove the ring
- how long the swelling has been present
- whether the ring is causing pain.

EXAMINATION

The examination is limited to inspection and palpation. Inspection involves checking whether swelling is present, and if there is a change in colour. A bluish-purple colour indicates congestion. The GP then checks whether the ring can be twisted or moved up and down. Any obvious infection, arthritis, and so on should be noted.

TREATMENT

The treatment depends on whether it is necessary to remove the ring. If there are no signs of vascular congestion and the swelling is expected to go down very soon (e.g. allergic swelling after an insect bite), removing the ring is not necessary. In this case, it is important to give the patient instructions to re-attend if there is an increase in swelling, pain or a change in colour of the finger.

The simplest way to remove the ring is to lubricate the finger. By rubbing liquid soap or Vaseline onto the finger, the friction with the skin is reduced and the ring can sometimes be slid off.

If this is not successful, a strip of cotton fabric (or similar) can be slid under the ring, and a turning and pulling movement can help ease the ring off. Massaging the finger in a proximal direction can sometimes reduce the swelling.

If it is not possible to slide the ring off the finger, ring saw pliers may offer a solution. The end of the pliers is put under the ring and slowly moved back and forth, until the ring is sawn through. The two cut ends of the ring are then pulled apart using two small sets of pliers. This procedure is usually performed in the casualty department.

PREVENTION AND ADDITIONAL INFORMATION

People who run the risk of trauma to the fingers, due to work or
leisure activities, should be advised to not wear rings during these
activities. In general, a single experience with a ring becoming stuck
will have a powerful preventive effect for the future.

Key points

- The main complication of a ring that has become stuck is possible
  or actual vascular occlusion.

- The simplest way to remove the ring is to lubricate the finger with
  liquid soap or Vaseline.

- People who run the risk of trauma to the fingers, due to work or
  leisure activities, should be advised to not wear rings during these
  activities.

Literature
Cresap CR. Removal of a hardened steel ring from an extremely swollen
finger. *Am J Emerg Med* 1995;**13**(3):318–20.

96
MALLET FINGER

DEFINITION

A mallet finger describes a flexed position of the distal phalanx of a
finger due to the loss of continuity of the extensor apparatus over the
distal interphalangeal joint. This may involve a tear of the tendon
itself or an avulsion of the tendon together with its insertion on the
terminal phalanx.

AETIOLOGY/PATHOGENESIS

The cause is a vigorous flexion of the extended terminal phalanx
against resistance. This typically occurs in ball sports, especially
basketball and volleyball. The injury usually happens when the ball
hits the top of the extended finger. Mallet finger can also occur due to
other acute stress to the ends of the fingers – the classic description
cites bed-making as a cause.

PRESENTATION

The patient consults the GP because he has noticed a deformity of
the finger; sometimes pain is also present. In nearly 50% of cases, the
patient does not recall any trauma. In some cases, the patient attends
only after the abnormality has been present for a long period of time.

EPIDEMIOLOGY

The average GP sees this abnormality less than once a year. The
injury occurs almost exclusively in adults.

HISTORY

The GP asks:

- how long the injury has been present
- how it occurred.

EXAMINATION

The GP will find that the terminal phalanx is flexed by 20–80°. The so-called 'swan-neck deformity' may also occur as a secondary effect due to compensatory hyperextension in the proximal interphalangeal joint. X-rays and referral are indicated if there is an open wound or if the patient is a child (when the epiphysis may be involved).

TREATMENT

The GP can treat most cases of mallet finger with an extension (or mallet) splint. The splint should be fixed with tape and worn continually for 6 weeks. Aluminium strips and self-made splints using a wooden spatula can also be used, but are slightly less convenient and also less reliable. After 6 weeks, active flexion can gradually be built up. If an extension deficit recurs or persists, the splint needs to be worn for a further 2 weeks.

Referral to a surgeon for further treatment is indicated if the injury has been present for longer than 6 months (and the patient requests treatment), in the case of an open wound with loss of skin and tendon, if the patient is a child and in the case of an intra-articular fracture.

PREVENTION AND ADDITIONAL INFORMATION

Because this injury is almost exclusively caused by sudden, excessive, unexpected stress on the extensor tendon of the end phalanx, prevention is not a realistic possibility.

Key points

- The disruption of the extensor mechanism in mallet finger may involve a tear of the tendon itself or an avulsion of the tendon together with its insertion on the terminal phalanx.

- In nearly 50% of cases, the patient does not recall any trauma.

- X-rays and referral are indicated if there is an open wound or if the patient is a child (when the epiphysis may be involved).

Literature

O'Connor JF. Mallet finger. *Can Fam Physician* 1997;**43**:1725–6.

Wang QC, Johnson BA. Fingertip injuries. *Am Fam Physician* 2001;**63**(10):1961–6

97

FISH HOOK IN FINGER

DEFINITION

A fish hook can pierce the skin in many places, but it usually does not penetrate any deeper than the skin. However, a hook can sometimes penetrate subcutaneous tissue or the underlying muscle.

AETIOLOGY/PATHOGENESIS

The cause of a fish hook in the skin is usually careless manipulation of a fish hook while baiting the hook or when trying to remove it from the mouth of the fish. The fish hook can also be pulled forcefully through the skin of the finger as a person is trying to cast the line.

PRESENTATION

The patient attends with a fish hook in the skin and explains the circumstances.

EPIDEMIOLOGY

No exact figures are available. Many patients will attend the casualty department rather than the GP.

HISTORY

The GP asks:

- about the shape of the fish hook
- about the presence of one or more barbs
- about the position of the barb in relation to the fish hook's shaft.

EXAMINATION

The GP must have a good idea of the shape and depth of the hook. If the fish hook has broken off and its position cannot easily be defined, an X-ray is necessary and removal should be performed in the local casualty department.

TREATMENT

An effective method for removal involves pushing the hook through the finger and then cutting off the hook's point and barb. This is the preferred method for a fish hook with one or more barbs. The shaft of the hook is pushed further as if it were a (curved) needle, until the hook is pushed up through the skin. Cut off the point (with the barb) of the fish hook with a wire cutter and then pull the hook backwards out of the finger. Anaesthesia is usually not necessary.

Another method is extirpation. Local anaesthesia (lidocaine 1%, without adrenaline) is needed in the area to be incised with the scalpel. The tissue is incised from the point where the fish hook entered the finger, in the same plane as the fish hook. The scalpel then cuts along the hook, using the hook as a guide. The hook is then held against the scalpel and these are pulled out of the finger together. This method reduces the risk of the point or barb of the fish hook being caught in the tissue again.

The wound almost always heals without scarring.

Tetanus vaccination should be given as appropriate.

PREVENTION AND ADDITIONAL INFORMATION

Providing information about the use of fishing gear falls outside the GP's area of expertise. The patient must therefore consult an experienced fisherman.

Key points

- If the fish hook has broken off and its position cannot easily be defined, an X-ray is necessary.
- An effective method for removal involves pushing the hook through the finger and cutting off the point and barb of the hook.
- Another method is extirpation, which requires local anaesthesia.

Literature

College of Medicine of the University of Iowa. Removing a fish hook. *Patient Care* 1990;**17**(4):77–80.

David SS. Fishhook removal. *Lancet* 1991;**338**(8780):1463–4.

Gammons MG, Jackson E. Fishhook removal. *Am Fam Physician* 2001;**63**(11):2231–6.

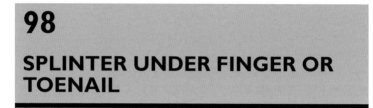

98

SPLINTER UNDER FINGER OR TOENAIL

DEFINITION

A splinter under the nail occurs when a small piece of wood, metal, glass, stone, bone or plastic becomes lodged between the nail plate and the nail bed.

AETIOLOGY/PATHOGENESIS

Certain activities increase the risk of acquiring a splinter of this sort: working with rough wood, metal or stone, gardening, cleaning up glass shards, etc. Due to direct contact of a hand or foot with the aforementioned materials, a small piece will tear or break off and become lodged between the nail plate and the nail bed. In healthy people, there is no space between the nail plate and the nail bed, which means that a splinter can easily become jammed in this area.

If a splinter remains under the nail for a period of time, a rejection reaction will occur, and inflammation will result. Spontaneous expulsion of this foreign body does not usually occur.

PRESENTATION

Patients with a splinter under the nail attend to ask the GP to remove it. The situation can be painful, especially if the splinter is moved, pressure is put on the nail or the end of the finger is touched.

EPIDEMIOLOGY

There are no data about the incidence of this ailment. Many patients will undoubtedly attend the local casualty department.

HISTORY

The GP asks:

- how long the splinter has been present
- what the splinter is made of and whether it is clean or dirty
- whether an attempt has been made to remove it and, if so, how this was done
- whether the presence of the splinter is causing pain.

EXAMINATION

The nail plate should be inspected. How deep is the splinter? What is the shape of the part of the splinter that is under the nail? Remember that the splinter will often be much larger than it appears.

TREATMENT

It is always necessary to remove the splinter. The instrument selected depends on the nature of the splinter; the presence (or lack) of a free end of the splinter determines the removal method.

The nail is cut as short as possible, so the GP has adequate room to work with. Choose an instrument that will be able to grip the splinter effectively: the smoother the splinter material, the more coarsely ribbed the ends of the instrument should be (e.g. tweezers). A wooden splinter can often be 'pricked' from the side with an injection needle; this involves a careful manipulation of the needle, perpendicular to the splinter. If the free end of the splinter cannot be gripped with sufficient traction, more space can be achieved by cutting a small wedge out of the nail. In this case, local anaesthesia (2% lidocaine administered with a very thin needle) in the end of the finger can help. Alternatively, a ring block may be necessary (see Chapters 102 and 115). The splinter is removed by pulling it out lengthwise.

Check that the splinter has been removed completely. Tape or bandage the area, depending on the size of the area treated. Tetanus prophylaxis should be arranged if appropriate.

PREVENTION AND ADDITIONAL INFORMATION

Point out the importance of protecting the fingers (and toes) by wearing work gloves (and proper shoes), especially if the patient often works with wood or metal in his free time or in his employment.

Key points

- It is always necessary to remove a splinter from under a nail.
- The presence (or lack) of a free end of the splinter determines the removal method.
- Cutting a small wedge out of the nail may be necessary to enable the splinter to be grasped properly.

Literature

Chan C, Salam GA. Splinter removal. *Am Fam Physician* 2003;**67**(12): 2557–62.

Schwartz GR, Schwen SA. Subungual splinter removal. *Am J Emerg Med* 1997;**15**(3):330–1.

99

NAIL-BITING

DEFINITION

Nail-biting is a common, repetitive, self-mutilating behaviour in children and young adults. It is bothersome, unattractive, socially undesirable, and can predispose to paronychia.

AETIOLOGY/PATHOGENESIS

Much has been published about the role of anxiety, tension and stress as an aetiological factor. It has been suggested that nail-biting serves to reduce tension in certain stressful situations. Some nail-biters show obsessive symptoms, such as excessive self-care rituals, which appear to be similar to the compulsive actions of patients with an obsessive–compulsive disorder. However, in the DSM-IV, nail-biting is not classified as a psychiatric diagnosis, nor is it named as an (additional) symptom in obsessive–compulsive disorders. The association between nail-biting and a psychiatric disorder has never been studied systematically.

Nail-biting may run in families. On the one hand, some children copy this behaviour from other family members. On the other, research indicates that this habit occurs around twice as often in monozygotic twins as compared to dizygotic twins, and that the closer the genetic relationship, the greater the chance that the family member is also a nail-biter.

It has also been suggested that nail-biting follows thumb sucking, and that the habit serves the purpose of oral satisfaction. This chron-ological relationship is supported by a longitudinal study of children aged 2–5 years. Although many thumb suckers later became nail-biters, the reverse of this hypothesis does not always hold true. Nail-biting can also be the result of poorly manicured nails – the irregular edges and rough ends can be a source of irritation.

Nail-biting occurs primarily on the fingernails, but sometimes also on the toenails. Most nail-biters bite all 10 nails to the same extent. The habit stimulates nail growth by approximately 20%, possibly because frequent manipulation of the nail stimulates the circulation to the germinal area in the nail root.

In most cases, the distal part of the nail is bitten off, which results in a short, uneven nail. Some nail-biters also bite the cuticles, the surrounding skin or other objects, such as pencils. Onychotillomania (compulsive picking at the nails) is a more serious disorder.

While nail-biting is usually not a serious problem in children, in rare cases severe nail-biting can cause medical and dental problems. If the patient also bites the cuticles and the skin on the fingers, local infections, scars, excoriations and possibly keloids can result. In nail disorders such as onychomycosis and paronychia, the infecting agent can spread to the mouth by nail-biting. The reverse can also occur – a nail-biter with oral herpes can spread this infection to the damaged finger.

PRESENTATION

In most cases, the patient will attend when complications occur, such as chronic subungual infections or recurring paronychia. Other reasons for consultation can include dystrophic nails, secondary bacterial infection, periungual warts, damage to the matrix resulting in scar tissue, and damage to the nail bed resulting in the loss of the nail.

EPIDEMIOLOGY

The problem usually begins at about the age of 3 years. The proportion of nail-biters increases to approximately 30% between the ages of 3 and 6 years. From ages 7 to 10 years, the prevalence remains about the same, but then increases to 45% during puberty. The prevalence reaches its peak between the ages of 10 and 18 years. In the late teenage years, the prevalence begins to drop and continues to fall steadily into adulthood. This fall with age continues, so that only about 10% of people above of 35 years old are nail-biters. The prevalence of nail-biting is approximately the same in both genders until the age of 10 years, after which the number of males that bite their nails is about 10% higher.

HISTORY

The GP asks:

- about the duration of the nail-biting and when it started
- about any increase in the severity of the problem and any apparent reason for this
- whether the patient bites the fingernails or toenails
- about previous infections or complications from the nail-biting.

EXAMINATION

Most nail-biters bite all 10 nails to the same extent. On inspection, short and rough nails are seen. The GP assesses whether the nail-biting has resulted in complications, such as chronic subungual infections and recurring paronychia, as well as nail dystrophy, secondary bacterial infection, periungual warts, damage to the matrix resulting in scar tissue, and damage to the nail bed leading to loss of the nail.

The cuticles and skin of the fingers that are bitten are examined to see if local infections, scars, excoriations and possibly keloids are present.

TREATMENT

Particularly in children, the approach must be aimed at identifying any factors causing stress. If no clear cause is found, attention must be focused on attempts to build the child's self-confidence and self-respect. Other important therapeutic factors include caring for the nails (filing them) and cuticles, behaviour-modifying techniques, positive reinforcement and regular follow-up.

Many behavioural therapies have been evaluated for the treatment of nail-biting, resulting in varying degrees of success. Changing the behaviour pattern has emerged as the best method in the studies published to date. This method concentrates on relaxation, self-control techniques, social support and looking back at difficult moments. In 84% of patients, nail-biting was reduced, and some 40% of patients stopped biting their nails altogether. Other methods have also proven that nail-biting can be eliminated: for example, by painting the nails with a bitter-tasting substance, learning competing responses (making a fist or holding an object) and negative reinforcement.

Only one randomized study has evaluated the pharmaceutical treatment of serious nail-biting. This study revealed that clomipramine is effective in severe cases.

PREVENTION AND ADDITIONAL INFORMATION

In mild forms, it is important to supplement the patient's request for help with an explanation and information about the risk of infection due to nail-biting. For more serious forms, it is very important that the patient is motivated to change the behaviour, in part by pointing out the complications.

Key points

- It has been suggested that nail-biting serves to reduce tension in certain stressful situations.
- During puberty 45% of children bite their nails to some extent. In the late teenage years the prevalence begins to drop and continues to fall steadily into adulthood.
- Complications include chronic paronychia and nail dystrophy.
- Sources of stress should be identified, especially in children.

Literature

Allen KW. Chronic nail-biting: a controlled comparison of competing response and mild aversion treatments. *Behav Res Ther* 1996;**34**:269–72.

Leonard HL, Lenane MC, Swedo SE, Rettew DC, Rapoport JL. A double-blind comparison of clomipramine and desipramine treatment of severe onychophagia (nail-biting). *Arch Gen Psychiatry* 1991;**48**(9):821–7.

Wagenaar I, Knuistingh Neven A. Nagelbijten [Nail-biting]. *Modern Med* 1998;**22**(10):93–5.

100
SUBUNGUAL HAEMATOMA

DEFINITION

A subungual haematoma is an effusion of blood between the nail and the nail bed.

AETIOLOGY/PATHOGENESIS

A subungual haematoma can be the result of: a blow with a hammer or other hard object to the nail; the end of a finger or toe becoming caught, for example, in a door; rapid stopping movements in the shoes, such as in people who jog or play tennis, basketball or squash; and shoes that are too narrow. The trauma causes pressure on the nail plate and bleeding between the nail and nail bed. This bleeding causes an increase in pressure on the nail bed, which can result in pain (although not always). The pain does not always occur immediately after the trauma; it may take several hours to develop, as the pressure under the nail increases.

PRESENTATION

Patients generally present with a painful blue nail. The reason for consulting is usually the pain. The patient almost always describes an injury to the nail, and many people know that a hole will have to be made in the nail to relieve the symptoms.

EPIDEMIOLOGY

There are no accurate figures about the incidence of this problem. A rough estimate is that an average general practice sees two to four cases a year, more often in men than in women. Some may attend the local casualty department.

HISTORY

A history does not usually need to be taken – the patient will volunteer how the subungual haematoma occurred. The exception is the situation resulting from shoes that are too narrow or from friction in shoes during sports, in which case the patient may not have worked out the cause.

EXAMINATION

Inspection is usually sufficient to make the diagnosis.

TREATMENT

If the haematoma is small and is not causing pain, it does not need to be treated. The affected nail may become detached after a while, but a new one will grow.

If the injury is very painful, a small hole can be made in the nail to release the unclotted blood and reduce the pressure between the nail and the nail bed. There are many ways of making a hole in the nail (e.g. using a scalpel, a small drill, or a disposable needle). The disadvantage of all these methods is that the nail bed is likely to be touched when the nail is pierced, which is very painful. The most convenient instrument remains a heated paperclip with a blunt end, which greatly reduces the risk of touching the nail bed after making a hole in the nail. No anaesthetic is needed for this simple procedure.

The paperclip should be straightened and held in a clamp. The free end of the paperclip is held in the blue part of a flame until it is red hot. The end of the hot paperclip is then applied to the site of the haematoma. Burning through the nail is painless, but touching the nail bed is very painful. Once the nail has been pierced, the blood will be released and the pain will quickly disappear. A plaster is sufficient to collect the rest of the exudate.

Clotted blood under the nail is not easy to remove.

PREVENTION AND ADDITIONAL INFORMATION

Recommendations about the use of well-fitting shoes when playing sports can be useful in preventing haematomas under the toenails.

Patients who have seen the paperclip technique can often carry this out themselves.

Key points

- A subungual haematoma may take several hours to develop.
- The history, and so the diagnosis, is usually obvious, except when the problem occurs in toenails via sport or ill-fitting footwear.
- A painless subungual haematoma does not require treatment.
- Relieving any pain involves making a hole in the nail to relieve the pressure.
- Using a heated paperclip greatly reduces the risk of painfully touching the nail bed after making a hole in the nail.

Literature

Helms A, Brodell RT. Surgical pearl: prompt treatment of subungual haematoma by decompression. *J Am Acad Dermatol* 2000;**42**(3):508–9.

Meek S, White M. Subungual haematomas: is simple trephining enough? *J Accid Emerg Med* 1998;**15**(4):269–71.

Wang QC, Johnson BA. Fingertip injuries. *Am Fam Physician* 2001;**63**(10):1961–6.

101

BRITTLE NAILS/FRAGILITAS UNGUIUM

DEFINITION

Brittle nails are characterized by increased fragility and an increased tendency for them to break or split. Similar problems include onychorrhexis (excessive lengthwise ridges) and onychoschisis (horizontal lamellar splitting of the distal nail plate accompanied by rough and irregular edges).

AETIOLOGY/PATHOGENESIS

Brittle nails lead to cracks in the nail plate. This is composed of three layers of keratin and its strength is determined by various factors, including the physical characteristics of the nail plate, its hydration and the presence of the matrix proteins. These proteins function as intercellular cement between the different layers of the nail plate.

There are two groups of causes of brittle nails. The first involves exogenous factors, which affect a normally formed nail plate. These are usually linked to work or hobbies, household tasks, or the use of nail cosmetics. Examples of substances that damage the nail plate are cement, detergents, caustic solutions, anilines, acids, paint substances, solvents, sugar solutions and hot water. While nail polish in itself protects the nail, the use of acetone-like nail-polish remover can cause damage and ultimately make the nails brittle. Fake nails, glued on for cosmetic reasons, can cause severe hypersensitivity reactions. They can also disturb the hydration of the nail plate (a relatively dry nail is less strong and elastic). Hydration is also affected by a dry, warm environment or by frequent washing. The adhesion between the different layers of the nail plate is particularly reduced if the nails are too frequently submerged in water and then allowed to dry. The fact that intercellular cement can dissolve in detergents may also be relevant.

Distal splitting, especially of long fingernails, can occur through trauma. Activities such as typing, manning a telephone and working with wood can be particular problems. Other injury may result from the incorrect use of the nail (e.g. as a screwdriver) or careless nail clipping. Finally, in this group, fungal infections (*Candida albicans*, dermatophytes) can damage the nail plate through proteolysis, and thereby cause brittleness.

The second group of causes disrupts the development of a healthy nail plate by the nail matrix. This group includes infections, anaemia, systemic disorders, circulatory disorders, poisoning with dangerous substances (e.g. arsenic), injuries and skin disorders (e.g. contact dermatitis, lichen planus, psoriasis).

There is also a group of patients for whom no cause can be established, even after extensive examination and investigation. If the nail abnormalities have been present for the patient's entire life, or if one or more family members also have brittle nails, this may be a congenital or hereditary disorder. Other patients suffer from brittle nails only during certain periods of their life – this idiopathic type is more common in women than men.

PRESENTATION

The patient explains that the nails break easily, tear or are brittle. The nail functions as an important aid in gripping and using objects, so the problem may be more than just cosmetic. In addition, pain (or an increased sensitivity to pain) can occur, as well as a decreased sense of touch. Rough nail ends often catch on clothing.

EPIDEMIOLOGY

A study conducted in various patient populations revealed that approximately one in five people suffer from brittle nails, with women being affected about twice as often as men.

HISTORY

The GP asks:

- how the symptoms have developed

- about the patient's profession, hobbies or other activities
- about contact with chemicals, cosmetics or hot water (e.g. when doing the washing up)
- about any injury
- about certain habits, such as nail-biting
- about other disorders, such as eczema, psoriasis, circulatory problems or endocrine disorders
- about whether brittle nails run in the patient's family.

EXAMINATION

When inspecting the nails, the GP examines the site and extent of the abnormalities, which nails are affected (one, several or all), the direction of the breaks (horizontal or lengthwise, lamellar or random), whether the nails are shiny or dull, and whether pits (psoriasis) can be seen. In addition, the GP checks for the presence of the remains of colouring agents, cosmetics or injury, and for signs of a mycosis. The skin is inspected to see if other skin disorders are present. A general physical examination is conducted if a systemic disorder is suspected – in practice, this is usually unnecessary.

Additional tests may be carried out if a mycosis (e.g. microscopy and culture) or a systemic disorder is suspected.

TREATMENT

The main aim is, if possible, to address any relevant causative or aggravating factors. For example, if relevant, can changes be made in the person's work or household activities, such as wearing gloves? Cotton gloves can be worn under rubber gloves to reduce perspiration (and therefore the risk of infection). Nail polish is not damaging and can even strengthen the nail; however, this is usually used in combination with nail-polish remover, which can seriously damage the nail. If a fungal infection is present, this can be treated with terbinafine 250 mg once daily for at least 2 months, or itraconazole pulse therapy 200 mg twice daily for 1 week followed by three medication-free weeks, the cycle repeated once for fingernails and twice for toenails. Underlying systemic disorders must be treated as appropriate – this can also improve the quality of the nail.

For the hereditary or idiopathic form, the following recommendations are helpful. The nails must be regularly clipped and then filed. Clipping dried-out nails increases the risk of damage, so it is better to cut the nails after a bath. The patient should wear gloves when washing up and afterwards apply a greasy cream to the nails.

PREVENTION AND ADDITIONAL INFORMATION

An explanation about the damaging effects of trauma, nail-biting, cosmetics, cleaning agents and other chemical substances can help to prevent the problem. The preventive use of gloves may be helpful.

Key points

- Brittle nails are caused by exogenous factors, which affect a normally formed nail plate, or endogenous factors, which disrupt the development of the nail plate.
- While nail polish protects the nail, the use of acetone-like nail-polish remover can cause damage, and ultimately make the nails brittle.
- In some patients no cause is found.
- Clipping dried-out nails increases the risk of damage, so it is better to cut the nails after a bath.

Literature

Scher RK, Bodain AB. Brittle nails. *Semin Dermatol* 1991;**10**:21–5.

Uyttendaele H, Geyer A, Scher RK. Brittle nails: pathogenesis and treatment. *J Drugs Dermatol* 2003;**2**(1):48–9.

Van de Klaauw JW, Gill K. Kleine kwalen in de huisartsgeneeskunde; brosse nagels [Minor ailments in general practice; brittle nails]. *Ned Tijdschr Geneeskd* 1989;**133**:1931–3.

102

PARONYCHIA/WHITLOW

DEFINITION

Paronychia or whitlow is an infection of the nail fold, which can develop into an abscess. The cause of acute infections is usually bacterial; the chronic forms are more often caused by fungi (see also Chapter 101).

AETIOLOGY/PATHOGENESIS

Paronychia probably begins with a minor injury to the nail fold, which can be caused by poor nail hygiene, nail-biting or picking, and the nails being clipped too short. This gives commensal skin bacteria (e.g. staphylococci) the opportunity to multiply. The infection may remain limited to a local infiltrate of the nail fold, but can spread beneath the nail in more severe cases. The fact that the nail is a relatively inert object contributes to maintaining the infection. When the big toe is involved, an ingrowing nail may be the underlying cause. Another type of acute paronychia of the fingers is the herpesvirus – this type of infection is sometimes seen in dentists.

Mycotic infections of the nail fold (usually *Candida*) often occur via a combination of frequent minor injuries and long-term exposure to moisture.

In infants, small 'abscesses' are often found on several fingers after birth. This appears to involve a sterile inflammation.

PRESENTATION

The GP probably only sees the more severe cases. In the acute situation, the patient usually presents with a painful, throbbing red patch proximal to the nail fold; a small local accumulation of pus is sometimes also visible. The patient may have trouble using the finger.

Pain is not a prominent symptom in chronic paronychia. In such cases, a larger area of the nail fold is red and swollen.

EPIDEMIOLOGY

The incidence is 3.5–4.5 new cases per 1000 patients per year. Paronychia occurs in people of all ages, slightly more often in men than in women.

HISTORY

The history can be brief because simply looking at the affected finger is usually sufficient to make the diagnosis. The GP asks:

- about the duration of the symptoms
- about the severity and character of the pain
- about any injury that might have caused the problem – such as nail-biting or pulling off small pieces of skin.

If the symptom is chronic, the GP also asks about work and leisure activities.

EXAMINATION

The examination can also usually be brief. In general, it is not difficult to distinguish between paronychia and other infections of the finger. If the symptoms are chronic, the GP also inspects the other fingers, and checks for other signs of mycotic infections.

TREATMENT

For acute paronychia, the GP explains about the nature and good prognosis of the problem. If there are no signs of an abscess, resting the finger and protecting it against being hit or bumped may be sufficient. A moist bandage may offer some relief, but has no effect on the outcome. Covering the finger with a 1.25 cm wide adhesive plaster will provide protection and prevents irritation. Antibiotics may help, unless the lesion obviously requires drainage.

Small superficial abscesses can be opened with a needle. If the infection has spread under the nail, a part of the nail base must be removed to achieve proper drainage.

After disinfecting the area, a ring block is performed. Depending on the spread of the infection, one or two lengthwise incisions can be made in the corners of the nail fold. The nail fold is loosened and the nail base exposed. The parts of the nail affected by pus are excised. The pus is then drained and a small piece of gauze is placed between the nail and the nail fold to keep the nail fold separate from the nail. A bandage is applied with pressure at the site of the incision. When the wound stops bleeding, a simple finger bandage is applied, possibly first covered with some gauze to prevent the bandage from sticking to the wound. The gauze is removed the next day, the wound is inspected and a dry dressing is then applied.

Chronic nail fold infections are treated with a local antifungal cream. The patient is advised to keep the hands out of water as much as possible and to avoid traumatizing the fingers and nails. If the fungus has also affected the nail bed and the nail, oral antifungal therapy can also be considered.

PREVENTION AND ADDITIONAL INFORMATION

Eliminating certain habits, such as biting the nails and the nail fold, not cutting the sides of the nails too short, and ensuring the hands have less frequent contact with water and chemicals, can play an important role in preventing paronychia.

Key points

- Acute paronychia is usually bacterial (occasionally herpes-simplex virus); chronic paronychia is usually fungal.
- Habits such as nail-biting and picking, and repeated contact with water, may be causative or contributory factors.
- Abscesses caused by paronychia require drainage.

Literature
Rockwell PG. Acute and chronic paronychia. *Am Fam Physician* 2001;**63**(6):1113–16.

Van den Bosch WJH, Voorn ThB. Kleine chirurgie in de huisartspraktijk [Minor surgery in general practice]. *Huisarts Wet* 1986;**29**:243–7.

Yates YJ, Concannon MJ. Fungal infections of the perionychium. *Hand Clin* 2002;**18**(4):631–36.

103

FUNGAL INFECTION OF THE NAIL

DEFINITION

A fungal infection of the nail produces characteristic abnormalities, and the diagnosis is confirmed by demonstrating the presence of fungal spores or yeasts. The typical abnormalities include a yellowish-white discoloration of the nail plate with distal onycholysis (the nail end becoming detached), subungual hyperkeratosis, total nail dystrophy and, in some cases, paronychia (particularly in *Candida* infections).

AETIOLOGY/PATHOGENESIS

Fungal nail infections occur mainly on the feet; only 20–30% involve the fingernails.

More than half of nail infections are caused by dermatophytes, of which *Trichophyton rubrum* infections are most common. Toenail infections are almost always caused by dermatophytes. When the fingernails are infected, 75% of cases are candidal.

Dermatophytes use keratin as a food source. As growth occurs, many spores form, which can remain contagious for years. These spores are released into the environment with skin flakes or breaking nails, and so can spread infection. Because the spores are well protected in the nail flakes, they are relatively insensitive to external influences. Spores are inactivated by temperatures above 80°C (so they remain intact in washing machine programmes of 40–60°C).

Some factors will promote infection. These include damp and damaged skin, poor hygiene (poorly ventilated shoes, insufficient drying of hands or feet), reduced cellular resistance, overly high skin pH, the use of antibiotics or corticosteroids, and diabetes mellitus (sugar provides a food source for yeasts, which are consequently not dependent on keratin).

If a yeast infection occurs, chronic paronychia may develop (see Chapter 102). This typically affects the middle or index finger. The nail fold becomes detached from the nail plate and there is red swelling of the surrounding tissue, which can spread around the entire nail. Over time, a greenish to black discoloration develops and crosswise ridges occur (washboard phenomenon). There is little pain.

Fungal infections usually begin on the free distal edge in one corner of the nail plate, often where the shoe exerts pressure. The fungus grows in or under the nail plate. The end of the nail becomes raised and whitish-yellow patches develop in the areas where the nail comes loose from the nail bed. The nail plate thickens, crumbles and separates from the nail bed, growth is disrupted and eventually the nail is destroyed.

Eczema or psoriasis could be considered in the differential. These skin diseases are usually also present elsewhere on the body and, unlike fungal infections, they tend to affect the nails symmetrically.

PRESENTATION

The patient may well have had nail abnormalities for years before consulting the GP. In many cases there are remarkably few symptoms: there is usually no pain (except in paronychia), but itching is some-times present. Patients usually present with a 'chalky nail', which is a late stage of the fungal infection. Alternatively, they may be concerned because the nail appears to be detaching.

The symptoms accompanying chronic paronychia (redness and swelling of the nail fold, washboard phenomenon) are also a reason for consulting.

EPIDEMIOLOGY

The prevalence is between 3% and 8% of the adult population. Toenails are affected four times as often as fingernails. At-risk groups include nursing-home patients and employees of swimming pools and cleaning services.

HISTORY

The GP asks:

- whether the fingernails, toenails or all the nails are affected
- about the site of the abnormalities
- whether there have been colour changes
- how long the abnormalities have been present
- about other illnesses (especially dermatological) or use of medication
- about hygiene measures
- about excessive use of soap
- about the patient's work.

EXAMINATION

Examination will reveal, in early cases, the sides of the nail affected by brown, white or yellow discoloration. In more advanced cases, the nail will be thickened and crumbly, and may be separated from the nail bed. Unlike with many cases of dermatological disease (e.g. psoriasis), the abnormalities are asymmetrical.

Blood tests are generally unnecessary. If there is doubt about the diagnosis, clippings may be taken for mycology. If negative, they may be worth repeating.

TREATMENT

Treatment of a fungal infection of the nail is not always necessary. Cosmetic abnormalities can be treated with nail varnish.

Mechanical discomfort resulting from the infection requires further treatment. There are three options: debridement to remove the infected keratin, the application of local medication, and oral medication.

Local treatment produces disappointing results: insufficient penetration of the medication (because the fungus is protected by the nail plate) means that relapse rates are high. Thus local therapy with antimycotics is helpful only for very superficial infections.

Itraconazole and terbinafine can be used as oral antifungals. Success rates of more than 80% have been reported with both remedies.

However, the GP should consider carefully whether such treatment (which may have to be prolonged) is desirable or necessary, for such a 'minor' complaint, partially in view of compliance problems. Both medications are well tolerated, but they are, rarely, hepatotoxic.

PREVENTION AND ADDITIONAL INFORMATION

Much practical advice can be provided. Patients should wear dry, well-ventilated shoes that do not pinch the feet, and, preferably, cotton socks. Walking bare-footed on floors in bathrooms and gyms is one of the commonest ways of becoming infected by fungi, and so should be avoided if possible. Excess soap should be avoided, and the skin should be rinsed well, especially after using alkaline soap.

If *Candida* is suspected as the cause of the infection, avoid contact with water as much as possible.

Antimyotic powder may be sprinkled in the shoes if there is an increased risk of infection, and to prevent reinfection.

Key points

- The differential diagnosis of fungal nail infections includes eczema and psoriasis. These conditions usually affect the nails symmetrically.
- Treatment of a fungal infection of the nail is not always necessary. Cosmetic abnormalities can be treated with nail varnish.
- Local treatment produces disappointing results.
- The GP and patient should consider carefully whether oral treatment (which may have to be prolonged) is desirable or necessary.
- Walking bare-footed on floors in bathrooms and gyms is one of the commonest ways of becoming infected by fungi, and so should be avoided if possible.

Literature
Bergman W, Rutten FFH. Orale behandeling van onychomycose van de teennagels; vergelijking van kosteneffectiviteit van griseofulvine, itraconazol,

ketoconazol en terbinafine [Oral treatment of onychomycosis of the toenails; a comparison of the cost-effectiveness of griseofulvin, itraconazole, ketoconazole and terbinafine]. *Ned Tijdschr Geneeskd* 1994;**138**(47):2346–50.

Crawford F, Hart R, Bell-Syer S, Torgerson D, Young P, Russell I. Topical treatments for fungal infections of the skin and nails of the foot. *Cochrane Database Syst Rev* 2000;**2**:CD001434.

De Kock CA, Duyvendak RJP, Jaspar AHJ, et al. NHG-standaard: dermatomycosen [NHG standard: dermatomycosis]. *Huisarts Wet* 1997;**40**:541–52.

Denning DW, et al. Fungal nail disease: a guide to good practice. *BMJ* 1995;**311**:12781.

Faergemann J, Baran R. Epidemiology, clinical presentation and diagnosis of onychomycosis. *Br J Dermatol* 2003;**149**(Suppl 65):1–4.

104

LEG-LENGTH DISCREPANCY IN CHILDREN

DEFINITION

A child is considered to have a discrepancy in leg length if the distance between the anterior superior iliac spine and the heel on the left side is different to that on the right. A single measurement is, of course, only a snapshot of a particular point in time, but it can indicate the need for further assessment. The measurement should be repeated periodically, particularly during the growth period in children.

AETIOLOGY/PATHOGENESIS

A discrepancy in leg length is caused by an acceleration or delay in growth in one of the legs. The legs grow independently of one another; there is no known compensation mechanism for growth that is too rapid or too slow on one side. A final leg-length difference of up to 2 cm should be considered physiological.

Growth can be adversely influenced by trauma and rare problems, such as infections, paralysis and tumours.

It is likely that epiphyseal circulation plays an important role. Damage to the epiphyseal plate leads to a delay in growth, and stimulation to an acceleration. So trauma can actually result in both shortening or lengthening, depending on the effect on the epiphyseal plate.

Infections such as osteomyelitis – which, fortunately, is rare – can inhibit growth in a young child by damaging the epiphyseal plate, which can lead to very significant shortening. Conversely, infection can also stimulate the epiphyseal plate, resulting in a stimulation of growth.

Congenital abnormalities, such as congenital hip dysplasia, can, if they occur on one side and do not receive correct treatment, lead to a considerable discrepancy in leg length, as can paralysis or paresis (poliomyelitis, spasticity).

Other causes of decreased circulation in the epiphyseal plate are avascular necrosis of the femoral head (Perthe's disease), tumours and X-ray radiation.

PRESENTATION

Children with a leg-length discrepancy may present at any age from birth until the end of the growth period. A difference in leg length may be evident in the routine examination of a neonate. In most cases, the parents or others will notice the difference and ask for advice, even though the child is not experiencing any symptoms. Children are very capable of adapting to differences in leg length, even significant ones. In most cases, they only experience symptoms if the leg is overburdened. Typical symptoms that result are walking with a pes equinus (the foot and ankle being held in plantar flexion) or a limp. In some cases, a difference in leg length is discovered because the child complains of pain in the leg or the back.

EPIDEMIOLOGY

There are few data available on prevalence. However, it is known that approximately 50% of adults have a (physiological) discrepancy in leg length of up to 2 cm. Of the demonstrable causes, trauma is probably the most common. A GP will see other causes infrequently – for example, a 'missed' congenital hip dysplasia (the average GP will see only two cases of congenital hip dysplasia in 40 years of practice).

HISTORY

The GP asks:

- about the child's symptoms and how long they have been present
- who noticed that one of the child's legs is longer than the other – the parent or the child
- about past leg fractures
- about any congenital hip disorder and/or whether congenital hip disorders run in the family
- whether the child has had osteomyelitis.

EXAMINATION

In order to properly assess a discrepancy in leg length, the child should be completely undressed.

In children who can stand, the GP first determines whether there is an actual length difference in the legs. First of all, with the child in a sitting position, the GP puts his thumbs on both anterior superior iliac spines and determines whether the height of the thumbs is the same. If not, the pelvis position is not straight, and there is probably no actual difference in leg length. Next, with the child standing, the GP determines the leg-length difference using the 'plank method': the space under the foot of the shortest leg is filled up with small pieces of wood, 0.5 or 1 cm thick, until the thumbs on the anterior superior iliac spines are level. The margin of error with this method is no larger than with X-ray measurement. If, after correction, the knees are at the same level, the difference is located in the lower leg; if the knees are not level, the difference can be either in the upper leg or in both the upper and the lower leg. Further assessment can take place as described below for younger children.

In children who cannot yet stand, the GP lays the child on its back with its hips and knees flexed 90°. In this position, a difference in the length of the upper leg is visible. If the child lies on its stomach with the knees flexed 90°, a difference in the length of the lower legs is visible.

It is important to examine newborns for congenital hip abnormalities. In some cases, a leg-length discrepancy will be visible. To assess for congenital dislocation of the hip, Ortolani's (for the reducible dislocation) and Barlow's tests (for the dislocatable hip) can be conducted. The specificity of these tests is high, but the sensitivity low. False-positive results lead to overtreatment and false-negative results are associated with a high late-presentation rate. Sensitivity is improved significantly with the use of experienced examiners.

Additional tests, such as X-rays, are not helpful. If congenital hip subluxation is suspected, an ultrasound scan can clarify the situation.

TREATMENT

In rare cases where the GP suspects a serious cause of leg-length discrepancy, the child should be referred. Referral is also necessary if the leg-length difference is more than 2 cm. If the discrepancy is less than 2 cm the GP can conduct two follow-up examinations at intervals of 6 months. If the leg-length difference does not increase, then any deterioration is unlikely, so further follow-up is unnecessary. In the case of (back) symptoms or the parents requesting cosmetic treatment, the leg-length difference can be corrected by an insole in the shoe (1 cm) or by raising the heel or sole of the shoe (if more than 1 cm). Also, it is important to reassure the parents and the child and not to place any restrictions on the child.

PREVENTION AND ADDITIONAL INFORMATION

Screening for congenital hip problems may detect abnormalities at an early stage. However, these tests are imperfect and caution should be exercised before coming to any conclusions that might cause unnecessary parental anxiety. As stated above, the GP should reassure that any small discrepancy in leg length is normal and harmless.

Key points

- A final leg-length difference of up to 2 cm should be considered physiological – this occurs in up to 50% of adults.

- Trauma is the most common pathological cause.

- In rare cases where the GP suspects a serious cause of leg-length discrepancy, or if the discrepancy is more than 2 cm, the child should be referred.

- If the discrepancy is less than 2 cm the GP can conduct two follow-up examinations at intervals of 6 months. If the leg-length difference does not increase, then any deterioration is unlikely, so further follow-up is unnecessary.

Literature

Diepstraten AFM, Van Linge B, Swierstra BA. *Kinderorthopedie* [*Paediatric orthopaedics*]. Utrecht: Bunge, 1993.

Eastwood DM. Neonatal hip screening. *Lancet* 2003;**361**(9357):595–7.

Paton RW, Srinivasan MS, Shah B, Hollis S. Ultrasound screening for hips at risk in developmental dysplasia. Is it worth it? *J Bone Joint Surg Br* 1999;**81**:255–8.

Rosendahl K, Markestad T, Lie RT. Congenital dislocation of the hip: a prospective study comparing ultrasound and clinical examination. *Acta Paediatr* 1992;**81**:177–81.

Visser JD. *Kinderorthopedie: pluis of niet pluis?* [*Paediatric orthopaedics: trustworthy or a scam?*] Groningen: Styx, 2003.

105

RESTLESS LEGS SYNDROME

DEFINITION

Restless legs syndrome (RLS) is characterized by unpleasant sensations, usually deep in the calves, sometimes in the upper legs or feet, and rarely in the arms. The sensations are almost never painful, but irritating. They occur during relaxation, while sitting and lying down, and are accompanied by an irresistible urge to move.

AETIOLOGY/PATHOGENESIS

The cause of RLS is unknown. There are suggestions that heredity may play a part. The disorder is seen more often in pregnant women, or in people with iron-deficiency anaemia or a polyneuropathy (e.g. in the case of uraemia); in dialysis patients, RLS disappears after a kidney transplant. Age also seems to be important: the incidence increases with age.

PRESENTATION

People with RLS usually consult the GP because their symptoms make it difficult to fall asleep. They may complain of a sensation of insects moving around in their calves, or of tingling, itching, piercing or cramping sensations – whatever description is used, the consensus is that RLS produces a very irritating feeling in both calves. The sensations are virtually always present in both legs. The feeling of an urge to move sometimes starts while the patient is sitting, but more commonly occurs on lying down. Moving the legs (e.g. walking) reduces the symptoms. Patients can usually live with the symptoms, but sometimes it can cause serious sleep problems and psychological disturbance.

RLS is often accompanied by involuntary muscle movements during sleep. These kicking movements, however, should not be considered a component of RLS. They are, in fact, a separate syndrome, 'periodic leg movements in sleep' (PLMS), which often occurs together with RLS.

EPIDEMIOLOGY

Approximately 5% of the population suffers from RLS. While it can affect people of all ages, it is most commonly seen in the elderly.

HISTORY

The GP asks:

- when the symptoms began
- whether the sensations in the legs are accompanied by an urge to move the legs
- whether the symptoms occur during relaxation in the evening or when trying to fall asleep
- whether the symptoms disappear when walking or moving
- whether the symptoms occur in one or both legs.

The following points are also important:

- pregnancy
- symptoms of anaemia or polyneuropathy
- whether there are other family members with the same problem
- whether the patient experiences involuntary muscle movements at night.

EXAMINATION

If necessary, examination and investigation should be conducted to rule out any underlying cause, such as anaemia, polyneuropathy or pregnancy. Physical examination and additional tests are otherwise not helpful.

TREATMENT

For many patients, reassurance and the recommendation to move the legs or walk a little when experiencing symptoms will suffice. However, if the patient is experiencing severe symptoms resulting in sleep problems, treatment with medication can be effective.

Quinine should not be used as part of the treatment. The preferred remedy is clonazepam, 0.5 mg tablet, a half or whole tablet at night. This can be increased to a maximum of 3 mg at night. If necessary, clonazepam 0.25 mg can also be given during the day.

If clonazepam does not offer sufficient relief, levodopa 100 mg plus carbidopa 25 mg (in a single tablet), one tablet at night may help. In extreme cases, codeine may be tried, but this obviously carries with it the risk of habituation.

PREVENTION AND ADDITIONAL INFORMATION

The effect of preventive measures, such as limiting the consumption of coffee and alcohol, exercising more during the day, stretching, taking a hot shower before retiring, using hotwater bottles or cold compresses in bed, has never been objectively demonstrated. The GP can explain that it is a harmless, albeit bothersome, disorder, but it should be remembered that the syndrome can sometimes cause considerable psychological stress for the patient.

Key points

- RLS causes unpleasant sensations in the legs, worse at rest, which result in an irresistible urge to move.

- The cause of RLS is unknown, although it can occasionally be associated with uraemia or iron deficiency.

- Reassurance may help some patients; if not, medication can be tried.

- There is little evidence to back up the often cited advice of stretching, avoiding alcohol, and so on.

Literature

Boot P, Eekhof JAH, Knuistingh Neven A. Restless legs-syndroom (minor ailments). *Huisarts Wet* 2003;**46**:573–5.

Earley CJ. Clinical practice. Restless legs syndrome. *N Engl J Med* 2003;**348**(21):2103–9.

Hening W, Allen R, Earley C, Kushida C, Picchietti D, Silber M. The treatment of restless legs syndrome and periodic limb movement disorder. An American Academy of Sleep Medicine review. *Sleep* 1999;**22**:970–99.

Phillips B, Young T, Finn L, Asher K, Hening WA, Purvis C. Epidemiology of restless legs symptoms in adults. *Arch Intern Med* 2000;**160**:2137–41.

Van Dijk JG, Caekebeke JFV, Roos RAC, Kamphuisen HAC. Het restless legs-syndroom [Restless legs syndrome]. *Ned Tijdschr Geneeskd* 1990;**134**:221–3.

106

MERALGIA PARAESTHETICA

DEFINITION

'Meralgia paraesthetica' is the term used to describe a compression mononeuropathy of the lateral cutaneous nerve of the thigh. The clinical picture comprises pain and troublesome paraesthesiae on the anterolateral aspect of the thigh. This disorder is usually unilateral.

AETIOLOGY/PATHOGENESIS

The lateral cutaneous nerve of the thigh originates from nerve roots L2 and L3, and runs under the inguinal ligament, approximately 2 cm medial to the anterior superior iliac spine, to the outside of the thigh.

This anatomical path can vary, making it more prone to compression. In some cases, the nerve does not run under, but through, openings in the inguinal ligament. An increase in mechanical stress on this ligament occurs in obesity, ascites and pregnancy, as well as due to tight belts, girdles, corsets or clothing. Heavy bunches of keys and a wallet worn in the front pockets of trousers can also cause the problem, as can sitting with the legs crossed for a long time and repeated extension of the upper leg (e.g. during skating). It is assumed that repeated pressure leads to irritation of the nerve.

In addition to the causes mentioned above, compression can also occur in retroperitoneal processes, pelvic tumours, direct trauma (fracture of the anterior superior iliac spine) or as a complication of surgical procedures. It can also represent an isolated metabolic neuropathy (diabetes mellitus, alcohol, lead intoxication) or result from underlying illnesses such as rheumatoid arthritis, multiple sclerosis and viral infections. Hereditary anatomical variations can result in a positive family history.

PRESENTATION

The patient presents with symptoms of pain accompanied by a tingling, burning sensation, and sometimes numbness, in a very specific area on the side of the thigh.

EPIDEMIOLOGY

Meralgia is the most common compression mononeuropathy. It occurs more often in men than women (3:1). Further epidemiological data are scanty. GPs probably only see a small proportion of actual cases.

HISTORY

The GP asks:

- when the symptoms began
- whether the symptoms are present continuously
- whether they are provoked by leg movements (radiating to the back)
- whether they radiate to the knee or ankle (which might suggest nerve root compression elsewhere)
- whether there is any weakness.

EXAMINATION

The clinical picture is so characteristic that the diagnosis can usually be made on this alone. Hyperextension of the thigh may increase the pain; the symptoms may also be elicited by firm palpation under or on the inguinal ligament.

If there is any doubt about the diagnosis, and a prolapsed disc is a possibility, power and reflexes should be tested, as these may be affected by a disc prolapse. It is usually not difficult to differentiate meralgia from other pain-causing disorders, such as arthritis of the hip, pelvic tumour and metabolic neuropathies. In doubtful cases, the patient may be referred to a neurologist. Additional tests might then include electromyography, electrophysiology and a computed tomography scan.

TREATMENT

The GP should explain the nature of the problem and the prognosis to the patient. In two out of three patients with meralgia, the symptoms spontaneously disappear within 2 years. Recommendations with regard to posture, movement and weight loss may be relevant. The value of other treatments (ice compresses, non-steroidal anti-inflammatories, local injections with corticosteroids/lidocaine) has not been established. Surgical intervention should be viewed with caution. Only in the case of persistent, severe pain should the GP consider referral for surgery; neurolysis results in total anaesthesia of the area supplied by the nerve.

PREVENTION AND ADDITIONAL INFORMATION

Some of the measures described above have a preventive effect; they may also prevent recurrences.

Key points

- 'Meralgia paraesthetica' is the term used to describe a compression mononeuropathy of the lateral cutaneous nerve of the thigh.

- It is usually caused by compression, but occasionally can represent an isolated mononeuropathy.

- The clinical picture is so characteristic that the diagnosis can usually be made on this alone.

- In two out of three patients with meralgia, the symptoms disappear spontaneously within 2 years.

Literature

Grossman MG, Ducey SA, Nadler SS, Levy AS. Meralgia paresthetica: diagnosis and treatment. *J Am Acad Orthop Surg* 2001;**9**(5):336–44.

MacNicol MF, Thompson WJ. Idiopathic meralgia paresthetica. *Clin Orthopaed* 1990;**254**:76–80.

Smid GJC, Hoekstra WM. Kleine kwalen in de huisartsgeneeskunde; meralgia paraesthetica [Minor ailments in general practice; meralgia paraesthetica]. *Ned Tijdschr Geneeskd* 1994;**138**:392–4.

107

KNOCK KNEES AND BOW LEGS/ GENU VALGUM AND GENU VARUM

DEFINITION

A specific definition is difficult, as the relevance and degree of knock knees and bow legs strongly depend on a child's age. At certain ages, physiological knock knees or bow legs can be observed in all children. In most, it resolves spontaneously. However, in a small number of cases, an underlying disorder is present.

AETIOLOGY/PATHOGENESIS

Knock knees and bow legs occur because of changes in the tibio-femoral angle during growth. Often, a varus or valgus position is accentuated by internal or external rotation of the tibiae, respectively. This rotation is due to the uneven growth of the tibia and fibula, and disappears spontaneously during normal development.

A varus position during a child's first 2 years is normal. A distance between the knees of 10 cm or less, measured with the child lying down, is considered within normal limits. The physiological varus position decreases around the child's second birthday. In young children, an underlying problem should be considered if the varus position does not decrease with age and if it has not resolved by around the child's second birthday.

Subsequently, a valgus position develops. This is at a maximum around a child's third birthday, and gradually decreases until the child's sixth year.

The anatomy of the hips creates a valgus angle of approximately 7° in a clinically straight leg position. This leg position and angle are usually achieved around a child's seventh birthday. At this age, the distance between the two medial malleoli, the intermalleolar distance, is normally less than 2.5 cm, with a maximum of 8 cm. A larger distance indicates a valgus position, which may require treatment.

Abnormal knee positions can be caused by physiological variation, rickets and Blount disease. The latter disorder involves a growth disturbance in the proximal metaphysis and epiphysis of the tibia. It occurs primarily in the Caribbean, West Africa and Scandinavia and leads to an increased varus position of the legs. Less likely causes are endocrine and metabolic bone disorders, epiphyseal dysplasia, treponematosis, post-traumatic, post-radiation or post-infection abnormalities, local congenital defects, tumours and abnormalities resulting from paralysis. In such cases, the disorder is often asymmetrical.

PRESENTATION

The reason for the consultation is usually worry on the part of the parents, or a question about whether the child has flat feet. In some cases, the reason for seeing the GP appears to be that the child trips over his own feet.

EPIDEMIOLOGY

Non-physiological knock knees or bow legs are diagnosed about once every 3–4 years per 1000 patients; so it is seen less than once a year in an average general practice. Physiological abnormalities are more common.

HISTORY

The GP asks:

- about the child's diet (in connection with rickets)
- about any diseases the child has suffered
- about any history of injury.

EXAMINATION

This mainly comprises measuring the distance between the knees or between the internal malleoli to determine the degree of varus or valgus, respectively. These distances are usually measured when the child is lying down flat with extended legs and knees or legs touching. Distances that do not fall within the aforementioned limits can be considered abnormal. Repeated measurements may be required to see how the situation develops. Hip examination should also be performed.

Additional tests, such as X-rays, are unnecessary before the child's second year, unless the abnormality is unilateral.

TREATMENT

An explanation and reassurance is usually all that is required. 'Treatment' of physiological varus with a splint or any other method is, of course, unnecessary. This would result in unnecessary bother for the patient, and would probably also exaggerate the physiological valgus occurring later.

It is also reasonable to wait and see in the later valgus phase, provided that the abnormality is symmetrical and the history does not give cause for concern. It should be explained that the leg position usually becomes normal in the child's seventh year, although it may take longer. Correction aids used at night and other forms of therapy are not helpful. An intermalleolar distance of up to 9 cm at 4 years of age will usually correct itself without treatment.

A valgus position even within the norm can give rise to problems, especially the complaint of clumsy walking. Wedge-shaped insoles can improve the child's walking, but do not influence the development of the leg position. A slight remaining valgus position does not necessarily cause problems in adulthood.

However, it cannot be expected that a valgus position with an intermalleolar distance of 8 cm or more at 7 years of age will still spontaneously disappear. Such children should be referred to a paediatric orthopaedic surgeon. Surgical techniques may then be used in an attempt to create a straight leg position.

PREVENTION AND ADDITIONAL INFORMATION

Providing information about the natural development of the knee position will prevent unnecessary worry. The knowledge that treatment can be delayed until puberty prevents unnecessary tests and unrealistic expectations before that time.

Key points

- At certain ages, physiological knock knees or bow legs can be observed in all children.

- A varus position during a child's first 2 years is normal. A distance between the knees of 10 cm or less, measured with the child lying down, is considered within normal limits.

- At 7 years of age, the intermalleolar distance is normally less than 2.5 cm, with a maximum of 8 cm. A larger distance indicates a valgus position, which may require treatment.

Literature

Oudshoorn P, Mulder Dzn JD. Kleine kwalen in de huisartsgeneeskunde: genu varum en genu valgum bij kinderen [Minor ailments in general practice: genu varum and genu valgum in children]. *Ned Tijdschr Geneeskd* 1987;**134**:11–12.

Raney EM, Topoleski TA, Yaghoubian R, Guidera KJ, Marshall JG. Orthotic treatment of infantile tibia vara. *J Pediatr Orthop* 1998;**18**:670–4.

Visser JD. *Kinderorthopedie: pluis of niet pluis?* [*Paediatric orthopaedics: trustworthy or a scam?*] Groningen: Styx, 2003.

108

CALF STRAIN/'TENNIS LEG'

DEFINITION

Calf strain, also known as 'tennis leg', is caused by a (partial) rupture of the gastrocnemius muscle. It is characterized by a sudden, severe pain in the calf accompanied by difficulty in walking, usually occurring during sports or when walking, but also sometimes when standing still.

AETIOLOGY/PATHOGENESIS

The gastrocnemius muscle is particularly vulnerable to injury because it covers two joints. When active plantar flexion of the foot and passive stretching by extension of the knee occur at the same time, the muscle is stretched to its maximum, and so may rupture. This movement happens, for example, when serving on the tennis court; it is also common during volleyball. The injury probably occurs more often in untrained people and in cold or damp weather. However, elite sportspeople can also develop the same problem. Overstraining may play a role in this. Bear in mind, though, that the injury can occur simply by walking slowly or even standing still.

PRESENTATION

The patient presents with a typical story. For example, while serving on the tennis court, the patient thought he was hit hard in the calf by a ball from another court, or, while running, by a stone. He may have even heard a 'snap'. Immediately after, he is unable to walk because of the searing pain in his calf. Some patients even collapse from the pain. Several hours or days after the injury, the patient attends with a typical clinical picture: he walks on the toes of one foot or limps, the foot on the injured side is in a twisted position, and it is impossible to put the foot on the ground in the normal position, as this aggravates the pain.

EPIDEMIOLOGY

The incidence is about 2.7 per 1000 patients per year for men and 1.6 for women. Many will attend the local casualty department rather than the GP.

HISTORY

The GP asks:

- how the injury occurred
- whether the patient was able to continue his activities
- whether the pain was acute or more gradual
- whether the patient leads an active (sports) life
- whether the patient had warmed up with stretching exercises.

EXAMINATION

On examination, the calf muscles will usually be slightly swollen. The injury sometimes gives the impression of an indentation, almost always just above the transition from the Achilles tendon to the medial muscle belly of the gastrocnemius muscle. This site is very tender on palpation. Plantar flexion of the ankle is possible, especially passively, but passive dorsiflexion is very painful. Plantar flexion against resistance is nearly impossible because of the pain. A haematoma is often visible one or several days after the injury occurs (distal from the injury).

To rule out a complete Achilles tendon rupture, Thompson's test can be used. In this test, the GP firmly squeezes the lateral and medial calf muscle groups (this is not always easy in tennis leg due to the severe pain), while the patient is lying on his stomach or kneeling on a chair. If there is a total rupture of the Achilles tendon, no plantar flexion of the foot will occur.

A Doppler assessment can be performed if deep vein thrombosis is suspected.

TREATMENT

Icing the area is helpful during the first 24 hours after the injury. It should be iced for 20 minutes four to five times daily (do not put the ice directly on the skin); cold water may also be used. Rest is important initially. This is aimed at limiting the bleeding, and therefore the tissue damage – the less damage that occurs, the less scar tissue develops.

If necessary, an oral non-steroidal anti-inflammatory drug can be prescribed for the pain.

Rest is particularly important during the acute phase; exercise may take place according to the pain. After the acute phase of 2–3 days, exercise can be increased. If there is difficulty with mobilization, the patient can be referred to a physiotherapist, who can begin with active and passive non-weight-bearing exercise.

In the absence of complications, the patient can begin walking and light stretching exercises after a week. Once the normal walking pattern has been restored, the patient may carefully start sport and stretching exercises. Complete recovery will occur after an average of 4–6 weeks.

PREVENTION AND ADDITIONAL INFORMATION

Although stretching and warm-up exercises are always advised, there is insufficient evidence to determine the effectiveness of stretching exercises for lower-limb muscle groups in reducing lower-limb soft tissue injuries.

Key points

- Calf strain is caused by a (partial) rupture of the gastrocnemius muscle.
- The history is typical: a sudden, severe pain in the calf accompanied by difficulty in walking, usually occurring during sports.
- Important differentials include a ruptured Achilles tendon and (less likely) a deep vein thrombosis.

Literature

Groeneveld Y, Eekhof JAH, Knuistingh Neven A. Kleine kwalen in de huisartsen-geneeskunde. Zweepslag van de kuit of 'Coup de fouet' [Minor ailments in general practice: calf strain]. *Huisarts Nu* 2003;**32**:190–2.

Herbert RD, Gabriel M. Effects of stretching before and after exercise on muscle soreness and risk of injury: systematic review. *BMJ* 2002;**325**: 468–70.

Sando B. Calf strain. *Aust Fam Physician* 1988;**17**(12):1060–1.

Touliopolous S, Hershman EB. Lower leg pain. Diagnosis and treatment of compartment syndromes and other pain syndromes of the leg. *Sports Med* 1999;**27**(3):193–204.

Yeung EW, Yeung SS. Interventions for preventing lower limb soft-tissue injuries in runners (Cochrane Review). *Cochrane Library*, Issue 3. Chichester: Wiley, 2004.

109

TROCHANTERIC BURSITIS

DEFINITION

Trochanteric bursitis is an inflammation of the trochanteric bursa, which is a fluid-filled sac separating the gluteus maximus from the posterior and lateral sides of the greater trochanter.

AETIOLOGY/PATHOGENESIS

In general, bursae are found in areas of the body where pressure and friction occur, particularly on bony protrusions just underneath the skin, and directly under the bony insertion sites of tendons (see also Chapter 93). There are a number of possible causes of trochanteric bursitis. These include biomechanical left–right differences in the legs (e.g. a leg-length discrepancy, which causes bursitis in the longer leg), abnormalities of the ipsilateral hip (e.g. arthritis), abnormalities of the lumbosacral spine, friction of the iliotibial tract over the greater trochanter in long-distance runners, rheumatoid arthritis and local injury.

PRESENTATION

Patients complain of vague, usually mild, fluctuating pain, which is at the level of, or around, the greater trochanter. The pain may radiate to the entire lateral side of the upper leg, and sometimes even to the knee. The symptoms disappear when the patient is at rest and increase during certain types of exercise, such as walking for a long time. The pain may cause the patient to limp. Sleeping on the affected side or putting on a seatbelt can also aggravate the problem.

EPIDEMIOLOGY

Trochanteric bursitis occurs much less often than bursitis of the shoulder or elbow. It is seen mainly in middle-aged women, often in combination with obesity, and in younger people who play sports.

HISTORY

The GP asks:

- about sporting activities
- about pre-existing hip symptoms
- about lower-back symptoms and rheumatoid arthritis.

EXAMINATION

The findings of the examination may be vague. Local tenderness is usually present. Some passive movements, such as flexion and external rotation of the hip, and sometimes also adduction, are painful. Active movement is usually painful, as is abduction against resistance.

The GP should look for any underlying problems, such as leg-length discrepancy or abnormalities of the ipsilateral hip or lower back. The diagnosis is reinforced if the symptoms disappear after infiltration of the bursa with a local anaesthetic. In terms of the differential diagnosis, the GP should consider nerve root entrapment (L4–L5) and overstretching of the iliotibial tract.

TREATMENT

Most cases of trochanteric bursitis resolve spontaneously. Standard analgesics can be used if necessary. If this fails, the bursa can be infiltrated with 2 ml lidocaine 1%. If this injection temporarily reduces the pain, a steroid can be injected into the bursa. The technique is as follows. The patient lies on his back and the most painful spot (usually slightly above and behind the greater trochanter) is located. The needle is inserted horizontally and the bursa infiltrated in a fan-like manner.

PREVENTION AND ADDITIONAL INFORMATION

The GP should look for and manage any possible underlying problems or contributory factors.

Key points

- Check for possible underlying causes, such as leg-length discrepancy.
- The diagnosis is likely if the symptoms disappear after infiltration of the bursa with a local anaesthetic.
- Most cases of trochanteric bursitis resolve spontaneously.

Literature

Bewyer DC, Bewyer KJ. Rationale for treatment of hip abductor pain syndrome. Iowa *Orthop J* 2003;**23**:57–60.

Butcher JD, Salzman KL, Lillegard WA. Lower extremity bursitis. *Am Fam Physician* 1996;**53**(7):2317–24.

Shbeeb MI, Matteson EL. Trochanteric bursitis (greater trochanter pain syndrome). *Mayo Clin Proc* 1996;**71**(6):565–9.

110

CHONDROMALACIA PATELLAE

DEFINITION

Chondromalacia patellae comprises the clinical picture of pain at the level of the patella and is a syndrome attributed to dysfunction of the patellofemoral joint. Synonyms are 'retropatellar chondropathy', 'patellofemoral pain syndrome' and anterior knee pain. While these terms suggest a lesion of the patella, arthroscopic examination reveals a discrepancy between the reported symptoms and the extent of problems affecting the patellar cartilage.

AETIOLOGY/PATHOGENESIS

The patella is part of the very powerful extensor apparatus of the knee. Symptoms are usually the result of excessive stress to this area, such that the balance between stress and load-carrying capacity is disturbed. Disturbance of the functional position of the patella causes friction, which leads to local microtrauma and, therefore, symptoms.

There is a primary form of chondromalacia, which mainly occurs in girls aged 12–16 years. Otherwise, a distinction is made between internal and external causes. The internal causes include, in a normal patellofemoral joint, a muscle imbalance between the quadriceps muscle and the hamstrings, or the domination of the vastus lateralis over the medialis.

Disorders occurring outside the knee can also be a cause: abnormalities of the foot position when standing (e.g. a pronated flat foot), limitations of dorsiflexion of the foot (compensated for by stronger pronation, with internal rotation of the tibia) and rotation stress in the knee resulting from a rotation disorder of the tibia (e.g. after a fracture).

External causes include unsuitable footwear (e.g. high heels, which increase the patellofemoral pressure) and sports that involve stress on the patellofemoral joint (e.g. lifting weights, cycling, volleyball, running up hills and stairs, in which the patellofemoral pressure is increased). Running and walking on convex roads, which pulls the patella out of position, are other possible causes. Obesity and immobilization are aggravating factors.

PRESENTATION

Patients usually complain of pain in the front of the knee, which increases when walking up or down stairs, cycling or after sitting a long time with the knees bent (e.g. after travelling in a car or visiting the theatre). In addition, somewhat misleadingly, pain in the back of the knee can be the presenting symptom – this can be viewed as referred pain. Other symptoms include 'pseudo-locking', crepitus and/or cracking, and a feeling of the knee giving way.

EPIDEMIOLOGY

In an average practice, the diagnosis of chondromalacia patellae is made approximately 10 times a year, and is seen more often in women (particularly in girls aged 12–16 years) than men (3:2). The explanation may be that women have a wider pelvis than men, so the angle between the longitudinal axis of the quadriceps and the longitudinal axis of the patellar tendon (the Q angle) is larger.

HISTORY

The GP asks:

- about any injury to the knee or patella, recently or in the past
- about the site of the pain
- about activities that cause the symptoms
- about sports, hobbies and work
- about known foot abnormalities and the use of arch supports

EXAMINATION

While the patient is standing, the GP examines the following in succession: the foot position (looking for overpronation), the tibia for rotation, and the Q angle (the normal measurement is 15° in women and 10° in men). While the patient is sitting, the GP assesses the course taken by the patella in flexion and extension, and checks for pain or crepitus when extending the knee against resistance, and pain when compressing the patella as the patient extends the knee. While the patient is lying down, the GP assesses the Q angle, the extent of any effusion (a slight effusion may be present), and looks for possible quadriceps wasting. The following should also be examined: the insertion of the vastus medialis, the shape of the patella, any restriction of dorsiflexion of the ankle, pain when tensing the muscles, and patella mobility (e.g. lateral hypermobility).

TREATMENT

The most important measure involves eliminating the cause: correcting an abnormal foot position, mobilizing a restricted ankle joint, and so on. Quadriceps training is important. In particular, the vastus medialis muscle should be exercised intensively for a significant period of time. These exercises should be done isometrically with an extended knee. After referral to a physiotherapist, a tape can be used to correct any abnormal positioning of the patella. With this correction, the quadriceps exercises can be practiced painlessly – the symptoms that occur when walking up stairs or cycling will usually disappear. Stretching exercises for the quadriceps, hamstrings and iliotibial tract can be helpful. Sport-specific recommendations include decreasing the pedalling stress for cyclists by choosing a lower gear and the correct seat height. Runners should pay close attention to their footwear and the surface they are running on – running on a hard surface, convex roads or loose sand should be avoided.

Severe cases with persistent symptoms that affect daily functioning and which do not respond to conservative measures should be referred to an orthopaedic surgeon. Little is known about the real value of orthopaedic interventions, such as plaster immobilization or arthroscopic techniques, versus watchful waiting.

PREVENTION AND ADDITIONAL INFORMATION

Make clear to the patient that the balance between the load-bearing capacity and the stress put on the joint is the underlying problem. Minor symptoms should be taken seriously to prevent deterioration:

measures should be taken immediately to reduce the stress on the joint. A change to the shoes may be required. If a sportsperson wants to increase his exertion level, the load-bearing capacity will also have to be increased through extra quadriceps training.

Key points

- Patients typically complain of pain in the front of the knee, which increases when walking up or down stairs, cycling or after sitting a long time with the knees bent.

- The most important aspect of treatment involves eliminating the cause, such as correcting an abnormal foot position and mobilizing a restricted ankle joint.

- Severe cases with persistent symptoms that affect daily functioning and do not respond to conservative measures should be referred to an orthopaedic surgeon.

- Minor symptoms should be taken seriously to prevent deterioration.

Literature

Cirkel JW, Klaassen WRC, Kunst JA, Aarns TEM, Plag ECM, Goudswaard AN, Burgers JS. *Guideline of the Dutch College of General Practitioners: non-traumatic knee disorders for children and adolescents*, 1998. http://www.nhg.artsennet.nl/upload/104/standaarden/M65/start.htm

Rondhuis GB. Het McConnell-programma voor patellafemorale klachten [The McConnell programme for patellofemoral complaints]. *Geneesk Sport* 1993;**26**:26–7.

Soren A, Fetto JF. Chondromalacia patellae. *Arch Orthop Trauma Surg* 1997;**116**:362–6.

Van de Lisdonk E, Kuik M, Bakx JC. Chondropathia patella in de huisartspraktijk [Chondromalacia patellae in general practice]. *Ned Tijdschr Geneesk* 1991;**135**:374–7.

Van Teeffelen WM, Van Ernst GC, Backx FJG. Chondromalacia patellae, een literatuur-overzicht [Chondromalacia patellae, a literature overview]. *Geneesk Sport* 1990;**23**:24–9.

III

FLAT FEET/PES PLANUS

DEFINITION

A flat foot involves a fallen medial foot arch. In most cases, the posterior part of the foot takes on a valgus position. A distinction can be made between flexible flat feet, which can be corrected during the examination, and fixed flat feet, which cannot be corrected.

AETIOLOGY/PATHOGENESIS

Up to the age of 2 years, most children have little or no lengthwise arch in the feet because of the presence of a lot of subcutaneous fat. The valgus position of the feet is also normal at this age. Children aged 2–8 years can have significant individual differences in the shape, size and development of the bones of the legs. Initially, the joints are weak and hyperextendable, and this, together with bone development, means that valgus feet and knock knees are not uncommon.

Any case of flexible, and therefore correctible, flat foot is usually caused by weak joint ligaments. In this case, the medial foot arch falls when stress is put on it, and the heel drops into a valgus position.

Conversely, a fixed flat foot is usually caused by an abnormal joint in the tarsus, usually between the calcaneus and the navicular, or sometimes between the talus and the calcaneus. The symptoms of fixed flat feet can start at the age of 8 years, as the (abnormal) ossification continues – these patients often suffer pain.

No relationship has been demonstrated between flat feet and early arthritis of the hip, knee, neck or back symptoms or chronic headaches.

PRESENTATION

Many parents are worried when they see what they think are abnormalities of the lower legs and feet in their growing children. Flat feet or apparent ankle abnormalities may prompt a consultation. Another complaint often presented by parents is the uneven wear on the child's shoes.

Pre-school children almost never complain about pain in the feet. In older children and adults, foot pain usually indicates a fixed abnormality.

EPIDEMIOLOGY

A GP regularly encounters symptoms or questions relating to flat feet: approximately one or two every 1000 consultations. Research has shown that 65% of cases of flat feet in 2 year olds resolve by the age of 5 or 6 years, and that slightly flat feet remain in 30% – so most foot problems in young children correct themselves. In adults, 3–4% have flexible flat feet, often without symptoms. Little is known about the incidence and prevalence of fixed flat feet, which are clearly only a small percentage of the total.

HISTORY

It is important to determine the reason for the consultation. The GP asks:

- about worry (on the part of the parents) about supposed abnormalities
- about foot pain
- about fatigue after standing for a long time.

If pain is present, the GP should suspect fixed flat feet.

EXAMINATION

The examination should be aimed at establishing whether the feet really are flat and, if so, whether they are flexible or fixed. When inspecting the feet at rest, abnormalities may immediately be apparent. Attention should be paid to whether the heel is in the valgus position, if the anterior foot is positioned in abduction compared to the axis of the posterior foot, and if the lengthwise arch has fallen. As the child walks back and forth, the GP can examine the gait and whether the child walks flexibly and normally, if equal stress is put on both legs, and so on.

Distinguish between a flexible and contracted flat foot as follows. For a flexible flat foot, the medial foot arch can spontaneously re-establish itself, in children aged 2–6 years, when sitting (on a person's lap), and in older children when standing on tip toes, or by passively hyperextending the big toe. The arch cannot be re-established in a fixed flat foot.

If clear foot abnormalities are found in infants, the GP should also check for other possibly serious abnormalities, such as club feet, spina bifida or hip problems. In the case of an obvious valgus position of the feet, leg length should be checked and the hips inspected for instability, or abnormal rotation. If external rotation is significantly limited and the internal rotation increased, this indicates possible congenital dislocation of the hip.

Genu varus or valgus may lead to compensatory abnormalities in foot posture. In children with a clear valgus position of the knees, it is a good idea to measure the intermalleolar distance, between the ankles, in a standing rest position. For a varus position, the distance between the knees is measured. This allows changes over time to be monitored accurately (see Chapter 107).

TREATMENT

If no serious abnormalities are found on examination, reassurance is required. The GP can point out that these harmless abnormalities are usually temporary and linked to the growth process. However, the GP should follow the child's development with 6-monthly checks.

Special footwear for children is generally not necessary. Abnormal wear on the inside of the shoes can be compensated for by recommending shoes with a sturdy heel. Wedges for the shoes are unnecessary and costly.

In children with flexible flat feet, correction of the feet with arch supports is only necessary if there are relevant symptoms: pain in the medial foot arches, or fatigue or cramps in the legs when standing. Arch supports for children should be replaced regularly to allow for growth. For adults, most of the same rules apply, but correction with arch supports will probably occur earlier if the patient's occupation requires a lot of standing.

Children with fixed flat feet must be referred.

PREVENTION AND ADDITIONAL INFORMATION

For children with uncomplicated flexible flat feet, information about the natural history is important. Special footwear for children is only necessary when there are relevant symptoms.

Key points

- If pain is present, the GP should suspect fixed flat feet.

- For a flexible flat foot, the medial foot arch can spontaneously re-establish itself, in children aged 2–6 years, when sitting (on a person's lap), and in older children when standing on tip toes, or by passively hyperextending the big toe. The arch cannot be re-established in a fixed flat foot.

- In children with flexible flat feet, correction of the feet with arch supports is only necessary if there are relevant symptoms: pain in the medial foot arches, or fatigue or cramps in the legs when standing.

Literature

Asirvatham R. Foot problems seen in children. *Practitioner* 2001;**245**(1626):756–9.

Churgay CA. Diagnosis and treatment of pediatric foot deformities. *Am Fam Physician* 1993;**47**(4):883–9.

Dereymaeker G. De platvoet [The flat foot]. *Bijblijven* 1993;**9**(1):19–25.

Visser JD. *Kinderorthopaedie. Pluis of niet pluis?* [Paediatric orthopaedics: trustworthy or a scam?] Groningen: Styx, 2003.

112

CALLUSES ON THE FEET

DEFINITION

A callus is a hyperkeratotic area on the soles of the feet. It is a natural reaction of the skin to regular or continued pressure or friction. Calluses are whitish-yellow, feel hard to the touch and sometimes have cracks. They are usually found on the ball of the foot or the heel, or in places where the skin puts pressure on bony protrusions. In contrast to corns, calluses do not have a core or a centre.

AETIOLOGY/PATHOGENESIS

Calluses occur on areas where the skin is subjected to excessive pressure and friction. As a protective reaction to this stimulus, the horny layer (the stratum corneum) thickens. In contrast to corns, the calluses do not grow deep into the skin. The heel, toes and the ball of the foot are the typical sites. Wearing shoes that are too wide or too narrow, or wearing high heels, puts excessive pressure on these points and calluses may result. Increased pressure due to intensive sports or walking on bare feet can also be the cause.

In addition to these external factors, local factors can lead to callus formation. Bony protrusions of the foot put pressure on a number of points. Anatomical abnormalities of the foot or its bones (congenital or after a trauma) can create an abnormal distribution of pressure. In overweight people, there is even more pressure on these areas (even if no foot abnormalities are present). In the elderly, there may be atrophy of the skin and the subcutaneous fat. This reduces the natural shock-absorbing effect of the foot, which leads to changes in the distribution of pressure. All these factors promote the formation of calluses.

The callus layer can crack if it dries out. These cracks can split open while walking, which is very painful. The cracks can also become infected, which increases the pain and prevents healing.

Patients with diabetes mellitus or circulatory disorders run a higher risk of foot problems. Neuropathy may result in patients being relatively insensitive to pain, and this can lead to necrosis due to the continuous pressure on the callus. Circulatory problems impair healing and promote infection.

A number of dermatoses also promote callus formation. In most cases, these are dermatomycoses (tinea pedis) which have been present for a long time (usually caused by *Trichophyton rubrum*). In addition, tylotic (hyperkeratotic) eczema and atypical psoriasis can also cause calluses, possibly accompanied by cracking. Tylotic eczema is accompanied by significant callus formation, either on both the hands and the feet, or on the feet alone. The exact cause of tylotic eczema is unknown. It is usually symmetrical and most severe on the pressure points of the feet.

In terms of the differential diagnosis, distinguishing calluses from plantar warts can sometimes be very difficult. When treating thick skin on the foot, the GP may discover that the problem is actually a plantar wart.

Because abnormal pressure on the foot and dermatomycoses occur very frequently, they may well co-exist: for example, patients may have a dermatomycosis and experience abnormal pressure on the foot, because their shoes are too small.

PRESENTATION

The patient presents with discomfort like having a 'pebble in the shoe'; alternatively, the pain may be described as 'burning' if cracks have formed. Cosmetic concerns are another reason for attending. Often, the symptoms have been present for weeks or even years, and, typically, are not troublesome at rest.

EPIDEMIOLOGY

Calluses occur very frequently in the population and most people do not consult the GP about them. The Transition Project [Transitieproject] of the University of Amsterdam revealed a prevalence of calluses and corns of 4.6 per 1000 patients. Excessive callus formation occurs relatively frequently in people over 75 years old. Many patients will self-treat or consult a chiropodist rather than the GP.

HISTORY

The GP asks:

- what kind of shoes the patient wears and whether they fit properly
- how long the symptoms have been present
- what problems are being experienced
- whether the patient plays sport, and if so, how intensively
- about complicating factors, such as diabetes mellitus or circulatory problems.

EXAMINATION

On inspection, the GP finds a rough, yellowish-white layer of callus (hyperkeratosis), which may also have cracks. The callus can be diffuse or localized. Examining and palpating the pressure points of the foot and any abnormalities in foot posture can give clues about the possible cause. The GP should also inspect the patient's shoes.

Certain disorders, such as warts, tinea pedis, tylotic eczema and atypical psoriasis, can be accompanied by excessive callus formation. Because these disorders require specific treatment, they need to be distinguished from calluses caused by pressure. In the case of calluses caused by fungi, the toenails and skin between the toes are also often affected – a useful discriminating point. However, demonstrating the presence of fungi does not prove this to be the cause, as fungal infection of the foot is very common in the general population.

TREATMENT

Initial treatment consists of removing the excess callus, using a callus file, pumice stone or scalpel. This is easiest after soaking the feet or applying salicylic acid. Salicylic acid softens the horny layer and, depending on the thickness of the callus, can be applied in the form of plasters or creams. The concentration of salicylic acid in the ointment can, if desired, be increased. After this has softened the area, the callus can easily be removed. Any cracks can be treated with a disinfectant ointment, such as povidone iodine. A plaster used to pull the edges of the wound together can accelerate healing. Secondary infections can also be prevented or treated in this way.

Symptoms resulting from bony protrusions and foot-posture abnormalities can be alleviated by various types of pads and insoles that decrease the pressure from the shoe. Patients can remove the callus with a file or pumice stone and then apply the pads themselves. If desired, a chiropodist can also help with callus removal. Surgically removing bony protrusions or adjusting the posture of the foot is only indicated if conservative treatment does not produce the desired results.

Other disorders accompanied by the formation of calluses require specific treatment. Dermatomycoses should be treated with a (local) antimycotic. Plantar warts can be treated with liquid nitrogen, curettage or salicylic acid application. Tylotic eczema and atypical psoriasis can be treated by applying 0.1% triamcinolon acetonide cream under occlusion.

PREVENTION AND ADDITIONAL INFORMATION

The key point is for patients to wear shoes that fit properly. High-heeled shoes should be avoided.

Key points

- In contrast to corns, calluses do not have a core or a centre.
- A number of dermatoses, such as fungal infection, tylotic eczema and atypical psoriasis, also promote callus formation.
- The most important aspect of prevention is to ensure that patients wear properly fitting shoes.

Literature
Degreef H, Oris S. Veel voorkomende dermatologische afwijkingen van de voet [Frequently occurring dermatological abnormalities of the foot]. *Bijblijven* 1993;**9**:43–9.

Freeman DB. Corns and calluses resulting from mechanical hyperkeratosis. *Am Fam Physician* 2002;**65**(11):2277–80.

Singh D, Bentley G, Trevino SG. Callosities, corns, and calluses. *BMJ* 1996;**312**:1403–6.

Van Randeraat RA, Eekhof JAH. Eelt, eeltknobbels en eeltkloven van de voet [Calluses, callus bumps and callus cracks of the foot]. *Modern Med* 2000;**8**:686–8.

113

PLANTAR FASCIITIS/ POLICEMAN'S HEEL

DEFINITION

Plantar fasciitis, which is sometimes accompanied by a bony spur on the calcaneum, is characterized by pain in the heel.

AETIOLOGY/PATHOGENESIS

The plantar aponeurosis and the intrinsic muscles of the foot attach to the calcaneal tuberosity; these promote stability when walking. The plantar fascia contributes to supination as a counterbalance to the pronating effect of the Achilles tendon. If the foot is unstable, more counterforce is needed from the intrinsic muscles; this puts a strain on the insertion on the calcaneus. The degree of strain is influenced by the thickness of the fat cushion under the foot, body weight and age (less muscle strength, stiffer connective tissue, and therefore less absorption of the forces).

Problems occur when there is excessive pronation or supination of the foot. This causes excessive stress, resulting in microbleeds at the insertion of the plantar fascia and the intrinsic muscles. This inflammation can cause pain, without an anatomically evident ' heel spur' being demonstrated. A real heel spur develops when microbleeds, metaplasia and new bone formation result in ossification at the insertion site.

When there is excessive stress on the insertion of fascia and muscles on the calcaneus, the surrounding space fills up with exudate. As the patient starts to walk, this area compresses the surrounding tissues, causing pain. If the patient walks for a while, the amount of inflammatory fluid decreases, as does the pain. If the patient walks even further, the stimulation increases again, and the production of exudate exceeds its drainage, so pain recurs. This explains the pattern of pain in plantar fasciitis.

If the syndrome has become chronic, the pattern changes, with the patient feeling constant irritation.

There are a number of differential diagnoses. In the relatively rare retrocalcaneal exostosis (Haglund's deformity), there is an exostosis on the back of the heel. When there is a history of extensive walking, a stress fracture should be considered. If paraesthesiae or hyper-aesthesia are present in addition to pain, tarsal tunnel syndrome (also known as 'burning feet') and other nerve entrapments should be considered. In athletes, apophysitis is a possibility. The pain is continuous, more severe, and radiates out over the foot. Systemic disorders are also included in the differential diagnosis: these include infections, gout, rheumatoid arthritis, spondylarthritis, psoriatic arthritis, Reiter's syndrome, Paget's disease, ischaemia and venous thrombosis.

PRESENTATION

The patient will volunteer that he experiences pain in the heel, which makes walking difficult. The acute phase features severe pain, which occurs when the patient starts to walk and then disappears after several steps. If stress is placed on the heel for a longer time, the pain can return. The attacks of pain can last from several days to years. The chronic stage is characterized by pain radiating to the inside of the lower leg and to the entire heel.

EPIDEMIOLOGY

There are few data available for prevalence and incidence. According to the literature, 15% of adult patients at a foot clinic had pain in the heel, and in 75% of these a 'heel spur syndrome' was present.

HISTORY

Taking a careful history can usually rule out other causes of heel pain. The GP asks:

- about the exact location of the heel pain

- about the duration, progression and possible radiation of the pain
- about the possible presence of a foreign body (e.g. a splinter)
- about orthopaedic problems (e.g. a flat foot, a club foot, an abnormality of the anterior foot)
- about arthritis symptoms
- about any trauma.

EXAMINATION

Local examination reveals tenderness over the site where the patient complains of pain. There is no redness or skin warmth. The physical examination may be extended if a systemic disorder is suspected. In extreme cases of plantar fasciitis, an X-ray may show erosions in the calcaneal tuberosity.

Additional tests should also be considered as appropriate (e.g. an X-ray if a stress fracture is possible, blood tests for systemic disorders).

TREATMENT

In 90% of cases, the pain will disappear spontaneously in 3–6 months; in the remaining 10% the symptoms will decrease. Non-steroidal anti-inflammatory drugs can be prescribed in the acute phase if necessary.

The following 'mechanical' measures may help: a heel pad to improve the absorption of the forces that cause the symptom; shoe modification to reduce the pressure on the heel; alternating hot and cold baths to reduce the oedema; weight reduction if the patient is overweight; and, in the elderly, strengthening the intrinsic muscles through physiotherapy, which results in less direct force being put on the calcaneus via the plantar fascia.

The local use of corticosteroids is debatable: the inflammatory reaction is inhibited, but tissue degeneration occurs and rupture of the plantar fascia is possible (although this will cure the pain). Surgical procedures should be avoided if there is any uncertainty about the diagnosis. However, if, the disorder has not spontaneously resolved after 6 months or the other forms of therapy have not been effective, a plantar fascia release may help.

PREVENTION AND ADDITIONAL INFORMATION

Most of the treatment measures described above can also be viewed as potentially preventive. In particular, it is important to prevent recurrences by addressing any underlying cause (e.g. unstable ankle, improper footwear) when the symptoms first appear.

Key points

- The acute phase of plantar fasciitis features severe pain, which occurs when the patient starts to walk and then disappears after several steps.
- The attacks of pain can last from several days to years.
- In 90% of cases the pain will disappear spontaneously in 3–6 months, and the symptoms will decrease in the remaining 10%.
- If symptoms persist beyond 6 months, surgery may help.

Literature

Crawford F. Plantar heel pain (including plantar fasciitis). *Clin Evid* 2002;**7**: 1091–100.

Dailey JM. Differential diagnosis and treatment of heel pain. *Clin Podiatr Med Surg* 1991;**8**:153–66.

Scherer PR. Biomechanics Graduate Research Group for 1988. Heel spur syndrome. Pathomechanics and nonsurgical treatment. *J Am Podiatr Med Assoc* 1991;**81**:68–72.

Tomczak RL, Haverstock BD. A retrospective comparison of endoscopic plantar fasciotomy to open plantar fasciotomy with heel spur resection for chronic plantar fasciitis/heel spur syndrome. *J Foot Ankle Surg* 1995;**34**: 305–11.

114
CHILBLAINS/PERNIOSIS

DEFINITION

Chilblains, also called 'perniosis' or 'erythema pernio', involve patchy redness and swelling, accompanied by itching, burning and pain, which occurs at cold times of the year. This mainly occurs on the extensor side of the toes and fingers, but also elsewhere on the body.

AETIOLOGY/PATHOGENESIS

Cold is the key factor. However, it is not so much the temperature, but the degree of humidity of the cold air, which is of prime importance. This is because of the higher 'cold conductivity' of a damp environment. Cold normally causes contraction of the arterioles and venules in the skin and dilatation of the capillary network; the reverse occurs in warmer conditions. In patients with chilblains, this regulatory mechanism of hypo- and hyperperfusion does not function properly under certain conditions – in particular, the venules react too slowly to temperature changes. As a result, stasis and congestion can occur at capillary level. Over time, this can lead to damage of the vascular endothelium, vasculitis and chronic inflammation of the subcutaneous tissue and the skin. The results of this are patchy redness, swelling, itching, a burning sensation and pain.

Factors that compromise the peripheral circulation can increase the likelihood of chilblains – these include insufficiently warm and/or excessively tight clothing and shoes, long-term exposure of non-moving body parts to low temperatures, underlying illnesses such as acrocyanosis, erythrocyanosis, Raynaud's disease, lupus erythematosus, collagen disorders and arteriosclerosis, and disorders that increase the viscosity of the blood, such as dysproteinaemias and chronic leukaemia. Genetic factors explain hereditary forms, and gender-related hormonal influences account for the higher incidence in women. It is also known that certain medications (beta blockers and sulindac) can promote chilblains, as can being over- or underweight.

PRESENTATION

The patient usually presents between autumn and spring with the fairly acute onset of itching, burning and pain. These symptoms become worse when the affected body part 'warms up'. Often, various bluish-red, oedematous, well-defined raised patches are visible in the affected area, which may cause anxiety in the patient. In serious cases, haemorrhagic bullae, ulcers or secondary infection may also be present. In the majority, the abnormalities are often bilateral and are located on the extensor side of the toes and fingers. However, chilblains can also occur on the instep, heel, ankle, lower leg, knee, lateral side of the upper leg, buttocks, hips, wrist, nose, outer ear and at the site of a lipoma. Chilblains on the fingers and toes can cause some functional impairment.

EPIDEMIOLOGY

Chilblains almost never occur in areas with a very cold climate, but in places with a moderate climate. In north-western Europe, and particularly the UK, approximately 10% of the population suffers from this disorder at some time. A clear drop in incidence has occurred in recent decades, as a result of better clothing and better heating in houses. There are no reliable data about the exact incidence of chilblains, but it is estimated that one to two people per 1000 patients per year visit their GP with this problem. It occurs primarily in older children and in women aged 20–40 years. People who are outside during the cold and damp morning hours are at particular risk. The symptoms can continue for 2–5 weeks and recur annually; the severity declines after 5–10 years. In rare cases, mainly in the elderly, a chronic form can occur.

HISTORY

The GP asks:

- about what time of year the chilblains occur

- whether there are other family members with the same or similar disorders
- whether the symptoms increase when the affected body part warms up (itching, burning, pain)
- about clothing and shoes (warm enough, not too tight)
- whether the disorder occurs in the case of repeated and long-term exposure to cold conditions
- about the use of medications (e.g. beta blockers).

EXAMINATION

The physical examination consists of close inspection of the body parts affected by the symptoms and where any abnormalities can be seen. The GP must check for actual or incipient ulceration and secondary infection. In the case of extensive chilblains on the lower limbs, it is sensible to assess the peripheral circulation. Evidence of any underlying connective tissue disorder should also be sought.

TREATMENT

The advice to avoid cold and damp conditions is obvious. The patient should wear warm, not too tightly fitting clothes and shoes. Regular exercise is beneficial. Careful massage of the affected body parts can be helpful, as can warming them up with an infrared lamp and alternating hot and cold baths (3 minutes in warm water, 30 seconds in cold water). Painkillers can be given if there is a lot of pain; salicylates are preferred. The GP should expressly advise the patient not to scratch the area, because of the risk of causing ulceration and secondary infection. It has not been proven that smoking is a significant factor.

The effect of the many local and systemic remedies has not been established. Furthermore, local therapy can easily irritate the skin. The effect of cholecalciferol (vitamin D_3) has not been scientifically proven. In one small trial, nifedepine 30–60 mg once daily was more effective than placebo.

PREVENTION AND ADDITIONAL INFORMATION

Many of the above factors have a preventive role. A clear explanation about the relationship between chilblains and cold conditions is

important; preventive measures can be taken on this basis. The
patient should also know that the disorder may return during cold
times of the year.

Key points

- With chilblains, it is not so much the temperature, but the degree of humidity of the cold air that is of prime importance.
- Complications include ulceration and secondary infection.
- The symptoms can continue for 2–5 weeks and recur annually; the severity declines after 5–10 years.

Literature

Carruthers R. Chilblains (perniosis). *Aust Fam Physician* 1988;**17**(11):968–9.

Goette DK. Chilblains (perniones). *J Am Acad Dermatol* 1990;**23**(2):257–62.

Rustin MH, Newton JA, Smith NP, Dowd PM. The treatment of chilblains with nifedipine: the results of a pilot study, a double-blind placebo-controlled randomized study and a long-term open trial. *Br J Dermatol* 1989;**120**(2):267–75.

van der Meer V, de Jong-Potjer LC, Eekhof JAH, Knuistingh Neven A. Fenomeen van Raynaud en wintertenen [Raynaud phenomenon and chilblains]. *Huisarts Wet* 2003;**46**(13):778–81.

115

INGROWING NAIL

DEFINITION

An ingrowing nail involves the distal lateral edges of the nail growing inwards and so damaging the skin.

AETIOLOGY/PATHOGENESIS

It is unclear why the nail loses its slightly curved form and develops a marked bend on the lateral edges. The problem may run in the family; excessive local pressure due to shoes that are too tight may also be an important cause.

While any of the nails can become ingrowing, the nails of the big toe are by far the most commonly affected. Either one or both sides of the nail are involved. Because of the increased bend, the nail edge puts pressure on the underlying skin. As a result, a small skin defect can develop, accompanied by secondary infection and granulation tissue. This process is aggravated if the affected nail is cut too short on the lateral side.

PRESENTATION

In most cases, the patient only presents if there symptoms such as pain, swelling and redness of the lateral part of the toe. Infection and granulation tissue can sometimes result in pussy discharge. The patient experiences pain when standing and walking, and may find wearing shoes difficult. In some cases, the patient will have tried self-help measures, such as removing pieces of the lateral nail edge, soaking the feet in a bath of washing soda or using various ointments.

EPIDEMIOLOGY

The incidence according to recent figures is approximately 8 cases per 1000 patients per year, evenly divided between the genders. Ingrowing nails are found in people of all ages, except small children. The highest incidence is found in young men and elderly women. In the last 20 years, the incidence in general practice has doubled. GPs see this complaint more in patients from the lower socio-economic classes. It should be borne in mind that many patients self-treat; others may visit the chiropodist rather than the GP.

HISTORY

The history can generally be brief. The GP asks:

- when the symptoms began
- whether the patient wears tight shoes
- about the nail-cutting method.

EXAMINATION

The examination can usually also be brief. In general, it is not difficult to distinguish this from paronychia and other infections. Although paronychia does involve local infection of the skin under and next to the nail, the site is usually proximal. It may also be accompanied by a very localized head of pus on the distal side and, rarely, by granulation tissue.

TREATMENT

In minor cases it is sufficient to provide an explanation and advice, and to pare off the central part of the nail until it is thin. The assistance of a chiropodist can be helpful. Some GPs have had good results with positioning wads of cotton wool or cut-open thin plastic tubes (e.g. a cleaned piece of a plastic ballpoint refill) under the lateral nail edge, designed to force the nail to grow over (and not into) the skin.

If active inflammation is present, more radical treatment is recommended. This involves not only removing the lateral part of the nail (after which a recurrence almost always occurs), but also excising the part of the nail bed where the extra bend in the nail originates. In the past, a wedge excision was used. This method was effective, but also resulted in a high morbidity. After the introduction of lateral nail excision with the application of phenol, wedge excision has been almost completely abandoned. The phenol method does not require a lot of time, causes very few residual symptoms for the patient and few recurrences, and is easy to perform in the GP's surgery. The first step involves carrying out a ring block, in which 1–2 ml lidocaine 1% is injected on both sides of the toe base. After waiting for at least 15 minutes, the toe is tied off (e.g. with a wide elastic band and a clamp). Next, one-quarter of the nail on the affected side is cut lengthwise to under the nail fold using heavy, sharp-pointed scissors. The nail fold is not cut. The lateral part of the nail is grasped with nail extraction tweezers and removed. Immediately afterwards, a cotton bud soaked in phenol is applied under the nail fold. This cotton bud is left in place for 3 minutes. After this has been removed, the remaining phenol is rinsed out. Any granulation tissue present can remain in place; this will disappear by itself. The toe is then bandaged with paraffin gauze. The patient is told that there may be discharge from under the nail fold for a certain amount of time.

PREVENTION AND ADDITIONAL INFORMATION

If the patient has otherwise asymptomatic bent nails, filing them (and thus making them thinner) can have a preventive effect. Otherwise, the main recommendations are to limit damage to the tissue around the nail as far as possible, to wear shoes that fit properly and to cut the nails straight across.

Key points

- In the last 20 years, the incidence of ingrowing toenails in general practice has doubled.

- The problem needs to be distinguished from paronychia, in which the infection is usually more proximal.

- In troublesome ingrowing toenails, phenol ablation produces good results and low morbidity.

Literature

Dieudonné M, Eekhof JAH, Knuistingh Neven A. Ingegroeide teennagel [Minor ailments: ingrowing toenail]. *Huisarts Wet* 2002;**45**:138–9.

Rounding C, Hulm S. Surgical treatments for ingrowing toenails. *Cochrane Database Syst Rev* 2000;**2**:CD001541.

Senapati A. Conservative outpatient management of ingrowing toenails. *J R Soc Med* 1986;**79**:339–40.

116
CORNS

DEFINITION

A corn is an area of local hyperkeratosis of a particular type: a sharply defined and wedge-like area of callus in the sole of the foot with a diameter of several millimetres, which is positioned adjacent to bone, exerts pressure under the surface of the skin and can become infected.

AETIOLOGY/PATHOGENESIS

A callus is a reaction of the skin to intermittent pressure and friction, which cause rapid growth and keratinization of the epidermis cells. For a corn to develop, this pressure must be limited to a small spot, and a hard underlying layer must be present just under the skin. Corns only develop on the feet because the keratinized epidermal cells cannot come to the surface due to the pressure of the shoes. These cells then nestle together deeper in the foot. The ingrowth of 'foreign' cells causes an inflammatory reaction, and a sort of 'bursa' can develop around the 'core'.

Corns also develop as a result of abnormal pressures on the feet, such as in the case of anatomical abnormalities (e.g. hallux valgus or claw toes) and wearing certain types of shoes (e.g. high heels). In the elderly, the lack of subcutaneous fat in the foot can contribute to the development of a corn. The combination of corns and diabetes mellitus is very common (due to associated neuropathy and postural abnormalities of the foot) and requires careful handling because of the high risk of infection.

PRESENTATION

In itself, a callus is not a reason for a patient to see a GP. However, corns are painful, which may well prompt a consultation. In some cases, a chiropodist may refer patients to the GP – particularly the elderly and those with diabetes.

EPIDEMIOLOGY

GPs often see corns. According to one study, 6 per 1000 patients per year attended the GP with this problem. It primarily affects older people; in particular, there is a high prevalence in those aged over 75 years. Many patients will self treat or attend the chiropodist

HISTORY

The GP asks:

- about the patient's footwear – whether it fits properly and is not too tight
- whether there are complicating factors, such as diabetes mellitus
- how long the patient has suffered from this problem and what action has been taken to date
- about the patient's foot-care habits and whether the patient visits a chiropodist
- about sports activities, because corns often occur in people who practice karate and in beginner runners.

EXAMINATION

The site of the corn is important, because this offers clues about how it developed. The usual sites are on top of the toes in the case of hammer-toes and shoes that are too small, on the sole of the foot near the metatarsophalangeal joints as a result of high heels or degenerative change related to ageing, and interdigitally in the case of wearing pointed shoes or insufficient care of the nails. The foot position and any postural abnormalities when standing are assessed. The shoes may also be checked with regard to the fit and pressure points. Signs of a possible (secondary) infection should be sought.

If no clear cause is found, an X-ray is sometimes helpful (to detect possible postural abnormalities while standing, exostoses or accessory sesamoid bones).

TREATMENT

A painful, bothersome corn must be removed. In principle, the treatment is conservative and consists of the local application of keratolytics (e.g. salicylic acid) and the careful removal of the horny mass. Pressure on the corn can be prevented with the use of felt or rubber rings.

Another option involves pretreatment with salicylic acid, after which the callus patch and the corn are carefully cut away with a narrow, razor-sharp knife. Under local anaesthesia, the corn is excised along the boundary between the corn and the surrounding tissue.

If the corn is caused by a certain type of footwear (high heels, shoes that are too tight), this must also be changed after treatment of the corn. Proper follow-up is essential if other foot disorders are present, or if the patient is diabetic.

PREVENTION AND ADDITIONAL INFORMATION

The GP should recommend that the patient wears shoes with sufficient space for the anterior foot and which surround the heel properly, combined with a sturdy instep to prevent excessive movement. If pathological pressure ratios due to static or dynamic abnormalities of the foot are the cause, the GP will have to advise or arrange appropriate footwear or ensure that the anatomical abnormalities are corrected to prevent recurrences.

Key points

- Unlike straightforward calluses, corns are painful and have a central core.
- They are the result of localized pressure on the foot – they do not occur elsewhere.
- The combination of corns and diabetes is very common and requires careful management.

Literature

Day RD, Reyzelman AM, Harkless LB. Evaluation and management of the interdigital corn: a literature review. *Clin Podiatr Med Surg* 1996;**13**:201–6.

Degreef H, Oris S. Veel voorkomende dermatologische afwijkingen van de voet [Frequently occurring dermatological abnormalities of the foot]. *Bijblijven* 1993;**9**:43–9.

Freeman DB. Corns and calluses resulting from mechanical hyperkeratosis. *Am Fam Physician* 2002;**65**(11):2277–80.

Richards RN. Calluses, corns and shoes. *Sem Dermatol* 1991;**10**:112–14.

Singh D, Bentley G, Trevino SG. Callosities, corns, and calluses. *BMJ* 1996;**312**:1403–6.

117

ATHLETE'S FOOT

DEFINITION

Athlete's foot is a common fungal infection, which usually develops in the narrow areas between the third and fourth, and fourth and fifth toes. Other interdigital areas may also be affected.

AETIOLOGY/PATHOGENESIS

Interdigital infections are caused by local factors, dermatophytes and bacteria. If the local conditions are favourable (warm and moist), dermatophytes (typically *Trichophyton rubrum* and *T. mentagrophytes*) penetrate the skin. They damage the stratum corneum, which encourages infection by bacteria. Dermatophytes produce a penicillin and streptomycin-like substance, which particularly promotes the presence of bacteria such as *Staphylococcus aureus*, *Brevibacterium epidermidis*, *Micrococcus sedantarius*, *Corynebacterium jeikeium*, *Pseudomonas* and *Proteus*. These bacteria cause tissue damage by producing various proteolytic enzymes. The areas between the toes that have not been invaded by dermatophytes can resist the bacteria, because of the intact barrier function of the stratum corneum. The disorder can spread to the area under the toes and cause significant itching. Chronic or regularly recurring infections are very common.

In some of the asymptomatic areas between the toes, culture may demonstrate the presence of dermatophytes. This can be explained by the fact that fungal spores can survive for a very long time and because, in these areas, the stratum corneum is 30–50 times as thick as elsewhere on the body. Small amounts of dermatophytes probably remain on the surface, without infiltrating deeply enough to cause symptoms. The asymptomatic carrier status, the chronic character of the problem and the presence of onychomycosis in about one-third of patients explain the high chance of recurring infections. Cultures of the floors at swimming pools as well as communal shower and changing rooms are usually positive.

In occasional cases, a patient develops an 'id reaction'. This is a reaction to the presence of dermatophytes, which can result in symmetrical pompholyx-like lesions on both hands. These vesicles do not show any signs of fungi.

EPIDEMIOLOGY

The prevalence of foot fungi (tinea pedis) is estimated to be 10–30%. In some groups, such as people who play sports, this percentage is much higher.

PRESENTATION

The GP is consulted because of an itchy rash between the toes, usually in the interdigital area between the fourth and fifth toes.

HISTORY

The GP asks:

- how long the rash has been present
- about previous symptoms in the affected area
- about nail problems
- about visits to swimming pools and foot hygiene after showering
- about treatment undertaken by the patient.

EXAMINATION

When the toes are spread, greyish-white macerated skin is visible. After removal of the macerated layers, fissures and moist erosions remain. There is also a group of patients with a non-serious, chronic, flaky form of tinea pedis, which causes few symptoms.

Making a potassium hydroxide preparation and taking a culture are not part of the GP's routine approach. A potassium hydroxide preparation is unreliable (45% of the results are false-negative) and impractical. A culture takes 3–5 weeks and only has moderate sensitivity.

TREATMENT

Local treatment involves the use of an imidazole preparation, or possibly terbinafine, twice daily for 4 weeks. If inflammation is present, a combination of imidazole and hydrocortisone 1% may be used temporarily.

If the patient has very frequent recurrences, or if onychomycosis is also present, systemic therapy is necessary. Itraconazole as pulse therapy (a pulse consists of 200 mg twice daily for a week, followed by three medication-free weeks; three pulses are given in total) or terbinafine 250 mg once daily for at least 3 months are approximately 70% effective.

PREVENTION AND ADDITIONAL INFORMATION

Prevention is intended to prevent recurrences and to create unfavourable conditions for the pathogens. It is very difficult to prevent the first stage (the colonization with dermatophytes) because a person can be a chronic asymptomatic carrier or be reinfected very quickly from the environment.

Good evidence to guide recommendations for shower mats and swimming pools is not available. In general, the advice is to rinse shower mats well and dry them thoroughly on a regular basis. Floors should be cleaned with solutions containing chlorine. Wearing bath slippers in public shower areas and swimming pools apparently reduces exposure. Because moist, warm areas encourage dermatophytes, excessive perspiration should be combated and the feet should be properly dried after washing. It is important to wear clean socks every day and regularly change shoes.

Key points

- Athlete's foot usually develops in the narrow areas between the third and fourth, and fourth and fifth toes.
- The prevalence of foot fungal infection is estimated to be 10–30%.
- If the patient has very frequent recurrences, or if onychomycosis is also present, systemic therapy is necessary.

Literature

Crawford F. Athlete's foot and fungally infected toe nails. *Clin Evid* 2002;**7**:1458–66.

Crawford F, Hart R, Bell-Syer SEM, Torgonson DJ, Young P, Russell I. Topical treatment for fungal infections of the skin and nails of the foot. *Cochrane Database Syst Rev* 2000;**2**:CD001434.

Crawford F, Hart R, Bell-Syer SEM, Torgonson DJ, Young P, Russell I. Athlete's foot and fungally infected toenails. *BMJ* 2001;**322**:288–9.

De Kock CA, Duyvendak RJP, Jaspar AHJ, Krol SJ, Van Hoeve JAC, Romeijnders ACM, Kolnaar BGM. NHG-standaard Dermatomycosen [NHG standard Dermatomycoses]. *Huisarts Wet* 1997;**40**(11):541–52.

Vermeer BJ, Staats CCG, Van Houwelingen JC. Terbinafine versus miconazol bij patients met tinea pedis [Terbinafine versus miconazole in patients with tinea pedis]. *Ned Tijdschr Geneeskd* 1996;**140**(31):1605–8.

118

FOOT BLISTERS

DEFINITION

A foot blister is a superficial subdermal or epidermal cavity on the foot, filled with clear fluid and found on areas exposed to abnormal friction.

AETIOLOGY/PATHOGENESIS

Blisters occur when an area of skin is subjected to an abnormal level of friction. First, painful local inflammation develops. If the friction continues, a fluid-filled cavity appears. Abnormal friction can occur due to ill-fitting shoes (shoes that are too large or too narrow), chafing and poorly fitting socks, anatomical abnormalities of the foot (e.g. exotoses and hammer-toes), and walking for long periods, especially on down-sloping terrain.

PRESENTATION

Many cases of foot blisters are presented to first-aid workers during sports events, such as walking races. Pain, and therefore the fear of not being able to continue walking, is the motivation for seeking help. A typical reason for visiting the GP is secondary infection of the blister, possibly accompanied by lymphangitis and regional lymphadenopathy. Occasionally, locomotor symptoms develop as a result of the abnormal gait the patient adopts to relieve a painful foot blister.

EPIDEMIOLOGY

There are no reliable data on the incidence of foot blisters. The fact that it is a common problem for walkers was demonstrated by the figures for foot-blister treatment during an annual 4-day walking event in Nijmegen, The Netherlands, in which more than 25% of the participants were treated – and this only reflects the number requiring medical treatment (probably only a fraction of the actual number of blisters).

HISTORY

The patient's story is usually clear: a blister developed while walking, jogging, skating or skiing. The blister caused more and more pain and may have discharged (clear yellow, sometimes bloody fluid).

EXAMINATION

The blister can occur on any part of the foot exposed to abnormal friction, such as the heel, the lateral side or the area under the metatarsophalangeal joints. Under the foot, blisters can develop along the longitudinal arch on the anterior third of the foot. These develop because the metatarsal bones rotate somewhat, causing friction in the skin. In the case of hammer-toes, the blisters are located on the front of the toes, or over the interphalangeal joints.

If there is possible secondary infection, the GP should check for lymphangitis and enlarged regional lymph nodes. Additional tests such as a culture of the wound fluid are only necessary in the case of seriously infected foot blisters or when appropriate treatment does not resolve the problem.

TREATMENT

Small, slightly painful blisters are best left intact. Large, painful blisters should be treated as follows. The blister and the surrounding skin are disinfected with 10% povidone iodine solution, then the blister is punctured on two sides with a sterile needle. The blister is emptied by pushing on it with a cotton bud (rolling motion) and dried off. Finally, the blister is covered with a hydrocolloid plaster (if available, otherwise a zinc oxide plaster). Have the patient put on dry socks (if available) and lightly sprinkle talc into the shoes.

Treating infected blisters with a moist bandage and immobilization is usually sufficient. Blister fluid or pus may be aspirated and antibiotics used as for any skin infection.

PREVENTION AND ADDITIONAL INFORMATION

In the 'serious' walker, it is essential to reduce the risk of friction to the foot. There are a number of areas worth considering. For example, shoes must fit properly at the walking temperature, be 'broken in' and have proper ventilation. Insoles may be helpful. Socks must be free of seams and mended areas – and, because folds and wrinkles in the socks encourage the formation of blisters, the socks must fit perfectly. It is best to wear socks that have already been properly tried and tested. These can be normal socks or thin seamless liner socks made from acrylic or polyester (these fibres prevent the feet from becoming macerated) worn under walking socks. Proper advance training can help the skin adapt to friction as a result of proliferation of epithelial cells. Obviously, proper care of the toenails is also important. Hard and thick calluses must be removed. Applying pieces of tape or hydrocolloid plaster on the areas where blisters tend to occur is a proven method of preventing the problem.

Key points

- Small, slightly painful blisters are best left intact. Large, painful blisters should be punctured and emptied.
- Reasons for attending the GP include pain, interference with activity and secondary infection.
- In the serious walker, prevention is important and should include attention to footwear, socks, toenails, calluses and blister-prone areas.

Literature

Herring KM, Richie DH Jr. Friction blisters and sock fiber composition. A double-blind study. *J Am Podiatr Med Assoc* 1990;**80**(2):63–71.

Herring KM, Richie DH Jr. Comparison of cotton and acrylic socks using a generic cushion sole design for runners. *J Am Podiatr Med Assoc* 1993;**83**(9):515–22.

Knapik JJ, Reynolds KL, Duplantis KL, Jones BH. Friction blisters. Pathophysiology, prevention and treatment. *Sports Med* 1995;**20**(3):136–47.

Knapik JJ, Reynolds K, Barson J. Influence of an antiperspirant on foot blister incidence during cross-country hiking. *J Am Acad Dermatol* 1998;**39**(2):202–6.

Reynolds K, Darrigrand A, Roberts D, Knapik J, Pollard J, Duplantis K, Jones B. Effects of an antiperspirant with emollients on foot-sweat accumulation and blister formation while walking in the heat. *J Am Acad Dermatol* 1995;**33**(4):626–30.

119

PLANTAR WARTS/VERRUCAS AND PLANTAR MOSAIC WARTS

DEFINITION

The plantar wart, or verruca, is a clearly defined thickening of the skin on the sole of the foot, a few millimetres in diameter, which may be yellowish-grey in colour and is often covered with a callus. Plantar mosaic warts are actually clustered groups of verrucas that have sunk into the sole of the foot due to the pressure from walking. Because there are several groups of warts, the surface looks like a mosaic.

AETIOLOGY/PATHOGENESIS

See Chapter 10 for more information about warts and the human papillomavirus (HPV). HPV-1 is the pathogen in verrucas; plantar mosaic warts are caused by HPV-2. As for warts elsewhere, local and general resistance are important factors in the occurrence and resolution of plantar warts.

PRESENTATION

See Chapter 10.

EPIDEMIOLOGY

In a normal practice, an average of six new cases of plantar warts per year can be expected; the figures will fluctuate, however, as small epidemics can occur. Plantar warts occur primarily in children and young adults. One study revealed a prevalence of 27% in those that used a communal shower room.

HISTORY

See Chapter 10.

EXAMINATION

The diagnosis is usually immediately clear. It is important to distinguish a plantar wart from a corn, because the treatment is different. A corn is a cone-shaped, smooth keratinization of the skin, which can develop on pressure points of the foot (see Chapter 116). A plantar wart has a rough surface and can occur anywhere on the sole of the foot. If the superficial layer of a corn is cut or scraped off, a transparent edge and a white core are revealed. If a plantar wart is scraped, small points of blood are visible.

TREATMENT

The majority of plantar warts clear up spontaneously within 2 years. For those patients who do not want to wait, there are various effective treatments. Together, the GP and the patient should assess the problems caused by the warts, and weigh these up against the anticipated side-effects of treatment. Treatment of both verrucas and plantar mosaic warts with liquid nitrogen is less effective than for other warts, because the adhesion of the epidermis to the dermis on the soles of the feet is very strong.

Pretreatment with keratolytics, in which the isolating callus layer is removed as far as possible, is usually necessary. There are various methods, such as self-treatment with salicylic acid gel once every 1 or 2 days.

After pretreatment for about 10 days, the wart becomes receptive to treatment with liquid nitrogen or with a curette, after being frozen with ethyl chloride. However, one systematic review found that topical salicylic acid alone versus placebo increases wart clearance after 6–12 weeks.

The more aggressive treatments have the disadvantage that the sole of the foot is very sensitive to pain. In general, the treatment of plantar mosaic warts is the same as that for plantar warts, but has a somewhat lower chance of success.

PREVENTION AND ADDITIONAL INFORMATION

Wearing sports shoes in gyms can probably limit the spread of the virus. For more information, see Chapter 10.

Key points

- It is important to distinguish a plantar wart from a corn, because the treatment is different.
- The majority of plantar warts clear up spontaneously within 2 years.
- Treatment is only necessary if the plantar wart is causing significant problems.

Literature

Gibbs S, Harvey I, Sterling J, et al. Local treatments for cutaneous warts: systematic review. *BMJ* 2002;**325**:461–4.

Gibbs S, Harvey I, Sterling JC, Stark R. Local treatments for cutaneous warts (Cochrane Review). *Cochrane Library*, Issue 3. Chichester: Wiley, 2004.

Koning S, Bruijnzeels MA, Van der Wouden JC, Van Suijlekom-Smit LWA. Wratten: incidentie en beleid in de huisartspraktijk [Warts: incidence and treatment in general practice]. *Huisarts Wet* 1994;**37**:431–5.

Stulberg DL, Hutchinson AG. Molluscum contagiosum and warts. *Am Fam Physician* 2003;**67**(6):1233–40.

INDEX

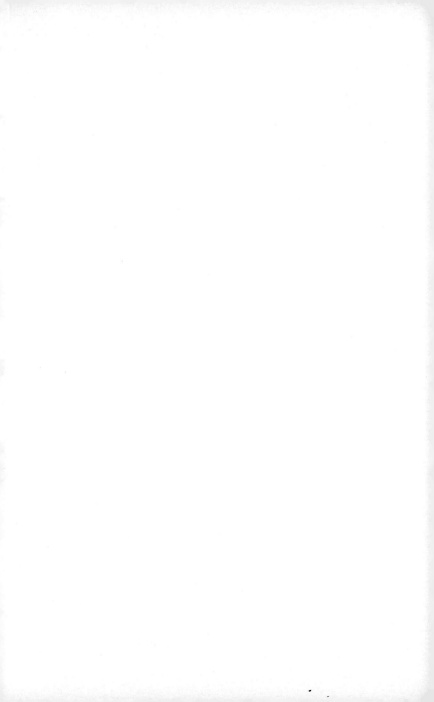